Theory, Practice, and Trends in Human Services

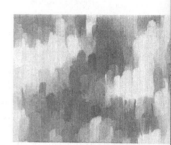

An Introduction

FIFTH EDITION

Ed Neukrug
Old Diminion University

BROOKS/COLE
CENGAGE Learning·

Australia • Brazil • Japan • Korea • Mexico • Singapore • Spain • United Kingdom • United States

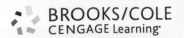

BROOKS/COLE
CENGAGE Learning·

Theory, Practice, and Trends in Human Services: An Introduction, Fifth Edition
Ed Neukrug

Publisher: Jon-David Hague

Acquisitions Editor: Seth Dobrin

Developmental Editor: Nicolas Albert

Assistant Editor: Naomi Dryer

Editorial Assistant: Suzanna Kincaid

Associate Media Editor: Elizabeth Momb

Marketing Communications Manager:
   Tami Strang

Art and Cover Direction, Production
Management, and Composition:
   PreMediaGlobal

Manufacturing Planner: Judy Inouye

Rights Acquisitions Specialist: Roberta Broyer

Photo Researcher: Susan Howard

Text Researcher: Pablo D'Stair

Cover Image: © brunoh/fotolia

For product information and technology assistance, contact us at
Cengage Learning Customer & Sales Support, 1-800-354-9706.

For permission to use material from this text or product,
submit all requests online at **www.cengage.com/permissions.**
Further permissions questions can be e-mailed to
www.permissionrequest@cengage.com.

Library of Congress Control Number: 2012930053

ISBN-13: 978-0-8400-2856-3

ISBN-10: 0-8400-2856-3

Brooks/Cole Cengage Learning
20 Davis Drive
Belmont, CA 94002-3098
USA

Cengage Learning is a leading provider of customized learning solutions with office locations around the globe, including Singapore, the United Kingdom, Australia, Mexico, Brazil, and Japan. Locate your local office at **www.cengage.com/global.**

Cengage Learning products are represented in Canada by Nelson Education, Ltd.

To learn more about Brooks/Cole, visit **www.cengage.com/brookscole**

Purchase any of our products at your local college store or at our preferred online store **www.cengagebrain.com.**

Printed in the United States of America
2 3 4 5 6   19 18 17 16 15

Dedicated to all the hard-working human service professionals in the world.

Contents

CHAPTER 5   **Development of the Person   135**

CHAPTER 6   Human Systems: Couples and Families, Groups, Organizational and Community, Administrative and Counseling Supervision   167

Preface

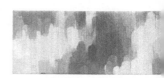

PURPOSE OF TEXT

When a book goes into its fifth edition, you would think that all that could be said about a profession has already been said. Not true in human services. As a relatively young profession, human services is changing quickly and redefining itself constantly. Thus, there has been much new material added to this text. From the recently developed credential called "Board Certified—Human Service Professional" to the spreading popularity and accreditation of human services programs, this is a field on the go. With as many changes being made in a profession, they must be reflected in any text that surveys this field. Thus, the purpose of this text is to offer the most up-to-date overview of the field of human services as possible. To do this, many changes have been made in this text, a large portion of which will be delineated in this preface. This preface will begin by providing an overview of the text, and will then suggest pedagogical aids that can be found throughout this text and online. Next, it will highlight some of the major changes to this text. It will conclude with ancillaries to this text and acknowledgments.

SECTIONS AND AFTERWORD

If you are familiar with former editions of this text, many of the chapter titles will seem familiar to you. However, there have been substantial changes in this text. For instance, we have removed the chapter called *The Human Service Professional and the World of Work* (formerly, Chapter 9). Some of the major points of this chapter have been moved to the *Afterword* where students can explore if this is the field they want to be in and find tips for applying to graduate school and to jobs in human services. Removing Chapter 9 allowed us to restructure Chapter 7, formerly called *Human Service Professionals in a Pluralistic*

Society. In past editions, this critical chapter explored theory and trends related to social and cultural issues in human services. Realizing the growing importance that this content area is to human service work, it was decided to expand this chapter into two distinct chapters, one that looks at advocacy, social justice, and multicultural issues from a theoretical perspective (Chapter 7) and a second chapter which specifically offers ideas for working with a wide range of diverse clients (Chapter 8). I believe this fills a gap from past editions by offering a more distinct focus on the work of the human service professional. The rest of the chapters have retained their primary focus although some of the titles have been changed and there is considerable content that was updated. The 10 chapters and the Afterword now are as follows:

Chapter 1.....Defining the Human Service Professional

Chapter 2.....The Human Service Profession: History and Standards

Chapter 3.....Theoretical Approaches to Human Service Work

Chapter 4.....The Helping Interview: Skills, Process, and Case Management

Chapter 5.....Development of the Person

Chapter 6.....Human Systems: Couples and Families, Groups, Organizational and Community, Administrative and Counseling Supervision

Chapter 7.....Diversity, Cultural Competence, and Social Justice

Chapter 8.....Working with Diverse Clients

Chapter 9.....Research, Evaluation, and Assessment

Chapter 10...A Look to the Future: Trends in the Functions and Roles of the Human Service Professional

Afterword.....Your Future in the Human Services

As in keeping with past editions, near the end of each chapter is a section called Ethical, Professional, and Legal Issues and this is followed by a section called "The Effective Human Service Professional" (formerly called, "The Developmentally Mature Human Service Professional"). Each of these sections refers back, in some manner, to the chapter content. At the very end of each chapter is a section called "Experiential Exercises" which offers a wide range of activities to do in and out of class that coincides with the chapter content. At the end of this section, is a separate section called "Ethical and Professional Vignettes" which offers ethical dilemmas and professional situations for students to ponder.

PEDAGOGICAL AIDS INCLUDING EXPERIENTIAL ACTIVITIES

Theory Practice and Trends in Human Services is filled with material that highlights the content of each chapter. These include:

1. Personal vignettes from the author and others concerning their experiences in the field of human services.
2. "Other" vignettes that highlight specific chapter content.
3. Testimonials from individuals in the field about their work.

4. Experiential exercises that are peppered throughout the chapters that students can do in class or at home.
5. A section called "Experiential Exercises" at the end of each chapter which offers activities that relate to the chapter content.
6. A subsection in the "Experiential Exercises" section called "Ethical and Professional Vignettes" where you will find ten to fifteen vignettes of an ethical and/or professional situation which students can ponder and discuss in class.
7. References to Web sites that can highlight specific course content.
8. Tables and graphs that elaborate what is in the chapter content.
9. For the instructor, there are numerous instructional aides (see "Ancillaries to Text" at the end of this preface).

SPECIFIC CHANGES TO THIS EDITION

If you've seen past revisions of this text, you'll know that I do not take a revision lightly. Thus, in an effort to keep the content updated and to better the quality of the text, there have been numerous changes to each chapter of this book. Some of the more substantive changes from the chapters follow.

Chapter 1: Defining the Human Service Professional. This chapter has updated information on the definition of the human service professional and the various related mental health professions. I have also reworked some of the information on the roles, functions, and competencies of the human service professional. More dramatically, based on the most recent research, I have updated the information on the characteristics that make for the effective human service professional. The eight characteristics now include the following: (1) relationship building, (2) empathy, (3) genuineness, (4) acceptance, (5) cognitive complexity, (6) embracing a wellness perspective, (7) competence, and (8) cross-cultural sensitivity.

Chapter 2: The Human Service Profession: History and Standards. You can't change history, but you should update information related to the recent past. Thus, in this chapter I have tried to ensure that the more distant history is presented in a palpable manner, and I have added or revised recent information on four standards in the profession: (1) Skill Standards, (2) credentialing, (3) ethical standards, and (4) program accreditation. In particular, the new credentialing standard in human services, Human Service—Board Certified Practitioner, is detailed.

Chapter 3: Theoretical Approaches to Human Service Work. Having recently written a book on counseling theories (*Counseling Theory and Practice*), I decided to do a major rewrite of this chapter. If you are familiar with past editions, I think you'll find this revised chapter has better flow. Besides defining counseling and psychotherapy and discussing what a "view of human nature" is, in this chapter I offer a quick look at twelve theories broken down into four conceptual approaches or schools: psychodynamic, existential–humanistic, cognitive–behavioral, and postmodern. The chapter also identifies some other, common, theoretical approaches and, as in previous editions, helps students understand what an integrative or eclectic approach means. You'll also find some new and interesting activities peppered throughout this chapter that will allow students to look at their own theoretical approach.

Chapter 4: The Helping Interview: Skills, Process, and Case Management. Although I've retained much of the information about basic counseling skills, I've added additional skills that have become increasingly important in recent years, such as the use of solution-focused questions and the importance of collaboration. In the section on "Case Management," I've updated the information on the *DSM*, noting that *DSM-5* will be coming out shortly. Here, I've also updated information on psychotropic drugs. Finally, in this section I've added information on the use of the soap format in writing case notes. This is an important addition to this chapter that many students will find useful at their internships and on the job.

Chapter 5: Development of the Person. Although the basic structure of this chapter has remained the same, I think you'll find much of the specific content of this chapter is updated and revised. In addition, I've added a section on post-modernism and social construction when talking about personality development (check out the section on "Color Therapy"—I think you'll find that fascinating). Finally, the last section of this chapter, on understanding different views of normality and abnormality, has been drastically changed and streamlined. I think you'll find it an interesting read.

Chapter 6: Human Systems: Couples and Families, Groups, Organizational and Community, Administrative and Counseling Supervision. Although the chapter title has changed somewhat, the basic focus of this chapter remains the same: systems. Despite the fact that the information about couples and family counseling is similar to previous editions, you'll find dramatic changes in how it is presented in this chapter as compared to past editions. The section on group work has remained fairly similar. However, I have added the traditional information on Tuckman's stages (forming, storming, norming, performing, and adjourning) which was lacking in past editions. I've streamlined the section on organization and community systems (working in agencies and working in communities for change), and in this chapter I've added a section on administrative and counseling supervision—two very important aspects of working in agencies.

Chapter 7: Diversity, Cultural Competence, and Social Justice. As noted earlier, this chapter underwent a more drastic revision than any of the chapters in this text. In fact, formerly called "The Human Service Professional in a Pluralistic Society," this chapter now has been expanded to two chapters—this one and Chapter 8. In this chapter we find information on cultural diversity in the United States and the world, the reasons why we need culturally competent human service professionals, some definitions of cross-cultural helping, the importance of social justice work which includes a model on advocacy, and some important definitions that all culturally competent professionals should know.

Chapter 8: Working with Diverse Clients. As just noted, this is the second chapter of what was formerly one chapter. In this chapter, we have offered some statistics that demonstrate how demographics in the United States have been changing dramatically. In addition, we have offered some models for the development of cultural competence, including the Multicultural Counseling Competencies model, the RESPECTFUL model, and the Tripartite model. This chapter follows up with specific guidelines for working with a number of clients from diverse groups, including cultural/racial groups; individuals from diverse religious backgrounds; men and women (gender-aware helping); gays, bisexuals, and lesbians;

the homeless and the poor; older persons; individuals who are HIV positive; the chronically mentally ill; and individuals with disabilities. This chapter also offers some ways of creating a human service program that effectively trains culturally competent professionals.

Chapter 9: Research, Evaluation, and Assessment. Formerly Chapter 8 and called "Research, Evaluation, and Testing," this chapter continues to distinguish between quantitative and qualitative research but offers new information on grounded theory not offered in the last edition. It also focuses a bit more on the importance of needs assessments in human service work. Although the section on assessment is fairly similar in overall content from past editions, since I have recently revised a testing and assessment book, I've made sure that this section included the most up-to-date information. In addition, I think you'll find some new, interesting vignettes in this chapter.

Chapter 10: A Look to the Future: Trends in the Functions and Roles of the Human Service Professional. One thing you can be sure of, what you expect to happen in the future, doesn't always happen. So, as usual, this chapter needed major revising from the last edition. Although many of the trends in client populations remain, I've updated the facts and figures pertaining to these populations. In addition, I've updated the information about four important standards in the profession: accreditation, credentialing, ethical codes, and the Skill Standards. Information on technology's impact on the human services has been greatly changed, and I've added information about the importance of crisis, disaster, and trauma training. The importance of having a developmental and primary prevention emphasis remains in this chapter, and I've updated the sections on managed care and medicine in human services. I've also added information on the importance of social justice and advocacy in human services and on obtaining an international perspective in the human service field. Finally, the section on stress, burnout, and cynicism and the section on wellness were significantly updated.

Afterword. This new addition to this text includes some information from Chapter 9 of the last edition: "The Human Service Professional and the World of Work." In this Afterword we discuss trends in jobs and earnings in the human services and whether or not your personality "fits" the human service profession. We identify a number of items to consider when choosing a graduate program or finding a job and discuss important aspects of the application process when applying for jobs or for graduate schools. How to write good résumé and the importance of a portfolio are discussed, and specific resources are given to help you find a job or a graduate program. We conclude the Afterword with a discussion on being chosen or being denied your ideal job or graduate program. Some interesting experiential activates are offered to help you explore your fit in the human service profession.

ANCILLARIES TO THE TEXT

For students: As already noted, throughout this text and at the end of each chapter, there are experiential activities that highlight the chapter content. I think you'll find many of these interesting and enlightening as you learn about the human service profession. Many of these activities can be completed on your own, while others may be facilitated by your instructor and completed with others in class. Also, your instructor can point out how to find sample test questions located within the instructor's companion site of this book on the Brooks/Cole Web site. The questions and answers are based on chapter content and will give you a feel for the types of questions that might be asked on an exam.

For the instructor: There are a number of ancillaries to ensure adequate student learning. These include the following:

1. *Activities Throughout Chapters and at the End of Each Chapter:* Exercises and activities that enhance student learning are found throughout many of the chapters and at the end of each chapter (called "Experiential Exercises). I believe these are an important add-on to your students' learning and, for the most part, will be fun and interesting for students.

2. *PowerPoint Slides:* Extensive PowerPoint slides that summarize each chapter's content are available from the instructor's companion site of the Brooks/Cole Web site.

3. *Test Bank:* An extensive test bank is available on the instructor's companion site of the Brooks/Cole Web site.

4. *Teaching Tips:* These suggestions, found on the instructor's companion site of the Brooks/Cole Web site, are based on the way I teach this course and may provide you with possible pedagogical suggestions as you navigate through the chapters.

5. *Sample Syllabus:* A sample syllabus is available on the instructor's companion site of the Brooks/Cole Web site.

ACKNOWLEDGMENTS

A lot of people go into the development of a book. First, a special thanks to all the people I know from the National Organization of Human Services who continue to make this a thrilling and challenging profession. You all inspire me! And, of course, a big shout out to my loving wife and children who put up with me as I "keep on writing."

From Brooks/Cole, I want to particularly thank Seth Dobrin, who is the Acquisitions Editor and Nic Albert, who is Associate Development Editor. Both Seth and Nic have continually supported me during the writing of this book and others. Others from Brooks/Cole that need mentioning include Matt Ballantyne, Production Manager; Brenda Carmichael, Art Director; Roberta Broyer, Rights Acquisition Specialist; Bob Kauser, Rights Acquisition Director; Naomi Dreyer, Assistant Editor; Suzanna Kincaid, Editorial Assistant; and Elizabeth Momb, Associate Media Editor.

For this edition, I also would like to thank Matthew Bonner, who worked laboriously on the subject index and my daughter, Hannah Neukrug, who assisted with the author index. I hope that this is just the beginning of a lifetime of scholarly publications for both of them.

In addition to those just noted, a special thanks goes out to my copy editor Jan Turner, and a big "cheers" and "thanks" to Jared Sterzer, Project Manager at PreMedia Global who keeps me on track and works with all of the crazy changes I make as I go through page proofs.

Defining the Human Service Professional

CHAPTER CONTENTS

I've been a human service professional for many years. For instance, I was a crisis and trauma counselor. I worked in agencies that provided services to individuals with developmental disabilities, assuring that they would be treated appropriately and adequately. I was a counselor at a substance abuse agency where I helped clients stop using and accompanied them to AA meetings and detox centers. I assisted therapists at an in-patient psychiatric center and saw some of the painful and unusual disorders that inflict people. For many of the jobs I've had over the years I was a caretaker to clients, helping them get through a particularly rough time in life. Other times, in my role as human service professional, I advocated for clients, helping them to find services and to connect with professionals. Additional roles I found myself in over the years included offering clients counseling so they could know themselves better, providing case management services to clients to facilitate a broad range of services for them, and even being an administrator at some agencies. The roles and functions of each of my jobs varied, and as you can see, the human service professional must have the knowledge and skills to conduct a wide range of activities and services.

My journey to becoming a human service professional, however, was very different than most people's today. In the early 1970s when I went to college, there were few human services program. Today, there are hundreds of programs offering associate's and bachelor's degrees, and even a handful of master's degrees in human services. No doubt, one's career path in the human services is different than it was when I went to school.

But what exactly is the human services professional of today? This chapter will begin to answer this question and define the professional identity of the human service professional. We will briefly discuss the beginning of human services in the United States and then describe some of what the human services professional does. Next we will contrast the human service professional with other mental health professionals and discuss associations that serve the various professionals. As the chapter continues, we will examine those characteristics that have been shown to be important in being an effective helper and discuss ways of acquiring such qualities. The chapter will conclude with a discussion about our professional relationships to related professions and the importance of being willing to continually examine ourselves as professionals.

IDENTIFYING THE HUMAN SERVICE PROFESSIONAL

The Beginning: The Human Service Professional Degree Emerges

Although human service work has been around for hundreds of years (see Chapter 2), a professional degree in human services didn't evolve until the mid-1960s. During this time, there was an increased sense of social responsibility toward the poor, minorities, women, and the mentally ill. This social awareness was one factor that led to President Johnson's **Great Society**[1] initiatives and resulted in the establishment of federal grants for a variety of social welfare programs (Fullerton, 1990a, 1990b; Osher, 1990). With the social safety net greatly expanding, it soon became apparent that the established graduate programs in counseling, psychology, and social work could not handle the increasing need for trained mental health professionals. Thus, we saw the beginning of the human service degree. Although both associate's and bachelor's programs in human services arose at this time, their orientations were somewhat different (McClam, 1997a). The associate's degree was geared toward training the mental health aide, or paraprofessional, whereas the bachelor's degree was seen as more broadly based and considered a professional degree (Fullerton, 1990a, 1990b).

As the need for **human service professionals** expanded, so did educational programs that would train such professionals. From these programs evolved a "human service curriculum" that borrows from other related fields, yet trains human service professionals in a unique way. Today, certificate programs as well as associate- and bachelor-level human service degrees are readily found throughout the country (McClam, Woodside, & Cole-Zakrewski, 2005; United States Department of Labor, 2010–2011a). A small number of graduate programs in human services are also available. It is clear that the human service profession has come into its own since the

---

[1] Words and terms in bold are listed in the glossary.

1960s. In this chapter and in Chapter 2, we will have the opportunity to take a closer look at the history of this relatively young profession, the roles and functions of human service professionals, and a number of standards that help to define the field today.

Who Is the Human Service Professional Today?

Generally, the human service professional is a person who has an associate's or bachelor's degree in human services or a closely related field (McClam et al., 2005). Although specific coursework varies from program to program, most human service degree programs offer a wide range of content that may include some or all of the following: history of human services; interviewing skills; interpersonal relationships; family guidance/counseling; group counseling; crisis intervention; policy development; human development; career development; research; assessment and evaluation; counseling theories; social and cultural issues; ethical, professional, and legal issues; special populations (e.g., substance abuse, intellectual disabilities, homelessness and poverty, and mental illness), funding and grant writing, leadership and administration, and field placement (Clubok, 1997; Council for Standards in Human Service Education, [CSHSE], 2010).

Today's human service professional is seen as a **generalist,** with interdisciplinary knowledge, who can take on a wide range of roles and often works side by side with a number of other professionals (Hinkle & O'Brien, 2010; National Organization of Human Services [NOHS], 2009a). Although the human service professional generally does not do in-depth counseling and psychotherapy, he or she is well equipped to facilitate client change and growth. One might find human service professionals in dozens of places, with some of the more common job titles listed in Table 1.1.

Table 1.1	Select Job Titles in Human Services	
Adult Day Ca Worker	Crisis Intervention Counselor	Neighborhood Worker
Alcohol Counselor	Drug Abuse Counselor	Parole Officer
Assistant Case Manager	Eligibility Counselor	Probation Officer
Behavioral Management Aide	Family Support Worker	Psychological Aide
Case Manager	Gerontology Aide	Rehabilitation Case Worker
Case Monitor	Group Activities Aide	Residential Counselor
Case Worker	Group Home Worker	Residential Manager
Child Abuse Worker	Halfway House Counselor	Social Service Aide
Child Advocate	Home Health Aide	Social Service Liaison
Client Advocate	Intake Interviewer	Social Service Technician
Community Action Worker	Juvenile Court Liaison	Social Work Assistant
Community Organizer	Life Skills Instructor	Therapeutic Assistant
Community Outreach Worker	Mental Health Aide	Youth Worker

Source: Adapted from: National of Organization of Human Services (2009b) and United States Department of Labor, 2010–2011a.

In addition to the curriculum, job titles, and job functions, another mechanism of recognizing the unique body of knowledge of a profession is through credentialing. In 2008, the **Center for Credentialing and Education (CCE)** in consultation with the **National Organization of Human Services (NOHS)** and with the **Council for Standards in Human Service Education (CSHSE)** developed a credential for human service practitioners entitled the **Human Services—Board Certified Practitioner (HS—BCP)**. In its relatively short existence, almost 2,000 individuals have obtained this credential, which will increasingly be used as a method of validating one's educational and professional knowledge (HS—BCP, 2011) (also see Chapter 2).

Roles, Functions, Competencies, and Skills of the Human Service Professional

What does the human service professional do? Broadly, this trained professional helps meet "human needs through an interdisciplinary knowledge base, focusing on prevention as well as remediation of problems, and maintaining a commitment to improving the overall quality of life of service populations" (NOHS, 2009a, About Human Services section). As far back as 1969, the **Southern Regional Education Board (SREB, 1969)** identified 13 roles and functions of the human service professional, most of which are still relevant to today's human service professional (Diambra, 2001; Hinkle & O'Brien, 2010) (see Box 1.1).

More recently, a large job analysis was completed to identify the competencies and skills that are necessary for the completion of human service work in a wide variety of human service jobs (Diambra, 2001; National Alliance for Direct

---

BOX 1.1 | **Thirteen Roles and Functions of the Human Service Professional (SREB, 1969)**

1. *Outreach worker* who might go into communities to work with clients
2. *Broker* who helps clients find and use services
3. *Advocate* who champions and defends clients' causes and rights
4. *Evaluator* who assesses client programs and shows that agencies are accountable for services provided
5. *Teacher/educator* who tutors, mentors, and models new behaviors for clients
6. *Behavior changer* who uses intervention strategies and counseling skills to facilitate client change
7. *Mobilizer* who organizes client and community support to provide needed services
8. *Consultant* who seeks and offers knowledge and support to other professionals and meets

with clients and community groups to discuss and solve problems
9. *Community planner* who designs, implements, and organizes new programs to service client needs
10. *Caregiver* who offers direct support, encouragement, and hope to clients
11. *Data manager* who develops systems to gather facts and statistics as a means of evaluating programs
12. *Administrator* who supervises community service programs
13. *Assistant to specialist* who works closely with the highly trained professional as an aide and helper in servicing

Support Professionals, 2008; Taylor, Bradley, & Warren, 1996). Known as the **Skill Standards**, the 12 identified competencies are as follows:

(1) participant empowerment

(2) communication

(3) assessment

(4) community and service networking

(5) facilitation of services

(6) community and living skills and supports

(7) education, training, and self-development

(8) advocacy

(9) vocational, educational, and career support

(10) crisis intervention

(11) organization participation

(12) documentation

These 12 competencies, and the skills needed to accomplish them, will be discussed in more detail in Chapter 2. Clearly, there is much overlap between the roles and functions, as identified by the SREB, and the more recent Skill Standards. However, there are also some significant differences, and perhaps what is more important, because the competencies are broken down into a large number of skills needed to accomplish them, is the competencies can greatly assist the human service professional in understanding his or her role and can be a guide for training programs.

Finally, how do the roles and functions of the human service professional differ from those of other related mental health professionals? Broadly, human service professionals help clients problem solve and do not facilitate personality reconstruction. Table 1.2 shows a visual representation of some differences in how

Table 1.2 | Comparison of Select Professionals' Orientation to Working with Clients*

	Human Service Professional	Counselor/ Social Worker	Psychologist
Supportive	High	Moderate	Low
Problem-focused	High	Moderate	Low/moderate
Works with conscious	High	Moderate	Low/moderate
Focused on present	High	Moderate	Low/moderate
Directive	Moderate	Moderate/low	Low
Facilitative	Moderate	Moderate/high	High
Nondirective	Moderate/low	Moderate/high	High
Insight-oriented	Moderate	Moderate/high	High
Works with unconscious	Low	Moderate/high	High
Focused on past	Low	Moderate	High

*These are generalizations, and professionals can be found doing any of the above as a function of the setting in which they find themselves working and their own personal style of conducting counseling.

human service professionals, counselors, social workers, and psychologists might approach working with a client.

RELATED MENTAL HEALTH PROFESSIONALS

Although there is some overlap in the training of the many different professionals in the social service fields, great differences also exist. Let's briefly review some of these different kinds of mental health professionals.

Psychiatrist

A **psychiatrist** is a licensed physician who generally has completed a residency in psychiatry, meaning that in addition to medical school, he or she has completed extensive field placement training in a mental health setting. In addition, most psychiatrists have passed an exam to become board certified in psychiatry. Being a physician, the psychiatrist has expertise in diagnosing organic disorders, identifying and treating psychopathology, and prescribing medication for psychiatric conditions.

Because psychiatrists sometimes have less training in conducting counseling and psychotherapy than other mental health professionals (including human service professionals), they are not always seen as experts in the delivery of such services. However, their expertise in conceptualizing client problems, in diagnosing clients, and in prescribing medication can be a great help to mental health professionals and the clients with whom they work. Psychiatrists are employed in mental health agencies, hospitals, private practice settings, and health maintenance organizations. The professional association for psychiatrists is the **American Psychiatric Association (APA)**.

Psychologist

Many different types of **psychologists** practice in a wide range of settings and are often found running agencies, consulting with business and industry, or serving in supervisory roles for all types of mental health professionals. Relative to the practice of psychotherapy, all states offer licensure in counseling and/or clinical psychology (American Psychological Association [APA], 2003), and many states now allow individuals with a "**Psy.D.**," a relatively new clinical doctorate in psychology, to become licensed as **clinical** or **counseling psychologists**. Licensed counseling and clinical psychologists obtain a doctoral degree in psychology, acquire extensive supervised experience after graduate school, and pass a licensing exam. Although some states grant psychologists prescription privileges for psychotropic medication (Johnson, 2009), currently it is psychiatrists, and in some cases psychiatric nurses, who take the lead in this important treatment approach.

In addition to counseling and clinical psychologists, human service professionals may work alongside **school psychologists**. A school psychologist generally has a master's degree in school psychology and has expertise in conducting testing and assessment and in assisting in the development and implementation of behavior plans for children. The professional association for psychologists is the **American Psychological Association (APA)**.

Social Worker

Those who obtain a bachelor's or master's degree from a social work program generally are called **social workers**. However, at times this term is generically applied to a wide range of jobs in the mental health field. Thus, you will sometimes find individuals with related degrees (e.g., human services, counselors) have a job title "social worker." Those who obtain a master's in social work are generally called "**MSWs.**"

Whereas social workers historically had been found working with the underprivileged and with family and social systems, today's social workers provide counseling and support services for all types of clients in a wide variety of settings. Some bachelor-level social workers have similar training to human service professionals. MSWs usually have extensive training in counseling techniques but less preparation in career counseling, assessment techniques, and quantitative research methods than counselors or psychologists. With additional training and supervision, MSWs can become nationally certified by the **Academy of Certified Social Workers (ACSW)**. In addition, all states have specific requirements for becoming a **Licensed Clinical Social Worker (LCSW)**. The professional association for social workers is the **National Association of Social Workers (NASW)**.

Counselor

For many years, the word **counselor** simply referred to any "professional who practices counseling" (Chaplin, 1975, p. 5). However, today, most individuals who call themselves counselors have a master's degree in counseling. These days, counselors are found in many settings and perform a variety of roles. For instance, they may serve as **school counselors, college counselors, mental health counselors, rehabilitation counselors**, and more. The counselor's training is broad, and we find counselors doing individual, group, and family counseling; administering and interpreting educational and psychological assessments; offering career counseling; consulting on a broad range of educational and psychological matters; and presenting developmentally appropriate guidance activities for individuals of all ages. Even though counselors do not tend to be experts in psychopathology, they do have knowledge of mental disorders and know when to refer individuals who need more in-depth treatment. The professional association of counselors is the **American Counseling Association (ACA)**.

Couple and Family Counselors

Couple and family counselors almost always have a master's or doctoral degree in counseling or a related field and are specifically trained to conduct counseling with couples and families. Found in a vast array of agency settings and in private practice, couple and family counselors tend to have specialty coursework in systems dynamics, couples counseling, family therapy, family life stages, and human sexuality, along with the more traditional coursework in the helping professions. The **American Association for Marriage and Family Therapists (AAMFT)** is one professional association for marriage and family counselors; another is the **International Association of Marriage and Family Counselors (IAMFC)**. Although all 50 states have some requirement for marriage and family licensure, these requirements can vary dramatically (United States Department of Labor, 2010–2011b).

Psychiatric-Mental Health Nurses

Primarily trained as medical professionals, **psychiatric-mental health nurses** are also skilled in the delivery of mental health services (American Psychiatric Nurses Association [APNA], n.d.). Most psychiatric-mental health nurses work in hospital settings, with lesser numbers working in community agencies, private practice, or educational settings. Psychiatric-mental health nursing is practiced at two levels. The registered nurse psychiatric-mental health nurse does basic mental health work related to nursing diagnosis and nursing care. The **Advanced Practiced Registered Nurse (APRN)** has a master's degree in psychiatric-mental health nursing and assesses, diagnoses, and treats individuals with mental health problems. Currently holding prescriptive privileges in all 50 states (Phillips, 2007), APRNs hold a unique position in the mental health profession. Psychiatric-mental health nurses can acquire certification in a number of mental health areas based on their education and experience (see American Nurses Credentialing Center, 2011). The professional association of psychiatric-mental health nurses is the **American Psychiatric Nurses Association (APNA)**.

Psychotherapist

Because most states do not have laws that regulate the term **psychotherapist**, individuals with no training, experience, or even a degree can call themselves psychotherapists. On a practical level, psychotherapists usually have advanced degrees in psychology, social work, or counseling and work in mental health settings or in private practice, providing individual, group, or marital counseling. However, if someone tells you he or she is a psychotherapist, it would be wise to inquire about the kind of degree(s), if any, he or she has obtained.

Other Professionals

The professionals just discussed represent a large part of the circle of mental health professionals. For instance, in addition to those already discussed, there are art therapists, play therapists, dance therapists, creative therapists, expressive therapists, body armor therapists, pastoral counselors, psychoanalysts, Jungian therapists, and more—each with their own professional association. Don't be surprised if in addition to the professionals highlighted, you find other kinds of mental health professionals in your professional journey.

PROFESSIONAL ASSOCIATIONS IN HUMAN SERVICES AND RELATED FIELDS

Purpose of Associations

In order to protect the rights of their members and support the philosophical beliefs of their membership, professional associations have arisen over the years for each of the professional groups discussed in this chapter. A few of the many benefits that these associations tend to offer are as follows:

- Sponsoring national and regional conferences to discuss training and clinical issues
- Publishing newsletters and journals to discuss topics of interest to the membership
- Hiring lobbyists to protect the interests of the membership
- Providing information on cutting-edge issues in the field
- Providing opportunities for mentoring and networking
- Developing codes of ethics and standards for practice
- Initiating advocacy for mental health concerns
- Providing access to malpractice insurance
- Advocating for accreditation of programs
- Providing grants for special projects
- Supporting credentialing efforts
- Providing job banks

Most of you who are reading this text are likely to be interested in joining NOHS and its divisions, which will be discussed in detail shortly. However, to broaden your professional knowledge and acquaint you with related associations you might want to join, some of the other major associations within the social service fields will also be highlighted. Keep in mind that there are dozens of professional organizations in the social services, and this section of the text features only a few of the more well-known ones.

The Associations

All of the following associations provide most of the benefits just noted to their membership. We will start with a lengthier description of NOHS, our professional organization. This will be followed by brief descriptions of related mental health associations.

National Organization for Human Services (NOHS) (www.nationalhumanservices. org) The major association in human services, the National Organization for Human Service Education (NOHSE), was founded in 1975. In 2005, the organization removed the word *education* from its name and became the National Organization for Human Services (NOHS). The mission of NOHS is to "strengthen the community of human services by: expanding professional development opportunities, promoting professional and organizational identity through certification, enhancing internal and external communications, advocating and implementing a social policy and agenda, and nurturing the financial sustainability and growth of the organization" (NOHS, 2009a, Our Mission section). NOHS is mostly geared toward undergraduate students in human services or related fields, faculty in human services or related programs, and human service practitioners. NOHS publishes one journal, the *Journal of Human Services* (formerly, *Human Service Education*), which focuses on enhancing research, theory, and education for practitioners and educators in the field of human services (Haynes & Sweitzer, 2005; T. Milliken, personal communication, May 5, 2011).

NOHS has an active student membership and six regional associations (Mid-Atlantic, Midwest, Northeastern, Northwest, Southern, and Western). Each region holds its own professional meetings, and they operate somewhat independently, offering workshops, conferences, and other professional activities. Membership in NOHS provides access to a number of benefits, including the following:

- Access to information on ethical codes, accreditation, credentialing and other standards
- Professional development workshops and conferences
- Scholarships and grants for professional development
- Resource directory of consultants in human services
- Access to six regional associations (see Box 1.2)
- Subscription to the *Journal of Human Services*
- Subscription to *The Link* (NOHS newsletter)
- Information and referral services
- Networking and mentoring
- Recognition awards

If you are interested in becoming more involved professionally as a human service professional, you should join NOHS and your regional chapter.

The American Counseling Association (ACA) (www.counseling.org)   Today, with more than 45,000 members, ACA is the world's largest association for master's- and doctoral-level counselors. ACA is an umbrella organization that serves the needs of all types of counselors in an effort to "enhance the quality of life in society by promoting the development of professional counselors, advancing the counseling profession, and using the profession and practice of counseling to promote respect for human dignity and diversity" (ACA, 2011, Mission Statement section, para. 1). ACA publishes one journal, the *Journal of Counseling and Development*, although most of its 19 divisions also publish journals. Although geared toward master's- and

---

BOX 1.2   **The Six Regions of NOHS**

"Because human services has a strong base in local communities, NOHS actively supports regional organizations across the country. These regional organizations offer separate annual conferences to address the distinct needs within each region, while also interfacing with the national organization through participation on the national board" (NOHS, 2009c, Regions section, para. 1). The six regional organizations are the following:

1. Mid-Atlantic Consortium for Human Services
2. Midwest Organization for Human Services
3. New England Organization for Human Service
4. Northwest Human Services Association
5. Southern Organization for Human Services
6. Western Region of Human Service Professionals

(click "About" then "Regions" at NOHS Web site*)
   (http://mwohs.webs.com/index.htm)
   (http://newenglandhumanservices.com/)
(click "About" then "Regions" at NOHS Web site*)
(http://www.sohse.org/)
(http://westernregionofhumanservice.org/)

---

*www.nationalhumanservices.org

doctoral-level counselors, counselor trainees, and counselor educators, undergraduates who are interested in the counseling field are welcome.

The National Association of Social Workers (NASW) (www.naswdc.org)
NASW was founded in 1955 as a merger of seven membership associations in the field of social work. Servicing both undergraduate- and graduate-level social workers, NASW has nearly 145,000 members (NASW, 2011). Its stated purpose is to "enhance the professional growth and development of its members, to create and maintain professional standards, and to advance sound social policies" (NASW, 2011, About NASW section, para. 1). The association publishes five journals and other professional publications. Only practitioners with an undergraduate or graduate degree in social work or social work students are allowed to join as regular members.

The American Psychological Association (APA) (www.apa.org)   Founded in 1892 by G. Stanley Hall, the APA started with 31 members and now maintains a membership of 150,000. Undergraduate and graduate students can join as affiliate members. The main purpose of this association is to "advance the creation, communication and application of psychological knowledge to benefit society and improve people's lives" (APA, 2011, Mission Statement section). The association has 53 divisions in various specialty areas and publishes numerous psychological journals.

The American Psychiatric Association (APA) (www.psych.org)   Founded in 1844 as the Association of Medical Superintendents of American Institutions for the Insane, today the American Psychiatric Association (which has the same acronym as the American Psychological Association, APA) has about 38,000 members. The association's main purpose is to "ensure humane care and effective treatment for all persons with mental disorders, including mental retardation and substance-related disorders" (American Psychiatric Association [APA], 2011, para. 1). The APA publishes journals in psychiatry and is responsible for the development and publication of the *Diagnostic and Statistical Manual-IV-Text Revision* (*DSM-IV-TR*; soon to be *DSM-5*), a major publication for mental health diagnosis.

The American Association of Marriage and Family Therapists (AAMFT) (www.aamft.org)   The AAMFT, with its 24,000 members, has become prominent in the field of marriage and family counseling. AAMFT was established in 1945 to develop standards for its field and to offer an association that could bring together people with varying professional backgrounds who had an interest in marriage and family therapy. Today, AAMFT plays a major role in representing "the professional interests of more than 24,000 marriage and family therapists throughout the United States, Canada, and abroad" (AAMFT, 2002–2011, About AAMFT section). AAMFT publishes the *Journal of Marital and Family Therapy*. Although geared toward licensed marriage and family therapists, AAMFT invites others to join.

The American Psychiatric Nurses Association (APNA) (www.apna.org)
Founded in 1986 with 600 members, today the APNA has over 7,000 members. APNA is "committed to the specialty practice of psychiatric mental health nursing,

health and wellness promotion through identification of mental health issues, prevention of mental health problems and the care and treatment of persons with psychiatric disorders" (APNA, n.d., Mission section). APNA provides advocacy for psychiatric nurses to improve the quality of mental health care delivery and publishes the *Journal of the American Psychiatric Nurses Association.*

Other Professional Associations As you can well imagine, in addition to NOHS and perhaps some of the associations we just mentioned, there are a number of other professional associations which you might be interested in joining. Just a few of these include the American Art Therapy Association (AATA), the American Dance Therapy Association (ADTA), the American Music Therapy Association (AMTA), the Association of Play Therapy (APT), the American Association of Pastoral Counselors (AAPC), the National Rehabilitation Counselor Association (NRCA), and more.

CHARACTERISTICS OF THE EFFECTIVE HUMAN SERVICE PROFESSIONAL

Whether you are thinking about entering or have already decided to enter the human services field, you probably have some intuition that this field fits your sense of who you are. You may have formed some image of the human service professional. Perhaps you think he or she is an altruistic person—a person who wants to help others; a person who cares about people and the state of the world; a person who is introspective, intuitive, and social; or a person who has other similar qualities. On the other hand, you probably also think that the human service professional is *not* an aloof person, is not pushy and dogmatic, and is *not* narcissistic or overly concerned about himself or herself. In point of fact, the qualities of the helping professional have been researched over the years (Wampold, 2010a, 2010b, 2010c). Based on these studies and others, I have generated eight characteristics that seem to be empirically or theoretically related to effectiveness as a helper. They are (1) **relationship building**, (2) **empathy**, (3) **genuineness**, (4) **acceptance**, (5) **cognitive complexity**, (6) **wellness**, (7) **competence**, and (8) **cross-cultural sensitivity**. (see Figure 1.1). As we take a look at these characteristics, keep in mind that as research becomes more refined, some of these characteristics might change.

Relationship Building

The relationship between the helper and client, sometimes called the **working alliance,** may be the most formidable factor in creating client change (Baldwin, Wampold, & Imel, 2007; Beutler et al., 2004; Marmarosh et al., 2009; Orlinsky, Ronnestad, & Willutzki, 2004; Whiston & Coker, 2000). Relationship building is closely related to the ability of the client and helper to build an emotional bond and to work on setting attainable goals. The impact of the helper's ability to build an emotional bond is felt throughout the helping relationship, regardless of whether it is acknowledged by the helper and the client (Gelso & Carter, 1994).

The well-known family therapist Salvador Minuchin (1974) has always stressed the importance of building an alliance with clients. Using the term **joining**

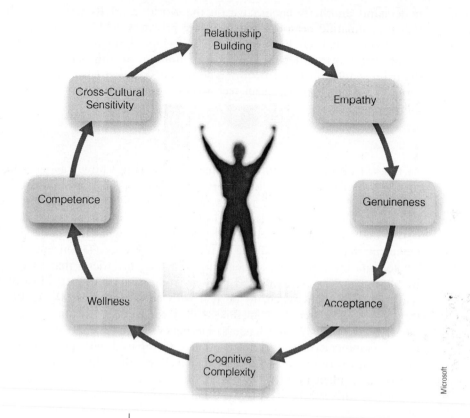

Figure 1.1 | Eight Characteristics of the Effective Helper

to describe the building of the client-helper relationship, he says that the helper must join with the family if therapeutic goals are to be reached. Although Minuchin has his own characteristic manner of joining with a family, all helpers must build an alliance based on their unique ways of helping. The challenge for all human service professionals is to have the emotional fortitude to build strong relationships, to know how to build such bonds within the context of their theoretical framework, and to be able to understand how these bonds dramatically affect work with clients.

Empathy

Perhaps as important as building a strong helping relationship, the quality of empathy, or the ability to understand the inner world of another, is the second critical element of an effective helping relationship (Bohart, Elliot, Greenberg, & Watson, 2002; Norcross, 2010). Empathic persons have a deep understanding of another person's point of view. These people can "get into the shoes" of another. If you have ever seen *Star Trek: The Next Generation*, you may be familiar with the "counselor," the epitome of the empathic person with a highly tuned ability to understand another's perspective on the world. **Carl Rogers** (1957) liked to say that the empathic person could sense the private world of clients as if it were his or her own, without losing the "as if" feeling. Empathic individuals can accept people with their differences and can communicate this sense of acceptance. For the helping relationship, empathy is seen as a skill that can build rapport, elicit information, and help the client feel accepted (Egan, 2010; Neukrug & Schwitzer, 2006).

Genuineness

At times, I find myself acting in a manner that is not how I actually feel. At these times, I often think, "Should I express my true feelings, or should I hide them to protect another person—or perhaps, more accurately, to protect myself?" For instance, should I tell my boss that I am angry at him or her and take the chance that I might get fired? Should I tell my client that what he or she shares with me makes me feel sad and take the chance that such a revelation might make him or her feel uneasy? Do I risk a friendship by telling my friend that I feel manipulated by him or her? These conflicts I have are indicative of a battle most of us struggle with—whether, and when, to be real with others. Rogers (1961, 1980) felt that genuineness, or what he sometimes called **congruence**, meant being in sync with one's own feelings and behaviors. He believed that such realness was critical to the development of healthy relationships. Compared with genuine people, nongenuine people are out of sync with their feelings, thoughts, and actions. How they feel is not evident in what they say or how they act. These individuals are fake—living life with subtle deceptions, often deceiving themselves. Although it may be prudent at times *not* to share certain feelings with your boss, friend, or client, a relationship that emphasizes nongenuineness can have little substance and, in the case of the helping relationship, will be less likely to promote growth in clients (Beutler et al., 2004; Klein, Kolden, Michels, & Chisholm-Stockard, 2002).

Research by Gelso (Gelso & Carter, 1994; Gelso et. al., 2005) suggests that regardless of one's theoretical orientation, there exists an ongoing *real relationship* in which the client, to some degree, will see the helper realistically. This real relationship has at its core the ability of the client to recognize the genuine (or nongenuine) self of the counselor. As you might expect, genuineness has been shown to be one more quality that is sometimes related to positive outcomes in the helping relationship (Beutler et al., 2004; Klein, Kolden, Michels, & Chisholm-Stockard, 2002; Norcross, 2010).

Acceptance

Acceptance, sometimes called **positive regard**, is another component likely related to successful helping relationships (Norcross, 2010). Acceptance is an attitude that suggests that regardless of what the client says, within the context of the counseling relationship, he or she will feel accepted. People who have high regard for others can accept people regardless of dissimilar cultural heritage, values, or belief systems. In a helping relationship, individuals with a high regard for others are able to accept the helpee unconditionally, without having "strings attached" to the relationship. Rogers (1957) referred to this quality as **unconditional positive regard**. Others have called it "responsible love":

> Responsible love is accepting and understanding ... [L]ove helps us to accept the fact that the other individual is behaving only as he [or she] is able to behave at the moment. (Buscaglia, 1972, p. 119)

Showing acceptance and positive regard for others does not mean that one necessarily likes everything a person has done. For instance, one would most certainly not like the actions of a convicted murderer or rapist; however, the person who is accepting can come to understand how the felon came to commit those actions. This deep understanding comes from being empathic and is like having a window that leads deep inside the soul of the other individual—a window that allows the helper to see the hurts and pains of the other.

Cognitive Complexity

Helpers who are cognitively complex are able to understand the world, and ultimately their clients, in multifaceted and abstract ways (Kegan, 1982, 1994; King, 1978). Such helpers are likely to be more empathic, more open-minded, more self-aware, more effective with individuals from diverse cultures, able to examine a client's predicament from multiple perspectives, and better able to resolve problems in the helping relationship (Deal, 2003; McAuliffe & Eriksen, 2010; Milliken, 2004; Norcross, 2010). Such individuals view learning as a mutual and reciprocal process whereby individuals can share knowledge and learn from one another. These helpers are willing to integrate new approaches into their usual way of helping and don't believe their way of helping is the "only" way (Wampold, 2010a). So, ask yourself, do you have this quality? Are you able to self-reflect, question truth, take on multiple perspectives, and evaluate situations in complex ways? Training programs are environments that seek to expand this type of thinking (McAuliffe & Eriksen, 2010). Hopefully, in your program, you'll be exposed to such opportunities.

Wellness

Stress, burnout, compassion fatigue, vicarious traumatization, and unfinished psychological issues can all hinder any helper's ability to have a working alliance (Lawson, 2007; Norcross, 2010; Roach & Young, 2007). Such concerns can prevent one from being empathic, lower the ability to show acceptance, lead to incongruence, and increase **countertransference**, or "the unconscious transferring of thoughts, feelings, and attitudes onto the client" (Neukrug, 2011).

All helpers need to attend to their own wellness if they are to be effective. One method of assessing your level of wellness is by examining what Myers and Sweeney (2008) identify as the **Indivisible Self**. This model views wellness as being composed of five factors and also takes into account an individual's context. The factors (creative self, coping self, social self, essential self, and physical self) and contexts are described at the end of this chapter, and you can have an opportunity of examining each of them for yourselves.

Finally, although many avenues to wellness exist, one that must be considered for all helpers is attending their own counseling. Counseling helps helpers (1) attend to their own personal issues, (2) reduce the likelihood of countertransference, (3) examine all aspects of their lives so they can increase their overall wellness, and (4) understand what it's like to sit in the client's seat. It appears that mental health professionals understand the importance of being in counseling as 85% of helpers have attended counseling (Bike, Norcross, & Schatz, 2009). However, some counselors resist, perhaps for good reasons (e.g., concerns about confidentiality, feeling as if family and friends offer enough support, or believing they have effective coping strategies) (Norcross, Bike, Evans, & Schatz, 2008). So, have you attended counseling? If not, have you found other ways to work on being healthy and well?

Competence

Helper expertise and mastery, otherwise known as competence, has been shown to be a crucial element for client success in counseling (Wampold, 2010a, 2010c; Whiston & Coker, 2000). Competent helpers have a thirst for knowledge. They continually want to improve and expand their expertise at delivering their theory. Such professionals exhibit this thirst through their study habits, their desire to join professional associations, through mentoring and supervision, by reading their professional journals, through their belief that education is a lifelong process, and through their ability to view their own approach to working with clients as something that is always broadening and deepening.

Competence is consistently acknowledged as a crucial ethical concern by most professional associations (Corey, Corey, & Callanan, 2011) (see also NOHS ethical code—Appendix A, Statements 26, 27, 30, and 31.) The legal system reinforces these ethical guidelines by stating that helpers "commit professional malpractice if they are visibly less competent than the average of their peers ..." (Swenson, 1997, p. 166). Therefore, having the desire to learn skills as well as the specific techniques needed to work with certain problems is essential for the effective human service professional.

Cross-Cultural Sensitivity

If you were distrustful of helpers, confused about the helping process, or felt worlds apart from your helper, would you want to be in a helping relationship? Assuredly not. Unfortunately, this is the state of affairs for many diverse clients. In fact, it is now assumed that when clients from nondominant groups work with majority helpers, there is a possibility that the client will frequently be misunderstood, often misdiagnosed, find the helping relationship less helpful than their majority counterparts, attend counseling and therapy at lower rates than majority clients, and terminate counseling more quickly than majority clients (Evans, Delphin, Simmons, Omar, & Tebes, 2005; Sewell, 2009; United States Department of Health and Human Services, 2001). Unfortunately, it has become abundantly clear that many helpers have not learned how to effectively build a bridge—form a working alliance with clients who are different from them.

Clearly, the effective helper needs to have cross-cultural sensitivity and be **culturally competent** if he or she is going to connect with his or her clients (Anderson, Lunnen, & Ogles, 2010; Neukrug & Milliken, 2008). Although some rightfully argue that all counseling is cross-cultural, when working with clients who are from a different culture than one's own, the schism is often great (Brinson & Denby, 2008). Therefore, cross-cultural sensitivity and competence is a theme we will visit and revisit throughout this text, and I will offer a number of ways for you to lessen the gap between you and your client. One model that can help bridge that gap is D'Andrea and Daniels's (2005) **RESPECTFUL Counseling Model,** which highlights ten factors that counselors should consider addressing with clients:

R—Religious/spiritual identity

E—Economic class background

S—Sexual identity

P—Psychological development

E—Ethnic/racial identity

C—Chronological disposition

T—Trauma and other threats to their personal well-being

F—Family history

U—Unique physical characteristics

L—Language and location of residence, which may affect the helping process. (p. 37)

Final Thoughts

The eight characteristics—relationship building, empathy, genuineness, acceptance, cognitive complexity, wellness, competence, and cross-cultural sensitivity—are qualities to which human service professionals should aspire. Few, if any, of us are already there. More likely, these qualities can be nurtured and developed as we travel our own unique paths through life. But how do we begin to acquire some of these qualities? Let's examine some possible ways.

BECOMING THE EFFECTIVE HELPER

Are some of us born with the previously described characteristics that lead us toward the human service field, can they be learned, or do these qualities reflect a combination of genetic and acquired traits? Many theorists and philosophers have struggled with trying to understand how one comes to acquire these characteristics. **Carl Rogers** and **Abraham Maslow** (1954), two of the founders of the field of humanistic counseling and education, thought we were born with a natural actualizing tendency and that if we were reared in a nurturing environment, many of the described characteristics would naturally develop. They also thought that even if the nurturing environment had not been present in early childhood, the qualities could still develop if such an environment was available later in life. On the other

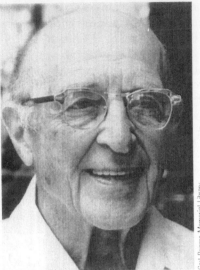

Carl Rogers, one of the founders of the field of humanistic counseling and education.

hand, **Sigmund Freud,** the founder of psychoanalysis, thought that people constantly struggled with instinctual aggressive and sexual drives and that these drives, in combination with early childhood experiences, determined each person's temperament. Therefore, he would have believed that a human service professional's personality had been formed in early childhood. Others, such as **B. F. Skinner** (1953), the famous behaviorist, and **Albert Ellis** (Ellis & Harper, 1997), the well-known cognitive therapist, believed that although we might not be born with these qualities, we could develop them through certain experiences.

An Adult Development Approach

Robert Kegan (1982, 1984) and **William Perry** (King, 1978) suggest that over a lifespan, if placed in an environment that is conducive to the development of the characteristics of the effective helper, just about anyone can develop such qualities. Their adult development approach suggests that through a supportive and challenging environment, many of the eight qualities noted earlier would be more fully embraced and individuals would become more empathic, less critical, less dogmatic, more accepting, increasingly open to other points of view, increasingly complex thinkers, and so forth.

More specifically, Kegan (1982, 1994) suggests there are six stages of adult development (Stages 0 through 5), with Stages 3, 4, and 5 representing ways in which most adults view the world. Kegan's **incorporative, impulsive,** and **imperial stages** (Stages 0, 1, and 2) deal mostly with child development and focus on how the individual moves from total self-involvement toward the beginning awareness of a shared world with other people. These stages will be examined in more detail in Chapter 5.

Kegan's third stage, the **interpersonal stage,** represents the individual who is embedded in his or her relationships. Individuals in this stage cannot truly separate their sense of who they are from their families, friends, or community groups. Kegan's fourth stage, the **institutional stage,** represents the person who has separated his or her values and sense of self from parents, peers, or community groups. These individuals have a strong sense of personal autonomy and self-reliance. Kegan's final stage is the **interindividual stage.** Here, individuals are able to maintain a separate sense of self and have the capability to incorporate feedback from others—feedback that allows for growth and change. They are not embedded in their autonomous, self-reliant way of living, as are Stage 4 institutional persons.

The Woody Allen comedic movie called *Zelig* clearly shows an individual in transition from Stage 3 to Stage 4. Zelig is the epitome of Stage 3, the interpersonal person. He takes on the persona of whomever he is around. He is afraid to be himself. If he's around an African-American, he becomes African-American; if he's around a Chinese person, he speaks fluent Chinese. He becomes obese when he is around someone who is obese, and he becomes a psychiatrist attempting to treat the psychiatrist who is treating him. What seems to be a lighthearted movie soon becomes serious when we see the reasons why Zelig becomes whomever he is around. Under hypnosis, Zelig reveals the reasons he becomes the person he is with—he is afraid to be himself. A lifelong history of ridicule every time he expressed his own opinion made him too scared to be himself. After intensive therapy, Zelig is "cured." Finally, the big day arrives when Zelig is to meet a number of renowned psychiatrists who will examine him to see if he is actually cured. At first, things seem successful because Zelig does not take on the persona of the psychiatrists. But as the meeting continues, one of the psychiatrists remarks that it is a beautiful day, and Zelig, who has become his "own person," assertively states, "It is not a nice day." Indeed, Zelig has become too much of his own person because he soon starts a fight with the psychiatrist to prove his point. Although Zelig has changed and grown, he is now embedded in another developmental level—Kegan's Stage 4, the institutional stage.

If this film were to show Zelig moving into Kegan's final stage, the interindividual stage, we would see him being able to hear other points of view and incorporate them into his view of the world, if he chose to do so. In Maslow's terms, he would then be the **self-actualized** person—a person who is in touch with himself, can hear feedback from others, is nondogmatic, is empathic, accepting, genuine, and introspective—in other words, an individual who embodies many of the characteristics of the effective human service professional. Zelig can even understand why the psychiatrist thinks it's a beautiful day—and maybe even decide himself that it is a beautiful day by hearing and understanding the psychiatrist's point of view. Although Zelig represents a comedic example of movement through the Kegan stages, finding a real-life illustration is not difficult, as there are many individuals who have dramatically changed and matured over their lifetimes (see Box 1.3).

As the Woody Allen and Malcolm X examples describe, change can occur if a person is in a supportive yet challenging environment. In Zelig's case, it was personal counseling that supported yet challenged him to change. In Malcolm X's case, it was initially the Nation of Islam, and later other experiences he had in life. As you might expect, college is another avenue that can offer an environment conducive for growth, with the classroom as the necessary supportive environment that is also challenging to the student. The classroom environment can assist students in

BOX 1.3 | The Story of Malcolm X

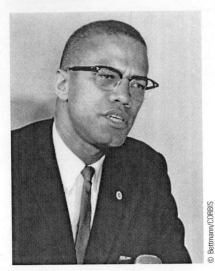

© Bettmann/CORBIS

The life of Malcolm X reflects movement through Kegan's stages of development.

As a young adult, **Malcolm X** found himself involved in a life of crime and drug addiction (X & Haley, 2001). While serving a ten-year prison sentence for robbery, he was introduced to the Nation of Islam, the Black Muslim religion headed by Elijah Muhammad. Malcolm readily gave up his former lifestyle and became embedded in the values of the Nation of Islam. He lived, slept, and breathed their values, and

his identity became the values held by the Nation of Islam (Kegan's interpersonal stage). However, as he developed and found new individuals to support him and learn from, he realized that he did not agree with some of the ideas of the Nation of Islam, and he moved from embeddedness in their values to a strong sense of his own religious, cultural, and moral values. Still somewhat closed to other points of view, Malcolm X had matured to the point where he could now embrace his own set of values (Kegan's institutional stage).

Following a pilgrimage to Mecca, he changed his name to **Al Hajj Malik al-Shabazz** and again modified his views "to encompass the possibility that all white people were not evil and that progress in the black struggle could be made with the help of world organizations, other black groups, and even progressive white groups" (Encyclopedia of Black America, 1981, p. 544). Clearly, Al Hajj Malik al-Shabazz was moving toward Kegan's interindividual stage. He now could hear other points of view, be open to feedback, and yet have a clear sense of his own uniqueness in the world. Unfortunately, as with many great people like Martin Luther King, Gandhi, and Jesus, he was killed because others were upset that he had grown beyond the rigid and dogmatic beliefs he had left behind.

their development as successful human service professionals and who embody many of the eight characteristics listed earlier (Diambra, McClam, Woodside, & Kronick, 2006). For instance, in class, you may want to now do Activity 1.1.

Because Activity 1.1 and similar exercises are important in helping you to cultivate the human service professional's characteristics, there will be experiential exercises at the end of each chapter to facilitate your own personal growth while you learn some basic facts and principles of the human service field.

ETHICAL, PROFESSIONAL, AND LEGAL ISSUES: KNOWING WHO WE ARE AND OUR RELATIONSHIP TO OTHER PROFESSIONAL GROUPS

Human service professionals have a unique identity that is reflected through the field's body of knowledge. By knowing who we are, we also have a clear sense of who we are not. When we identify ourselves as human service professionals, we

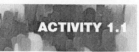

ACTIVITY 1.1 | Assessing Your Eight Characteristics

Using the following scale and following table, complete the first five or six items (Note: Item 6 can also be done at a different time if need be.

1. Of the eight human service professional characteristics, rate in Column 1 how important you think each characteristic is for the effective functioning of the human service professional.
2. Next, in column 2, rate how well you think you embody each of the eight characteristics.
3. Now, in column 3, rate whether you think you exhibited each of the eight qualities as you went through your life today.
4. In the Column 4, write what you can do to improve your scores of those areas where you have rated yourself lower.

5. Next, find a partner or have your instructor divide you into small groups to discuss your results. Talk about whether there are areas that you state you value but did not exhibit through your behavior. Discuss which areas you think you need to improve upon.
6. Finally, if you have the chance, ask another person who you know well and who will be honest with you, to rate you in column 5 on the eight characteristics. See if that person's ratings are similar to yours. Discuss that person's ratings and be open to his or her feedback.

_____ 1 _____ 2 _____ 3 _____ 4 _____ 5 _____ 6 _____ 7 _____ 8 _____ 9 _____ 10

Low Rating   Moderate Rating   High Rating

	Columns				
	1	2	3	4	5
	Importance	Self-Rating	Exhibited Today?	How to Improve Scores?	Others' Rating?
Relationship building					
Empathy					
Genuineness					
Acceptance					
Cognitive complexity					
Wellness					
Competence					
Cross-cultural sensitivity					

are able to clearly define our professional limits, know when it is appropriate to consult with colleagues, and recognize when we should refer clients to other professionals.

> Human service professionals know the limit and scope of their professional knowledge and offer services only within their knowledge and skill base. (Appendix A, Statement 26)

THE EFFECTIVE HUMAN SERVICE PROFESSIONAL: WILLING TO MEET THE CHALLENGE

The effective human service professional looks at his or her own behavior, risks obtaining feedback from others, and is open to change. This person views life as affording opportunities for growth and transformation. Although this individual's goal may be to embody the characteristics of the effective human service professional, he or she realizes that the "healthy" individual is always "in-process"—that is, he or she realizes that life is a continual, never-ending growth process. This person has a clear sense of his or her values relative to the human service profession and knows himself or herself. However, despite this firm sense of self, this person is willing to change if offered other ideas or concepts that make sense. "Firm yet flexible" is this person's credo. Finally, effective human service professionals are committed to excellence in themselves and in the profession. Therefore, they look for avenues of personal and professional growth and are willing to give of themselves to promote the profession (Evenson & Holloway, 2003).

SUMMARY

We began this chapter by defining the human service professional. We briefly discussed the early development of human service education and how it was a response to the need for more helping professionals during the 1960s. We highlighted the development of the associate's and bachelor's degrees in human services and discussed some of the typical kinds of courses one might today find in a human service curriculum. We noted that today's human service professional is a generalist, with interdisciplinary knowledge, who works side by side with other mental health professionals and takes on many roles in a variety of settings. This individual may have gained a credential as a Human Services—Board Certified Practitioner (HS—BCP). In defining specific roles, functions, and competencies of the human service professional, we delineated the 13 roles as identified by SREB, the 12 identified Skill Standards, and discussed some differences in how human services professionals,

counselors, social workers, and psychologist approach clients.

Comparing and contrasting the human service professional with related mental health professionals was another focus of this chapter. We gave brief explanations of some of the roles and functions of psychiatrists, psychologists, social workers, counselors, couples and family counselors, psychiatric-mental health nurses, psychotherapists, and also listed some "other" mental health professionals human services professionals might work with. We also highlighted their respective professional associations, including the American Psychiatric Association (APA), the American Psychological Association (APA), the NASW, the ACA, the AAMFT, and the APNA. We noted others. We paid particular attention to the professional association for human service students, educators, and practitioners: the National Organizations of Human Services (NOHS) and highlighted its regions and benefits.

The last half of this chapter emphasized the importance of the human service professional embodying the eight characteristics of the effective helper. These characteristics include relationship building, empathy, genuineness, acceptance, cognitive complexity, wellness, competence, and cross-cultural sensitivity. We described each of these characteristics and discussed the importance of continually embracing them throughout our careers. We noted that there are different theories of development that suggest how one's personality is formed. We suggested that an adult development approach, such as one that is described by Robert Kegan, is a good model for understanding how positive growth can occur. Using examples from the Woody Allen Movie *Zelig* and from Malcolm X's life story, we suggested that through support and challenge, individuals can grow and learn and become more empathic, less critical, less dogmatic, more accepting, increasingly open to other points of view, increasingly complex thinkers, and so forth. We also suggested that life opportunities, such as those through counseling and through education, can move us more toward embracing the eight qualities of the effective helper. We offered an activity to allow you to examine how much of each of these qualities you have and what you can do to increase some of the qualities.

As we neared the conclusion of this chapter, we stressed the importance of knowing our professional identity, for it assists us in defining who we are and in setting professional limits on ourselves. We noted that this ethical and professional issue is highlighted in the Ethical Standards of Human Service Professionals (see Appendix A). Finally, we concluded this chapter by examining what it means to be an effective mature human service professional, noting that such an individual is open to change and views life as a continual transformational process. Such human service professionals are personally and professionally committed to excellence and are willing to expend the energy needed to improve both themselves and the profession.

Experiential Exercises

I. Comparisons of Social Service Professionals

1. We often have varying perceptions of the training, education, and salary of the different social service professions. To see whether your perceptions are correct, fill in the items requested for the social service professionals listed in the following chart.

	Education	Coursework	Additional Training	Credential?	Salary
Human service professional					
Psychologist					
Psychiatrist					
Mental health counselor					
School counselor					
Social worker					
Psychotherapist					
Other					

2. Obtain a list of social service jobs (Sunday newspaper, online professional sites, professional newspapers) and identify all the classified ads that are social service oriented. In class, make a list of the types of jobs being advertised; the education, training, and experience needed for each job; and if available, the salary being offered. If the salary is not listed, you might want to consider contacting the agency and inquiring about the salary range.

II.   Interviewing Professionals in the Field

Using the following questions as a guideline, have one-fourth of the class interview a human service professional, one-fourth a social worker, one-fourth a psychologist, and the remainder, a counselor. Then, based on whom you interviewed, divide the class into groups of four representing each of the four disciplines. In your small groups, discuss the similarities and differences you find in the professions.

1. Why did he or she decide to enter the chosen profession?
2. What degree(s) was (were) obtained?
3. What is the theoretical orientation of the professional?
4. What are the job roles and functions as defined by the professional?
5. What was his or her entry-level salary?
6. What is his or her current salary?
7. What is his or her view on the differences among the four professions?

III.   SREB's 13 Roles and Functions

Using the 13 roles and functions of human service professionals as identified by SREB, describe an activity that might correspond to each role and function. Use the interview completed in Exercise II if you need some assistance in identifying specific activities.

1. Outreach worker
2. Broker
3. Advocate
4. Evaluator
5. Teacher/educator
6. Behavior changer
7. Mobilizer
8. Consultant
9. Community planner
10. Caregiver
11. Data manager
12. Administrator
13. Assistant to specialist

IV.   Discussing the Difference Between Counseling and Psychotherapy

In class, the instructor will write the words *counseling* and *psychotherapy* on the board. Students will free-associate to these words, and the instructor will write these associations on the board. Then, as a class, discuss the differences between the two terms. What do you think the counseling limitations are of the human service professional? Do you think the human service professional does counseling? Psychotherapy? Something else? Refer to Table 1.2 when discussing this question.

V. Joining Professional Associations

What professional association(s) do you want to join? Why might you join one association rather than another?

VI. The Characteristics of the Effective Human Service Professional

The following sets of activities have to do with the characteristics you think make an effective human service professional, as well as the qualities you possess that will make you an effective human service professional. To each question, write responses that you can bring to class. In class, you will be given the opportunity to discuss your responses in small groups.

1. Make a list of the personality characteristics you believe the effective human service professional should embody.
2. Make a list of the skills and techniques you think the effective human service professional should have.
3. What personality characteristics do you currently possess that will make you a successful human service professional?
4. What skills do you currently possess that will make you a successful human service professional?
5. Consider any differences between your list and the eight characteristics of the effective human service professional identified in this chapter.

VII. Acquiring the Characteristics of the Effective Human Service Professional

The following sets of questions concern ways of acquiring the qualities of the effective human service professional. Write responses for each question that you can bring to class. In class, you will be given the opportunity to discuss your responses in small groups.

1. How have the following influences affected your desire to enter the human service field? (If you are not entering the field, base your response on the field you think you will eventually enter.)
   a. Parents' education
   b. Parents' occupations
   c. Placement in family (e.g., middle child, youngest child)
   d. Educational experiences
   e. Work experiences
   f. Volunteer experiences
   g. Your values and beliefs
   h. Your gender and ethnic background
2. Often, individuals enter the helping professions because they have gone through their own painful experiences and want to assist others with theirs. What personal experiences have made you sensitive to other individuals' difficult life situations?
3. Many of the eight characteristics of the effective human service professional are developed through modeling the behavior of people who have significantly affected our lives. On the following chart, write the names of four people in your life who have affected you in a positive way.

These individuals can be friends, parents, religious leaders, politicians, movie figures, literary figures, and so on. Then fill in the chart, noting how the individuals modeled one or more of the characteristics. Finally, in class, share with another student how you have taken on some of the characteristics modeled by each person.

Significant Person

Characteristic ⇓	1.	2.	3.	4.
Relationship building				
Empathy				
Genuineness				
Acceptance				
Cognitive complexity				
Wellness				
Competence				
Cross-cultural sensitivity				

VIII. Assessing Your Wellness

Score yourself from 1 to 5 on all subfactors of the Creative, Coping, Social, Essential, and Physical Self listed in Table 1.3 (5 = the area you most need to work on). Then, find the average for each of the five factors. Next, write down the ways you can better yourself in any dimension or factor where your scores seem problematic (probably average scores of 3 or more).

Table 1.3 | Abbreviated Definitions of Components of the Indivisible Self Model

Wellness Factor	Definition
Total Wellness	The sum of all items on the 5F-Wel; a measure of one's general well-being or total wellness
<u>Creative Self</u>	The combination of attributes that each of us forms to make a unique place among others in our social interactions and to positively interpret our world
Thinking	Being mentally active, open-minded; having the ability to be creative and experimental; having a sense of curiosity, a need to know and to learn; the ability to solve problems
Emotions	Being aware of or in touch with one's feelings; being able to experience and express one's feelings appropriately, both positive and negative

Table 1.3 | Abbreviated Definitions of Components of the Indivisible Self Model (Continued)

Wellness Factor	Definition
Control	Belief that one can usually achieve the goals one sets for oneself; having a sense of planfulness in life; being able to be assertive in expressing one's needs
Work	Being satisfied with one's work; having adequate financial security; feeling that one's skills are used appropriately; the ability to cope with workplace stress
Positive humor	Being able to laugh at one's own mistakes and the unexpected things that happen; the ability to use humor to accomplish even serious tasks
Coping self	The combination of elements that regulate one's responses to life events and provide a means to transcend the negative effects of these events
Leisure	Activities done in one's free time; satisfaction with one's leisure activities; having at least one activity in which "I lose myself and time stands still"
Stress Management	General perception of one's own self-management or self-regulation; seeing change as an opportunity for growth; ongoing self-monitoring and assessment of one's coping resource
Self-Worth	Accepting who and what one is, positive qualities along with imperfections; valuing oneself as a unique individual
Realistic Beliefs	Understanding that perfection and being loved by everyone are impossible goals, and having the courage to be imperfect
Social Self	Social support through connections with others in friendships and intimate relationships, including family ties
Friendship	Social relationships that involve a connection with others individually or in community, but that do not have a marital, sexual, or familial commitment; having friends in whom one can trust and who can provide emotional, material, or informational support when needed
Love	The ability to be intimate, trusting, and self-disclosing with another person; having a family or familylike support system characterized by shared spiritual values, the ability to solve conflict in a mutually respectful way, healthy communication styles, and mutual appreciation
Essential Self	Essential meaning-making processes in relation to life, self, and others
Spirituality	Personal beliefs and behaviors that are practiced as part of the recognition that a person is more than the material aspects of mind and body
Gender Identity	Satisfaction with one's gender; feeling supported in one's gender; transcendence of gender identity (i.e., ability to be androgynous)
Cultural Identity	Satisfaction with one's cultural identity; feeling supported in one's cultural identity; transcendence of one's cultural identity

Continued

Table 1.3 | Abbreviated Definitions of Components of the Indivisible Self Model (Continued)

Wellness Factor	Definition
Self-Care	Taking responsibility for one's wellness through self-care and safety habits that are preventive in nature; minimizing the harmful effects of pollution in one's environment
Physical Self	The biological and physiological processes that compose the physical aspects of a person's development and functioning
Exercise	Engaging in sufficient physical activity to keep in good physical condition; maintaining flexibility through stretching
Nutrition	Eating a nutritionally balanced diet, maintaining a normal weight (i.e., within 15% of the ideal), and avoiding overeating
Contexts	
Local context	Systems in which one lives most often—families, neighborhoods, and communities—and one's perceptions of safety in these systems
Institutional context	Social and political systems that affect one's daily functioning and serve to empower or limit development in obvious and subtle ways, including education, religion, government, and the media
Global context	Factors such as politics, culture, global events, and the environment that connect one to others around the world
Chronometrical context	Growth, movement, and change in the time dimension that are perpetual, of necessity positive, and purposeful

Note: 5f-Wel = Five Factor Wellness Inventory
Source: Myers, J., & Sweeney, T. J. (2008). Wellness counseling: The evidence base and practice. *Journal of Counseling and Development, 86,* p. 485.

IX. Assessing Your Adult Developmental Level

Directions. The following inventory is designed to assess some of the qualities we discussed as important to being an effective counselor. It is extremely important to answer honestly and to *not fake good* on the instrument. After you have taken the instrument, have your instructor review the importance of these qualities in the helping relationship. The instrument has not been researched to show its validity and should be used only to give you a rough sense of your conglomerate score on these qualities.

Use the following scale when responding to each item.

1. Strongly Agree   4. Slightly Disagree

2. Slightly Agree   5. Strongly Disagree

3. Neither Agree nor Disagree

_____1. I believe that my opinions are almost always the correct opinions.

_____2. It is not unusual for people to seek me out to talk about their problems.

_____3. I find feedback from a professor enlightening.

_____4. The professor almost always has "the answer."

_____5. When making decisions, I usually gather information rather than making quick decisions from my "gut."

_____6. Usually, when I try to listen to someone, I interject my point of view.

_____7. The best type of learning takes place when the professor gives us the facts.

_____8. My church, synagogue, or mosque always espouses the right views.

_____9. When listening, I usually know from the opening statement what that person is going to say.

_____10. I rarely research answers to tough questions.

_____11. I can almost always determine the value of a person's belief system based on his or her appearance.

_____12. When considering important decisions, it is best to defer to specific figures (e.g., parents) rather than gathering information from multiple sources.

_____13. In coming to my views on life, I have spent a lot of time gathering information from others, reflecting, and being introspective.

_____14. In understanding other people with whom I am not familiar, I believe it is important to take the time to listen to them and understand their background.

_____15. My views are solid and no one can change them!

_____16. I have strong views and usually know what is best for another person when that person is struggling with a difficult situation in life.

_____17. I have chosen my values following deep reflection, and I am still open to examining them further.

_____18. Through conversations with others, I can change and see the world, differently.

_____19. When listening to someone, I usually disregard the person's feelings and listen more to "the facts" of the situation.

_____20. Generally, I think students can offer much to the knowledge base of a class.

_____21. I have rarely questioned the views of my parents.

_____22. When in a work group, in an effort to complete tasks efficiently, it is often necessary to make decisions with little or no collaboration.

_____23. Most clients need to be given strong advice and firm direction from the beginning of the counseling relationship.

_____24. The most important quality of the counseling relationship is understanding how the client comes to make sense of the world.

Scoring the inventory. For items 2, 3, 5, 13, 14, 17, 18, 20, and 24 give yourself *1* point if your response was a "5," *2* points if your response was a "4," *3* points if your response was a "3," *4* points if your response was a "2," and *5* points if your response was a "1." For all other items, give yourself the number of points that you rated the item. The highest score on this inventory is a 120. Higher scores (closer to 100 or more) are likely an indication that you are more empathic, accepting, competent, cognitively complex, and open to feedback. In class, your instructor might want you to anonymously hand in your score, so you can compare your score to the average score of your class. This will give you a sense of your score as it compares to your peers.

X.   Assessing Our Values

In class, divide into triads with each person taking the number "1," "2," or "3" (no repeats). Those who have been given the number 1 will be "pro," and those who have been given the number 2 will be "con." Number 3s are to help numbers 1 and 2 if they have trouble doing the task. Your task is to take one of the following situations (or come up with one of your own) and role-play your feelings about the situation. If you are pro, role-play the situation as if you are for it, even if you actually are against it. If you are con, role-play the situation as if you are against it, even if you are for it. It is important not to tell the members of your triad how you actually feel about the situation. Role-play for about 5 minutes. Then do the same thing, but this time take a new situation and rotate your positions; in other words, number 2 will be pro, number 3 will be con, and number 1 will be the helper. Finally, take a third situation, and this time number 3 will be pro, number 1 will be con, and number 2 will be the helper. Situations:

1. Abortion
2. Capital punishment
3. Opening an X-rated bookstore in your neighborhood
4. The War on Terrorism
5. National health insurance
6. Affirmative action
7. Increased tuition

Processing the exercise. In class, discuss how your values may have made it difficult to effectively listen to the other person at times. For instance, someone might say, "I was so upset that I just wanted to tell the other person how I felt." The instructor can put a list of "hindrances" to effective listening on the board. In class, discuss the following:

1. Why is it difficult to hear someone who holds differing values from your own?
2. How can you learn to be more accepting of differing values?
3. What techniques can you use to listen more effectively to an individual who holds values that vary from your own?
4. Why is acceptance of diversity important when you are in the role of helper?

XI.   Ethical and Professional Vignettes

Read the following ethical dilemmas. Using the Ethical Standards of Human Service Professionals in Appendix A, write a response to each dilemma.

1. A human service professional is making disparaging remarks about social workers, saying things like "They don't know what they're doing" and "Their training is inferior." Is this ethical? Professional? Legal? What should you do?
2. You are working with a client who is also seeing another human service professional at a different agency for the same problem. Is this ethical? Is this professional? What should you do?

3. You have heard one of your colleagues make racist remarks. What should you do? What can you do?

4. A colleague of yours seems to have rigid views about his clients and refuses to participate in continuing education activities. He says, "I've been in this field a long time; I know what I'm doing." Is he acting ethically? Professionally? What, if anything, should you do?

5. A client of yours is asking you to advocate for her child, who she suspects is learning disabled. Your client asks you to call the school and request testing for the child. The school has thus far refused such testing. Should you do this? Is this ethical? Is this professional?

6. A former classmate of yours finishes his degree and decides to advertise that he is a "psychotherapist." He sets up an office and sees clients using this title. Is this ethical? Professional? Legal?

7. A former classmate of yours finishes her degree and decides to advertise that she is a "life coach." She sets up an office and sees clients using this title. Is this ethical? Professional? Legal?

8. You decide to go to a pro-choice (or pro-life) rally despite the fact that you know some of your clients may see you and be turned off by your political affiliation. Is what you're doing ethical? Professional? Legal?

9. Your agency has implemented a new policy that states that all clients who are using illegal drugs will be reported to the police. You vigorously oppose such a policy and decide to ignore it. Are you acting ethically? Professionally? Legally?

10. A colleague of yours states that she is a credentialed human service professional. Actually, she has not obtained any credential. Is she acting ethically? Professionally? Legally? What, if anything, should you do?

The Human Service Profession: History and Standards

There I was, entering college as an idealistic, energetic young man trying to decide what major to pursue. I started out as a biology major, but after a couple of years realized that as much as I liked the sciences, this was not the direction I wanted to take in life. I wanted something where I would be helping people, or at least, engaged with people in some manner. I started asking around. I met with friends, met with professors, and met with advisors. I told them I wanted to be a helper in some fashion. I always got the same answer—switch your major to psychology. They offered no alternatives—there were no alternatives as far as they were concerned. I thought there must be some other options, so I went to the career center where I was given the same advice. In the early 1970s, these advisers felt there was only one choice for men going into the helping professions—psychology. Now I realize that these well-intentioned advisers were likely sexist, uninformed, and perhaps a little elitist in their views about the helping professions. For them, men became psychologists, and women went into social work. For those who couldn't make it into the few doctoral programs in psychology— well, they could become counselors. And at that time, few ever heard of this relatively new major and profession called human services. Fortunately, today there are many career options in the mental health professions, including human services.

In this chapter, we will explore the history of psychology, social work, and counseling; examine some of the stereotypes that have emerged based on their histories; and look at how these three fields have greatly affected the emergence of the human service profession. We will then examine the relatively short history of the human service profession and see what trends have taken place in this developing field. Finally, we will examine the emergence of standards in the profession and reveal how such standards are a mark of the maturity of a profession.

HISTORY

Why Look at History?

Can you imagine a woman being burned as a witch because she was mentally ill, or placed in a straitjacket and thrown into a filthy, rat-infested cell for the remainder of her life? Can you envision a man being placed in a bathtub filled with iron filings to cure him of mental illness, or bled to rid him of demons and spirits that caused him to think in "demonic ways"? What about having a piece of your brain scraped out to change the way you feel? These gruesome scenarios are a part of the history of our profession.

Unfortunately, I've taught long enough to know that when history is discussed, it is often not as interesting as what you just read. In fact, my experience has been that half the class mentally steps out. Why is this so? Learning names, dates, and a few facts is just plain boring for many people. If you're a student who is dreading this chapter, you may be asking yourself, "Why learn it?" To answer this question, let me introduce a concept that has helped me put historical events in perspective.

In 1962, **T. S. Kuhn** wrote a book called *The Structure of Scientific Revolutions*. This book had a profound effect on me because it helped put my ideas about knowledge and change in perspective. In particular, Kuhn's concept of the **paradigm shift**

Early treatment
of the mentally ill

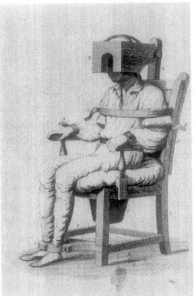

National Library of Medicine

intrigued me. He said that knowledge builds upon itself and that new discoveries are based on the evolution of past knowledge. However, Kuhn went on to note that sometimes current knowledge does not adequately explain the way things work. When this is the case, circumstances are ripe for a change in our understanding of the world—ripe for a paradigm shift. For instance, for hundreds of years individuals were at ease with the concept that the earth is flat. However, the advent of new scientific equipment seemed to contradict this model of viewing the world. A new explanation was needed. Thus, scientists hypothesized that the earth must be round. Similarly, in the social sciences, past theories worked adequately for a while. For instance, for many years **psychoanalysis** was the treatment of choice for mental illness. However, research on the effectiveness of treatments and the advent of new theories and new treatment procedures revealed that psychoanalysis often should *not* be the treatment of choice. In other words, a paradigm shift took place in the mental health field.

The human service field has undergone, and will continue to undergo, paradigm shifts. By studying the history of the field and by gaining knowledge about its roots, perhaps you will be the person to initiate the next paradigm shift!

Predecessors to Modern-Day Social Service Fields

Since the dawn of time, people have attempted to understand the human condition. Before the advent of religion, people used myths, magic, beliefs in spirits, ritualism, and sacred art as implements for thought and introspection and to make sense out of this complex world—"tools with which to think, talk, and know about self and world" (Ellwood, 1993, p. 20). Over the centuries, shamans, or individuals who had special status because of their mystical powers, were considered to be care-takers of the soul and were thought to have knowledge of the future. Later in history, the concept of soul paved the way for the concept of psyche.

The modern-day understanding of the psyche began to emerge in the last 200 years and has been applied by a number of mental health professions, including counseling, social work, and psychology. The human service profession emerged much more recently than these other professions and has drawn heavily from these three fields.

> The human service knowledge base is derived as much from psychology, guidance and counseling, nursing, etc., as it is from social work. (Clubok, 1984, p. 3)

Today, we can see that from the field of psychology, the human service profession has borrowed an understanding of the counseling process and a rich appreciation for testing and research; from the social work field, a deep caring for the underprivileged and an awareness of the power of social and family systems; and from the counseling profession, a holistic and wellness approach that attempts to understand the individual within the context of his or her career, love relationships, and group interactions. Although, today, these fields share much in common, their somewhat divergent histories have strongly affected the roles of human service professionals. In the following sections, we will briefly examine the history of these three fields, discuss how they affect today's human service professionals, and then examine the recent history of the human services.

A Brief History of the Psychology Profession

The field of psychology has a rich history founded in religion, philosophy, and science, and the concepts that have evolved from psychology are often seen as representing the underpinnings of many, if not all, of the social service fields today. As you review the following condensed history of the field of psychology, consider how much of what you read may have affected the work of today's human service professional.

Hippocrates (BCE 460–377) was one of the first individuals in recorded history to reflect on the human condition. Whereas many of his contemporaries believed that possession by evil spirits was responsible for emotional ills, Hippocrates had a different view, and some of his suggestions for the treatment of the human condition might even be considered modern by today's standards. For instance, for melancholia he recommended sobriety, a regular and tranquil life, exercise short of fatigue, and bleeding, if necessary. For hysteria, he recommended marriage—an idea with which many in today's world would certainly argue.

As with Hippocrates, one might think that some of **Plato's** (BCE 427–347) ideas came right out of a text on modern psychoanalysis. He believed that introspection and reflection were the keys to understanding knowledge and reality and that dreams and fantasies were substitutes for desires not satisfied. In addition, he considered problems of the human condition to have physical, moral, and spiritual origins. Although Plato's views were enlightening, some consider his student, **Aristotle** (BCE 384–322), to be the first psychologist because he attempted to objectively study knowledge and his writings were psychological in nature (Iannone, 2001; Wertheimer, 2000). In fact, he wrote essays on how people learn through association and the role that the senses play in learning.

Although individuals such as **Augustine** (354–430 CE) and **Thomas Aquinas** (1225–1274 CE) highlighted consciousness, self-examination, and inquiry as philosophies that dealt with the human condition, there is very little written of a psychological nature during the 800 years between the dates that they lived. This was partly the result of the rise of Christianity, which renewed the focus on the supernatural and advanced a movement away from any attempts to view the person objectively, as Aristotle had proposed. Following this quiet period in the history of science, the Renaissance and the era of modern philosophy arose in Europe. Here was a rediscovery of the Greek philosophies and a renewed interest in questions regarding the nature of the human condition.

Soon after the Renaissance, we saw the beginning of modern psychology. In the early to mid-1800s, individuals like **Wilhelm Wundt** (1832–1920) and **Sir Francis Galton** (1822–1911), two of the first experimental psychologists, developed laboratories to examine physical differences among people for such things as height, head size, and reaction time (Neukrug & Fawcett, 2006). The natural outgrowth of this movement was the testing era, where individuals' traits and abilities were compared using assessment instruments. The rise of the testing movement saw individuals like **Alfred Binet** (1857–1911) develop the first individual intelligence test, which was used to help the French Department of Education separate those children who were of average intelligence from those who were "feeble-minded" (intellectually disabled) (Binet & Simon, 1916; Neukrug & Fawcett, 2010). Later, ability tests such as school achievement tests and personality tests were developed. Today, tests are found everywhere and are often an important vehicle for obtaining a deeper understanding of our clients.

The beginnings of the testing movement paralleled the rise of psychoanalysis, the first comprehensive approach to doing therapy. Developed by **Sigmund Freud (1856–1939)**, psychoanalysis held the view that an individual's problems may in part have psychological origins. Freud was greatly influenced by people like **Franz Mesmer (1734–1815)** (from whom the word *mesmerize* was derived), who were practicing a new phenomenon called hypnosis. Until this time, mental illness was generally thought to be of a physical nature, and treatments for mental illness often were quite odd (see Box 2.1). However, when some individuals with certain kinds of physical illnesses were placed under a hypnotic trance, their ailments would disappear, suggesting the illness had psychological origins. Freud later gave up the use of hypnosis and developed psychoanalysis, which attempted to explain the origins of human behavior. His new view on mental health and mental illness was revolutionary and continues to profoundly affect the ways in which we conceptualize client problems (Neukrug, 2011).

Freud's theory, which tended to be somewhat pessimistic concerning the nature of the individual and the ability of people to change, emphasized instincts and early

---

BOX 2.1 | The Beginnings of the Modern Mental Hospital

In 1773, the "Public Hospital for Persons of Insane and Disordered Minds" admitted its first patient in Williamsburg, Virginia. The hospital, which had 24 cells, took a rather bleak approach to working with the mentally ill. Although many of the staff of these first hospitals had good intentions, their diagnostic and treatment procedures left much to be desired. For instance, some of the leading reasons that patients were admitted included masturbation, womb disease, religious fervor, intemperance, and domestic trouble—hardly reasons we'd use today for admission to a mental institution. Normal treatment procedures were to administer heavy dosages of drugs, to bleed or blister individuals, to immerse individuals in freezing water for long periods, and to confine people with straitjackets or manacles. Bleeding and blistering were thought to remove harmful fluids from the individual's system (Zwelling, 1990). It was believed important to cause fear in a person, and even individuals like **Dr. Benjamin Rush**, known for his innovative and relatively benign treatment of the mentally ill, spoke of the importance of staring a person down:

> The first object of a physician, when he enters the cell or chamber of his deranged patient, should be, to catch his EYE.... The dread of the eye was early imposed upon every beast of the field.... Now a man deprived of his reason partakes so much of the nature of those animals, that he is for the most part terrified, or composed, by the eye of a man who possesses his reason. (cited in Zwelling, 1990, p. 17)

Although many believed in the value of these rather extreme procedures in treating the mentally ill, some tirelessly tried to employ more humane methods. For instance, **John Minson Galt II**, the hospital's administrator from 1841 to 1862, believed that comfortable surroundings, social interaction, and job-related activities could help the mentally ill get better. **Dorothea Dix** also fought for humane treatment of the mentally ill and helped to establish 41 "modern" mental institutions.

child-rearing patterns in understanding personality development. Partly in response to Freud's bleak views concerning the individual's development, his contemporaries and students such as **Alfred Adler** (1870–1937) and **Erik Erikson** (1902–1994) developed theories that were humanistically based and stressed the influences of social forces on the development of the individual. Today, there are many approaches to psychotherapy, a good number of which are an outgrowth of or a reaction to Freud's psychoanalytic approach. (See Chapters 3 and 5 for a further discussion of Freud and psychoanalysis.)

The twentieth century saw a great expansion in the field of psychology. Today, we still find experimental psychologists working in laboratories trying to understand the psychophysiological causes of behavior and clinical psychologists working directly with clients doing therapy. In addition, we find other highly trained psychologists doing testing in schools, working for business and industry on organizational concerns, and applying their knowledge in many other areas.

The **American Psychological Association (APA)**, which was founded by **G. Stanley Hall** more than 100 years ago, has expanded dramatically and today is a major force in the social service field (Sokal, 1992). For instance, APA offers divisions for individuals who have an interest in just about any aspect of psychology, lobbies for a wide array of mental health concerns, and publishes numerous research journals through which an attempt is made to understand human behavior (Pepinksy, 2001; Routh, 2000). APA has continually given feedback to the American Psychiatric Association in its continued refinement of the *Diagnostic and Statistical Manual of Mental Disorders IV–Text Revision* (**DSM-IV-TR**) (APA, 2000). This manual, soon to be in its fifth edition (**DSM-5**), is instrumental in helping the clinician understand the individual, and insurance companies use the clinician's diagnosis when processing mental health claims.

Although the field of psychology was initially dominated by white men, in recent years we have seen the emergence of women and minorities as prominent psychologists. Together with the field of psychiatry, psychology has attempted to unravel some of the mysteries toward the understanding of mental health and mental illness. Today, the field of psychology continues to lead the way in the development of new theories of working with the individual and of attempting to explain normal and abnormal behavior.

Psychology's Impact on the Human Service Field.   For the human service professional, the field of psychology has had many practical implications. From providing the theoretical underpinnings that help us understand the nature of the person, to assisting us in our understanding of human behavior, to helping us find better ways of working with our clients, the field of psychology has been a major force in the social sciences. Psychologists are often our employers, our supervisors, our colleagues, or individuals with whom we consult. Acknowledging how psychology impacted human service work is critical to understanding our profession.

A Brief History of the Social Work Profession

The emergence of the social work field grew out of concern for the underprivileged and deprived in society. In contrast with psychology, which focused more on understanding the nature of the person, social work originated with the desire to help the destitute.

In England prior to the seventeenth century, providing relief to the poor was voluntary and was usually overseen by the church. However, given the dismal social conditions that prevailed, the English government under Henry VIII established one of the first systems of social welfare (Burger, 2011). Known as the **Poor Laws** of 1601, this government-initiated social welfare system established local "overseers of the poor" within each parish. These individuals were responsible for finding work for the poor, aiding those who could not work, and providing shelter or almshouses for those who were incapable of taking care of themselves. Although crude in its initial establishment, this law later became a model for social welfare programs. As a carryover from the English system, during the colonial period, local governments in the United States enacted laws to help the poor. During the same time, organized charities, usually affiliated with a religious group, arose in the United States.

During the 1800s, as populations in cities grew, an increasingly large underclass developed in the United States. Because the traditional charitable organizations could not meet the needs of these individuals, politicians applied mounting pressure to create specialized institutions. Thus, "reform schools," "lunatic asylums," and other specialized institutions were established.

Two major movements arose to help the underprivileged who were not institutionalized. **Charity Organization Societies (COSs)** maintained a list of volunteers who would enter the poorer districts of cities, become acquainted with the people, aid in educating the children, give economic advice, and generally assist in alleviating the conditions of poverty. Usually, the poor were not given money but were given advice, support, and, at times, a few "necessities." The volunteers, who were often called **friendly visitors**, also stressed moral judgment and religious values. Sometimes these friendly visitors would spend years assisting one family. The COSs are seen as the beginning of **social casework**, which is the process by which the needs of a client are examined and a treatment plan is designed.

In contrast to the COSs, the **settlement movement** had staff members who actually lived in the communities in which they sought to help the poor and immigrants:

> The settlements claimed to deal in brotherhood, not philanthropy; their spirit was fraternalistic, not paternalistic.... The settlement worker ... learned not alone from firsthand observation and the compiling of evidence but from sharing the common lot of the disinherited; the resident must "have genuine sympathy and continued relations with those who work day after day, year after year." Through a shared life, the settlement workers would come in time, not to speak for the slum dwellers, but to help them "express themselves and make articulate their desires." (Chambers, 1963, p. 15; quotes by Addams as cited in Chambers)

These idealistic young staff members believed in community action and tried to persuade politicians to provide better services for the poor. One of the best-known settlement houses was **Hull House**, established by **Jane Addams** in 1899 in Chicago (Addams, 1910; Macht, 1990). Addams, the first American woman to receive the Nobel Peace Prize, was known for her compassion, social activism, feminist views, and progressive ideas (Dieser, 2005).

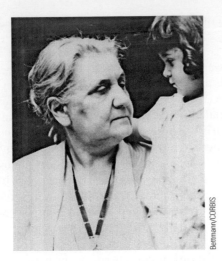

Jane Addams, one of the first "modern day" social workers, was a social activist known for her humane and liberal ways.

Bettmann/CORBIS

Out of this involvement with the underprivileged came articles and books concerned with methods of adequately meeting the needs of the underclass. Following the development of these "casebooks," and spearheaded by **Mary Richmond** at the turn of the century, the first social work training program was established at Columbia University. By 1919, there were 17 such programs in the country. During the next 30 years, the social work field grew in many different directions, with some of its main areas focusing on social casework, social group work, and community work.

Starting in the 1940s and continuing to the present, an increased emphasis on understanding social and family systems emerged in this country. Because social workers had already been intimately working with social systems and with families, this increased emphasis on the functioning and dynamics of these systems became a natural focus for many social work programs. Such programs were the first to view the individual in a contextual or systems framework, rather than seeing the individual in isolation as did many of the early philosophers and psychologists. One social worker in particular, **Virginia Satir** (1967), was instrumental in reshaping some of the practices of the mental health profession by including a greater systems focus.

In 1955, a number of social work organizations combined to form the **National Association of Social Workers (NASW)**. In 1960, NASW established the **Academy of Certified Social Workers (ACSW)**, which sets standards of practice for master's-level social workers. Today, NASW has 145,000 members, the vast majority of which hold a credential in the state in which they work (NASW, 2011a, 2011b). Social workers can be found in a variety of social service settings ranging from hospitals, to mental health centers, to homeless shelters—the roots of the social work profession. In addition, although many social workers today do individual psychotherapy and family therapy, some work in community settings, doing advocacy work, and others administer social service organizations.

Because the social work field grew out of charity organizations and volunteerism, and because women in the 1800s did not work outside the home, many women found their sense of meaning through these charitable efforts. Thus, for many years the field had the reputation of being a "woman's occupation." Recently, this has dramatically changed as the field and American values have transformed.

Social Work's Impact on the Human Service Field. The field of social work brings much to the human service profession. The beginning of the social work field in many ways echoes the essence of much of what today's human service professional does. Like the early social worker, today's human service professional helps the poor, the deprived, the underprivileged, and the mentally ill. And, like the early social worker, much of the human service professional's major emphasis is on support, advocacy, and caretaking. On a more practical level, the social work field has taught us casework approaches, how to work with systems, how to advocate for our clients, and the importance of respect and caring for our clients. One might say that the human service professional of today has taken on many of the functions and roles that the social worker used to embrace. Today, like psychologists, social workers are often our supervisors, administrators, colleagues, or consultants. The human service field is clearly a cousin to the social work profession.

A Brief History of the Counseling Profession

The **Industrial Revolution**, which began in the United States after the Civil War, changed the social and economic structure of the country. Many rural Americans, as well as immigrants—most of whom came from Europe to escape oppression— were drawn to urban factory centers in search of a better life. By the turn of the twentieth century, we saw the spread of the use of tests. These events set the stage for the very beginning of the counseling profession, which at that time was focused on vocational guidance (Herr, Cramer, & Niles, 2004).

Teachers and administrators were soon using tests in the schools to help individuals understand their skills and abilities and to "guide" them to appropriate professions. One of the leaders of this guidance movement was **Frank Parsons,** often said to be the founder of vocational guidance (Jones, 1994; McDaniels & Watts, 1994; Parsons, 1909/1989; Pope & Sveinsdottir, 2005). These events led to the founding, in 1913, of the **National Vocational Guidance Association (NVGA),** considered the forerunner of the **American Counseling Association (ACA).** As early as 1911, Harvard offered the first graduate courses for guidance specialists, and soon after, in Boston and New York, counselors were certified (Gladding, 2009).

Until the 1940s, most "counselors" were still doing vocational guidance. But during that decade, **Carl Rogers** (1942, 1951) and his nondirective, humanistic approach greatly affected the field of counseling. This client-centered revolution dramatically changed the way counselors were working, and they soon were giving less advice, focusing more on the "here and now," doing less testing and evaluation, and doing more facilitating. This humanistic approach to counseling starkly contrasted with the psychoanalytic approach of Freud. With the advent of World War II came an increased need for counselors and psychologists to work with war veterans. Thus, we soon saw counselors working outside the schools and practicing this new humanistic approach to counseling.

Probably the decade that most affected the counseling field was the 1950s (Neukrug, 2012). The *National Defense Education Act* (**NDEA**) of 1958 was a direct response to the Soviet Union's launching the world's first satellite, *Sputnik*, and funded the expansion of school counseling programs to identify gifted students. As a result, school counselors at the middle and secondary levels proliferated. The **American Personnel and Guidance Association (APGA)** was also founded during that decade. APGA was formed out of NVGA and other related counseling associations that were prevalent at that time.

In the 1960s, President Johnson's **Great Society** initiatives funded many social service programs (Kaplan & Cuciti, 1986). Partly in response to the growing need for counselors, the field diversified and counselors were increasingly found working in mental health, rehabilitation, higher education, and other related disciplines. In that decade, the **Association for Counselor Education and Supervision (ACES)**, a division of APGA, delineated standards for master's-level counseling programs (Sweeney, 1992). Also in that decade, differing types of group counseling were developed.

The end of the 1960s and the beginning of the 1970s saw a new approach to training counselors, known as **microcounseling skills training** (Carkhuff, 1969; Egan, 1975; Ivey & Gluckstein, 1974). These packaged ways of training helpers focused on learning specific skills, one at a time. It was quickly shown that learning basic helping skills in this manner could be accomplished in a relatively short amount of time and that the practice of such skills would positively affect the counseling relationship (Neukrug, 1980).

During the 1980s and into the 1990s, the counseling field continued to expand and eventually changed its name to the **American Association for Counseling and Development (AACD)** to stress the importance of how development impacts the person and on how prevention and education can be used to assist clients through normal developmental crises. Then, the association again changed its name to the more streamlined **American Counseling Association (ACA)**.

In recent years, there has been a push to stress the importance of cultural competence and social advocacy in the counseling relationship (D'Andrea & Heckman, 2008; Niles, 2009). Today, counselors can be found in almost any setting in which there are mental health professionals, and ACA now has 19 divisions that represent a number of specialty areas in counseling (ACA, 2011).

Counseling's Impact on the Human Service Field.   The counseling field has had a major impact on the human service field. The humanistic approach to the individual, which tends to be the focus of most counseling programs, is also pervasive in human service education. The concept that counseling skills or techniques can be taught in a systematic and focused manner is now a common method of training in most human service programs. In addition, counseling programs and many human service programs have stressed the importance of career as a major life force. Finally, other concepts which human services have borrowed from counseling include a developmental focus in understanding clients, the importance of prevention and education, and a focus on cross-cultural issues and social advocacy.

A History of the Human Service Profession

The Emerging Need for Human Service Practitioners.   In 1946 Congress passed the *National Mental Health Act*, which led to the creation of the **National Institute of**

Mental Health (NIMH) (Grob, 1996). This was the first real effort by the federal government to examine mental health issues, and it resulted in increased research and training in the mental health field. On the heels of the creation of NIMH came the **Mental Health Study Act of 1955**, which was a broadly based effort to study the diagnosis and treatment of mental illness. One result of the research from this act was the passage of the **Community Mental Health Centers Act of 1963** by the Congress. This bill greatly changed the delivery of mental health services in the United States by providing federal funds for the creation of comprehensive mental health centers across the country.

Although mental health centers may seem commonplace in today's society, the concept of having treatment centers available to the general public for mental health concerns is relatively new. Community mental health centers have greatly changed the face of mental health services across the country by supporting the associate- and bachelor-level professionals in the delivery of some services, by advocating for deinstitutionalization and the care of the chronically mentally ill within local municipalities, and by supporting the concept of primary prevention, which involves educating the public about mental health problems before they arise. Today, we often find human service professionals working at community mental health centers.

The 1960s saw great upheaval in the American society. There was unrest in the ghettos and a country in bitter turmoil over the Vietnam War. The civil rights movement was growing in momentum. Martin Luther King, Jr., Robert Kennedy, and others were advocating new directions for the country. Both were slain. It is often said that change cannot occur without pain. The death of some of our greatest leaders is perhaps a sad acknowledgment of this truth. Out of the turmoil of the 1960s came landmark civil rights and social change legislation (Diambra, 2001; Osher, 1990). As a result of President Johnson's **Great Society** legislation, civil rights laws and economic and social laws were passed:

> Service programs were intended to provide the resources and skills that would allow many poor and near poor individuals to compete for jobs effectively. Much of the emphasis was on youth and on education and training programs. Some of the key legislative changes included the Manpower Development and Training Act, Job Corps, Elementary and Secondary Education Act, Head Start, and the Work Incentive Program. The effort at reshaping the environment extended to the social and economic fabric of the community as well as its physical contours. Various types of discrimination were outlawed.... Key legislative actions included the ... Economic Opportunity Act of 1964, the Public Works and Economic Act of 1965, the Civil Rights Act of 1964, the Voting Rights Act of 1965, and the Model Cities Program of 1966. (Kaplan & Cuciti, 1986, p. 3)

As you can imagine from the large list of social service agencies that were developed during the 1960s, professionals were quickly needed to work at those agencies. Thus, there was the development of the associate- and bachelor-level human service programs (Diambra, 2001; McClam, 1997b).

Associate- and Bachelor-Level Human Service Programs Arise.   The creation of NIMH and the social changes of the 1960s were the impetus for the development of the human service field. With the development of comprehensive mental health services and dozens of new social service agencies, not only was there a need for highly trained master's- and doctoral-level professionals but there was

BOX 2.2 | A Conversation with Dr. Harold McPheeters

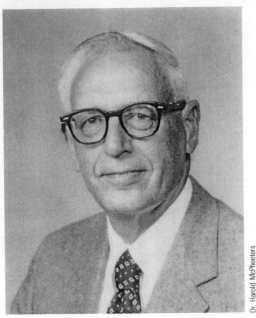

Dr. Harold McPheeters

Question: I think what is particularly interesting is that when the movement started it really was related to several factors that appeared to be unrelated.

McPheeters: Well, there were several things that made it an opportune thing to do. There was rampant professionalism that said "it's got to be done this way or it won't be right." The "great society" with its pressure for more manpower was clearly in conflict with that approach. There were a lot of other things that also came together. The new careers movement, the "hire now, train later" movement, was strong at that point. The movement was seen as a way for minorities and persons from deprived backgrounds to make it into human services. Otherwise, those groups tended to be excluded from the education programs and from the professions. There were civil rights issues that added to the pressure of the development of human services. (McClam & Woodside, 1989, pp. 3–4)

---

also a demand for associate-level human service professionals. Around this time **Dr. Harold McPheeters** (see Box 2.2) of the **Southern Regional Education Board (SREB)** applied for and received a grant from NIMH for the development of mental health programs at community colleges in the southern region of the country (McPheeters, 1990). This was the beginning of the associate-level human service degree in the United States. Therefore, some consider McPheeters to be the "founder" of the human service field.

During the 1980s and early 1990s the Reagan administration oversaw the reduction or elimination of some social service programs and a move toward federal block grants. Instead of the federal government designating which programs states should fund, **block grants** gave a "block" of money to the states and allowed *them* to decide which programs to fund (Hershenson, Power, & Waldo, 2003). In addition, during this period there was a stress on volunteerism, and many suggested that business and industry address some of the social woes of the country. Although some suggested that block grants would do away with many social service agencies, many of the social programs of the 1960s and 1970s lasted (Osher, 1990). And, despite the recession of the 1980s, associate degrees in human services became increasingly popular. In fact, there soon came a cry for more highly trained human service professionals.

During the mid-1970s funding from NIMH and SREB became available that offered workshops and conferences to explore the possibility of offering a bachelor's degree in human services. Then, during the 1980s we began to see the spread of bachelor degrees in human services. These degrees offered professional training in human services that borrowed from the knowledge base of psychology, social work, and counseling services (Clubok, 1984, 1997; Diambra, 2001; Fullerton, 1990a, 1990b). Although each of these three fields had explored the possibility of offering a bachelor-level degree in the mental health professions, ACA and APA ultimately moved toward training graduate-level professionals only, and the bachelor-level social worker degree offered by NASW simply did not fill the existing need for bachelor-level mental health workers. Thus evolved the bachelor's degree in human services (Fullerton, 1990a, 1990b).

Quickly, it became evident that whether trained at the associate or bachelor level, the human service professional was a generalist who drew from all the major mental health fields (Diambra, 2000, 2001; McPheeters, 1990). As defined by McPheeters and King in 1971, this definition still holds:

> The human service professional works with a limited number of clients or families in consultation with other professionals to provide "across the board" human services as needed; is able to work in a variety of agencies and organizations that provide mental health services; is able to work cooperatively with all of the existing professions in the field rather than affiliating directly with any one; is familiar with a number of therapeutic services and techniques rather than specializing in one or two areas; and is a "beginning professional" who is expected to continue to grow and learn ... (as cited in Clubok, 1984, p. 2)

Professional Organizations in Human Services Arise.   With dozens of human service programs being established throughout the country, a professional organization was needed to meet the needs of these new professionals. Thus, in 1975, the **National Organization for Human Service Education (NOHSE)** (now, the **National Organization of Human Services, or NOHS**) was founded with its mission being to strengthen the community of human services by:

- Expanding professional development opportunities
- Promoting professional and organizational identity through certification
- Enhancing internal and external communications
- Advocating and implementing a social policy and an agenda
- Nurturing the financial sustainability and growth of the organization

Soon after NOHS was founded, in 1979, the **Council for Standards in Human Service Education (CSHSE)** was formed "to give focus and direction to education and training in mental health and human service throughout the country" (CSHSE, 2011a, History section, para. 5). Today, this council offers a variety of services for associate-, bachelor-, and master-level human service programs. Some of the major functions of this council are as following (DiGiovanni, 2009):

- Maintaining national standards in human service education
- Accrediting associate-, bachelor-, and master-level human service programs
- Providing a directory of human service education programs
- Providing special reports and a monograph series in the human services
- Providing workshops and conferences for human service education
- Helping to establish credentialing processes for human service professionals

Recent History and a Look Toward the Future. The early 1990s were ushered in with promises by President Clinton to "focus like a laser beam" on the economy. And indeed, the economy flourished in the mid- to late-1990s. Then, during the first decade of the twenty-first century, we were faced with a series of new problems. As terrorism struck the American homeland, President Bush committed the United States to the War on Terrorism. Then, late in that decade, a serious economic recession hit our country and the world. With these events, many now ask, "Will these events deplete resources for human services and what will be the results of such an economic impact on services for the poor, destitute, mentally ill, and on the potential for employment for human service professionals?"

Today, we are still faced with a large number of homeless people, high poverty rates, the lack of or poor health care for a substantial number of citizens, and violence that seems to permeate our society. These problems tend to differentially affect individuals from nondominant groups (minorities and people of color). Clearly, the role of the human service profession is as important as ever, and the field has responded to the differential effects by stressing the importance of cultural competence and advocacy, among other things. In addition, with technology making us an interconnected world, the human service profession will increasingly need to take on a global focus and be facile with technological advances if it is to help all people (Gray, 2005; Kincaid, 2004).

Finally, the most recent accomplishment in the human services has been the adoption of a credentialing process for human services professionals. Started in 2008, there are already close to 2,000 **Human Services—Board Certified Practitioners** (HS—BCPs).

STANDARDS IN THE PROFESSION

The development of professional standards is an indication that a profession has matured and has taken a serious look at where it's been, where it is, and where it wants to go. As standards evolve, professions can reflect upon, revise, and sometimes even eliminate their standards. Standards in the profession can take many forms, with four of the more prominent ones in the human services being: (1) **Skill Standards,** (2) **credentialing,** (3) **ethical standards,** and (4) **program accreditation.** Let's examine how these professional standards in the human services have been established and how they affect the delivery of services in the profession.

Skill Standards

The primary purposes of the Skill Standards Project are to foster the adoption of national, voluntary skill standards for direct service workers; to increase both horizontal and vertical career opportunities for human service personnel; and to create a foundation for a nationally recognized, voluntary certification of direct services practitioners. The project is based on the assumption that the development of skill standards in the human service field is a critical step toward strengthening educational and training programs, improving responsiveness to service participants, increasing the marketability of workers, and enhancing the effectiveness and quality of services (Taylor, Bradley, & Warren, 1996, p. 1).

During the 1990s, a massive effort was undertaken to identify the job characteristics of the human service professional and develop a list of skills that would reflect these characteristics. To develop these Skill Standards, an in-depth job analysis was undertaken of human service professionals in four locations across the United States and was validated through a national survey of more than 1,000 individuals involved in human services. The result of this effort was the identification of 12 competency areas that are typically performed by human service professionals, a set of skills or job functions related to each competency, and activity statements or tasks that the human service professional would undertake to fulfill the job functions (Taylor, et al., 1996).

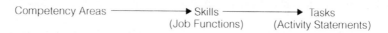

Competency Areas ⟶ Skills ⟶ Tasks
(Job Functions)   (Activity Statements)

As one example, for the competency of "communication," one skill would be to use "effective, sensitive, communication skills to build rapport" (Taylor et al., 1996, p. 26) and one activity (task) to accomplish this skill would be to use active listening skills. Box 2.3 defines the 12 competency areas. Can you identify possible skills and tasks that might be used for each of these competency areas?

The Skill Standards have become critical as they help educators define what needs to be taught in human service programs and they lend direction for accrediting and credentialing bodies in assessing what programs need to teach and what students who have graduated from such programs should have learned.

Credentialing

One method of ensuring that professionals are competent is through credentialing. Although credentialing in the mental health professions is a relatively new phenomenon, regulating occupations began as far back as the thirteenth century when the Holy Roman Empire set requirements for the practice of medicine (Hosie, 1991). Today, credentialing is common in many professions and can be found in many different forms. Usually, credentialing offers many benefits to the profession, the consumer, and the helper (Bloom, 1996; Corey, Corey, & Callanan, 2011), including the following:

- *Increased professionalization.* Credentialing increases the status of the members of a profession and clearly identifies who those members are.
- *Parity.* Credentialing helps professionals achieve parity in professional status, salary, and other areas with closely related mental health professions (e.g., social workers).
- *Delimiting the field.* The process of passing legislation to enable human service professionals to obtain credentials assists the profession in clearly defining who the human service professional is and what he or she is capable of doing.
- *Protection of the public.* Credentials help identify, to the public, those individuals who have the appropriate training and skills to do counseling.

Although credentialing takes many forms, three of the most common types are **registration, certification,** and **licensure.**

BOX 2.3 | Competency Areas for Skill Standards

Competency 1: Participant Empowerment
The competent community support human service practitioner (CSHSP) enhances the ability of the participant to lead a self-determining life by providing the support and information necessary to build self-esteem and assertiveness, and to make decisions. (p. 21)

Competency 2: Communication
The community support human service practitioner should be knowledgeable about the range of effective communication strategies and skills necessary to establish a collaborative relationship with the participant. (p. 26)

Competency 3: Assessment
The community support human service practitioner should be knowledgeable about formal and informal assessment practices to respond to the needs, desires and interests of the participants. (p. 29)

Competency 4: Community and Service Networking
The community support human service practitioner should be knowledgeable about the formal and informal supports available in his or her community and skilled in assisting the participant to identify and gain access to such supports. (p. 35)

Competency 5: Facilitation of Services
The community support human service practitioner is knowledgeable about a range of participatory planning techniques and is skilled in implementing plans in a collaborative and expeditious manner. (p. 40)

Competency 6: Community and Living Skills and Supports
The community support human service practitioner has the ability to match specific supports and interventions to the unique needs of individual participants and recognizes the importance of friends, family, and community relationships. (p. 45)

Competency 7: Education, Training, and Self-Development
The community support human service practitioner should be able to identify areas for self-improvement, pursue necessary educational/training resources, and share knowledge with others. (p. 51)

Competency 8: Advocacy
The community support human service practitioner should be knowledgeable about the diverse challenges facing participants (e.g., human rights, legal, administrative, and financial) and should be able to identify and use effective advocacy strategies to overcome such challenges. (p. 54)

Competency 9: Vocational, Educational, and Career Support
The community support human service practitioner should be knowledgeable about the career and education related concerns of the participant and should be able to mobilize the resources and support necessary to assist the participant to reach his or her goals. (p. 57)

Competency 10: Crisis Intervention
The community support human service practitioner should be knowledgeable about crisis prevention, intervention, and resolution techniques and should match such techniques to particular circumstances and individuals. (p. 60)

Competency 11: Organizational Participation
The community-based support worker is familiar with the mission and practices of the support organization and participates in the life of the organization. (p. 63)

Competency 12: Documentation
The community-based support worker is aware of the requirements for documentation in his or her organization and is able to manage these requirements efficiently. (p. 67)

Source: Taylor, Bradley, & Warren, 1996. Reprinted by permission of the Cambridge Human Services Research Institute.

Registration.   Registration is the simplest form of credentialing and involves a listing of the members of a particular professional group (Sweeney, 1991). Registration, which is generally regulated by each state, implies that each registered individual has acquired minimal competence, such as a college degree and/or an apprenticeship in his or her particular professional area. Registration of professional groups usually implies that there is little or no regulation of that group. Generally, registration involves a modest fee. Today few states provide registration for professionals, instead opting for the more rigid credentialing standards of certification and/or licensure.

Certification.   Certification involves the formal recognition that individuals within a professional group have met certain predetermined standards of professionalism. Although more rigorous than registration, certification is less demanding than licensure. Generally, certification is seen as a protection of a title (Remley & Herlihy, 2010); that is, it attests to a person's attainment of a certain level of competence but does not define the scope and practice of a professional (what a person can do and where he or she can do it). A yearly fee is usually paid to maintain certification.

Certification is often overseen by national boards, such as the **Center for Credentialing and Education (CCE,** n.d.). Although national certification suggests that a certain level of competence in a professional field has been achieved, unless a state legislates that the specific national certification will be used at the state level, such certification carries little or no legal clout. Many individuals will nevertheless obtain certification because it is an indication that they have mastered a body of knowledge, which can sometimes be important for hiring and promotion. Certification often requires ongoing continuing education for an individual to maintain his or her credential.

Licensure.   The most rigorous form of credentialing is licensing. Generally regulated by states, licensure denotes that the licensed individual has met rigorous standards and that individuals without licenses cannot practice in that particular professional arena (ACA, 2010b). Whereas certification protects the title only, licensure generally defines the scope of what an individual can and cannot do. One major advantage of licensure is that licensed mental health professionals generally can obtain third-party reimbursement (insurance reimbursement) for providing counseling and psychotherapy to clients. States generally set the standards for this most rigorous form of credentialing, which often requires a minimum educational level, passing a state or national exam, and additional documentation of expertise such as evidence of posteducation supervision. States may vary considerably on their requirements for licensure, so be sure to contact the licensing board of your state if you ever become license eligible. As with certification, licensure generally involves a yearly fee, and often continuing education requirements are mandated.

Credentialing in the Human Services

In 2008, the Center for Credentialing and Education (CCE), in consultation with NOHS and with CSHSE, developed a certification process for human service professionals. This certification has quickly certified close to 2,000 **Human Service—Board Certified Practitioners** (HS—BCPs) (CCE, n.d)

Table 2.1 | Number of Years' Experience Needed and Hours Needed as a Function of Degree to Become Certified

	Minimum Number of Post Years' Experience	Minimum Number of Hours
Technical certificate	5	7,500
Associate's degree	3	4,500
Bachelor's degree	2	3,000
Master's degree	1	1,500

The CCE certifies any individual who has a technical certificate or an associate's, bachelor's, or master's degree in human services or a related field. However, for those who have degrees in related fields, they must show that they have obtained 15 semester credits in courses traditionally offered in human service programs, and they must have two semester credits "in each of the following: interviewing and intervention skills, case managements, and ethics in the helping professions" (Hinkle & O'Brien, 2010, p. 25). In addition, based on the degree you have, the number of years of postdegree experience varies (see Table 2.1)

After showing that the person has achieved the necessary education and experience, the individual can take the national certification exam. This exam is developed by CCE in consultation with experts in human services and assesses knowledge in the following areas: "assessment, treatment planning and outcome evaluation; theoretical orientation/interventions; case management, professional practice, and ethics; administration, program development, evaluation, and supervision" (CCE, 2011, p. 4).

Those who pass the exam must obtain 60 clock hours of continuing education credits every 5 years in human service competence areas. In addition, those who obtain the HS—BCP are expected to abide by the HS—BCP code of ethics, which is different from the NOHS code of ethics. The NOHS code is an aspirational code, covering a large array of ethical concerns related to human service work. However, the CCE code is shorter and is focused more on the monitoring "the functioning of certificants and to adjudicate infractions" (Wark, 2010, p. 20).

This new credential in human services has "taken off" and is an important addition to standards in the field. It is a statement of how much the profession has developed in a relatively short amount of time and helps to delineate the professional identify of human service professionals.

Select Credentials in Related Helping Professions

Credentials abound in the mental health professions, and each credential makes a statement about a mental health specialist's body knowledge and expertise. The following highlights some of the more well-known credentials, but many others also exist.

Credentialing as a Substance Abuse Counselor and Other State Credentials. Some states have certifications for substance abuse counselors that require little or no educational experience, while other states require a master's degree for this credential. In addition, there are national master's-level certifications in addictions counseling (e.g., **Master Addiction Counselor (MAC)**, **National Board for Certified Counselors (NBCC)**, 2011). If you're interested in this growing field, contact your state health or credentialing office and see what the requirements are in your state. In addition, depending on the state you live in, there are likely other kinds of certifications available to you (e.g., child abuse, coaching, and mediation). Check with your state health or credentialing office to discover other areas of potential credentialing.

Credentialing for the Master's Degree in Counseling. There are many kinds of counselors, so as you might expect, there are many kinds of credentials available. Briefly, one can become a **certified** or **licensed** (depending on the state) **school counselor.** This credential is usually given by the State Board of Education after the attainment of a master's degree in school counseling. Also, rehabilitation counselors can obtain a credential as a **Certified Rehabilitation Counselor (CRC)**. All 50 states now have licensure for professional counselors **Licensed Professional Counselor (LPC)**, and any master's-level counselor can become a **National Certified Counselor (NCC)**, a certification sponsored by the NBCC. Subspecialities of the NCC include certifications in mental health counseling, school counseling, and addictions counseling. Finally, some counselors with a specialty in couples and marriage counseling can become a nationally **Certified Family Therapist (CFT)** and a state **Licensed Marriage and Family Therapist (LMFT)**.

Credentialing for the Master's Degree in Social Work. On the national level, a number of credentials exist for the many master's-level social workers. Experienced social workers can hold a credential as an ACSW from the **Academy of Certified Social Workers**. Those who have more clinical experience can become **Qualified Clinical Social Workers (QCSWs)**, and advanced clinicians can become **Diplomates in Clinical Social Work (DCSW)**. In addition, many clinical social workers become licensed in their states as **Licensed Clinical Social Workers (LCSWs)** (NASW, 2010).

Credentialing as a School Psychologist, and Counseling or Clinical Psychologist. One can generally become a **certified or licensed school psychologist** (states use different credentialing terms) after graduating from a state-approved school psychology program. The first push for credentialing of doctoral-level psychologists came during the 1950s (Cummings, 1990). Today, every state offers licensure for doctoral-level psychologists, generally in the areas of counseling and/or clinical psychology. In addition, many states now offer hospital privileges for **licensed psychologists**, which give them the right to treat those with serious mental illness. Psychologists have recently sought, so far with very limited success, to gain the right to prescribe medication for emotional disorders (Johnson, 2009).

Credentialing for Couples and Family Therapy.   Today, every state in the country has enacted some credentialing law for marriage and family counselors or therapists. In some cases, state marriage and family licensure boards have followed the guidelines set by the **American Association for Marriage and Family Therapists (AAMFT)**. In other cases, such marriage and family licensure has been subsumed under the counseling board or the boards of other related mental health professions. In addition to licensure, in 1994, the **International Association of Marriage and Family Counselors (IAMFC)**, a division of ACA, developed a certification process through the **National Credentialing Academy (NCA)** that enables a marriage and family therapist to become a **Certified Family Therapist (CFT)** (NCA, n.d.).

Credentialing as a Psychiatrist.   Because licensure as a physician is not specialty specific, individuals are licensed as medical doctors, not pediatricians, psychiatrists, surgeons, and so forth. Therefore, a physician who obtains a license within a state can theoretically practice in any area of medicine. However, because hospital accreditation standards generally require the hiring of **board-certified physicians**, almost all physicians today are board certified in a specialty area. Board certification means that the physician has had additional experience in the specialty area and has taken and passed a rigorous exam in that area. Thus, most psychiatrists are not only **licensed physicians** within the state where they practice but are also board certified in psychiatry (B. Britton, M.D., personal communication, March 10, 2010).

Credentialing as a Psychiatric-Mental Health Nurse.   There are two levels of **psychiatric-mental health nurses**—the basic and the advanced. Basic psychiatric-mental health nurses generally do not have advanced degrees and can work with clients and families doing entry-level psychiatric nursing. In contrast, advanced psychiatric-mental health nurses are generally registered nurses with a master's degree in psychiatric-mental health nursing. These **advanced practice registered nurses (APRN)** can do a wide range of mental health services, can prescribe medication, and can receive third-party reimbursement in many states (American Psychiatric Nurses Association, n.d.).

Ethical Standards

The Development of Ethical Codes.   The establishment of ethical guidelines in the helping professions began during the midpoint of the twentieth century, when, in 1953, the American Psychological Association (APA) published its code of ethics. Not long after, in 1960, the NASW adopted its code, and in 1961, the ACA developed its ethical code. Because ethical standards are to some degree a mirror of change in society, the associations' guidelines have undergone a number of major revisions over the years to reflect society's ever-changing values (see ACA, 2005; APA, 2003; NASW, 2008). Today, these codes serve a number of purposes, including all of the following (Corey et al., 2011; Dolgoff, Loewenberg, & Harrington, 2009):

- They protect consumers and further the professional standing of the organization.
- They are a statement about the maturity and professional identity of a profession.

- They guide professionals toward certain types of behaviors that reflect the underlying values considered to be desirable in the profession.
- They offer a framework for the sometimes difficult ethical decision-making process.
- They can be offered as one measure of defense if the professional is sued for malpractice.

Although ethical codes can be of considerable assistance in a professional's ethical decision-making process, there are limitations to the use of such codes (Corey et al., 2011; Dolgoff et al., 2009; Remley & Herlihy, 2010):

- Codes do not address some issues and offer no clear way of responding to other issues.
- There are sometimes conflicts within the same code, between the code and the law, and between the code and a counselor's value system.
- It is sometimes difficult to enforce ethical violations in the codes.
- The public is often not involved in the code construction process, and public interests are not always taken into account.
- Codes do not always address "cutting-edge" issues.

In the development and revision of ethical codes, deciding what might be included in a code can be a difficult task. For instance, it is sometimes difficult to decide which societal values should be reflected in codes (Gert, 2005; Ponton & Duba, 2009). Even when societal values are included, they are often not reflective of all individuals within American culture. As an example, codes have traditionally included the importance of client "self-determination." However, this is not a value held by all individuals in society, especially those who strongly value the opinions of extended family or authority figures when making important decisions. In addition to societal values, universal truths are often reflected in a code. However, people also debate the universality of universal truths. For example, the idea that "thou shall not kill" seems to be universal, yet many would hold that killing is ethical during war. Or, if someone is dying and in the last, very painful stages of cancer, and that person wishes to take an overdose of morphine and asks for your help—is that "killing." And, if it is, what about *that* person's right for "self-determination." You can see why the development of ethical codes and how to respond to ethical dilemmas can sometimes be a difficult task.

Ethical dilemmas come in many shapes and sizes. Take a look at Table 2.2, which surveyed all members of NOHS and asked them to decide whether each of the behaviors was ethical. See what you think. If time allows, discuss some of the more difficult situations in class.

Resolving Ethical Dilemmas Through Ethical Decision-Making.   In view of the practical limitations of ethical guidelines noted earlier, and in search of additional ways of resolving ethical dilemmas, **ethical decision-making models** have been devised (Cottone & Claus, 2000; Welfel, 2010). Three such approaches include **problem-solving models, moral models,** and **developmental models,** none of which is exclusive of each other; that is, they can be used in conjunction with one another.

Problem-Solving Models.   Problem-solving models provide the helper with a step-by-step, practical approach to ethical decision-making. One such approach,

Table 2.2 | Percentage of NOHS Members Who Believed Situations to Be Ethical

% Ethical	Behavior
100	Informing clients of the purpose of the helping relationship
100	Keeping information confidential
99.2	Respecting client self-determination
98.4	Breaking confidentiality if the client is threatening harm to others
98	Breaking confidentiality if the client is threatening harm to self
97.6	Being an advocate for clients
91.8	Referring a client due to interpersonal conflicts between you and your client
91.4	Using an interpreter when a client's primary language is different from yours
90.2	Addressing your client by his or her first name
90.2	Having clients address you by your first name
88.6	Sharing confidential client information with your supervisor
86.6	Engaging in two helping relationships with a client at the same time (e.g., individual counseling and group counseling)
85.8	Showing unconditional acceptance even when opposed to a client's behavior/values
85.8	Consoling your client by touching her/him (e.g., placing hand on shoulder)
85	Publicly advocating for a controversial cause
81.1	Providing services to an undocumented worker (sometimes called illegal immigrant)
80.9	Keeping client records on your office computer
70.9	Self-disclosing to a client
67.2	Counseling a pregnant teenager without parental consent
66.7	Hugging a client
64.8	Attending a client's wedding, graduation ceremony, other formal ceremony
63.8	Not being a member of a human services professional association
62.7	In a professional manner, telling your client you like him or her
61.1	Making a diagnosis (e.g., based on *DSM-IV-TR* or on client symptomology)
58.6	Counseling a terminally ill client about end-of-life decisions including suicide
57.4	Guaranteeing confidentiality for couples and families
54.9	Guaranteeing confidentiality for group members
54.7	Referring a client who is unhappy with his/her homosexuality for reparative therapy (therapy focused on converting sexual identity from homosexual to heterosexual)
51.2	Sharing confidential client information with your employer
51.2	Sending holiday and/or birthday cards to clients
50.8	Providing counseling over the Internet
49	Withholding information about a minor client despite the parents' request for information
48.4	Sharing confidential client information with your colleagues
47.2	Accepting a gift from a client that's worth less than $25
46.7	Not allowing clients to view your case notes about them
46.3	Viewing your client's personal web page (e.g., myspace, facebook, blog) without informing your client
45.9	Telling your client you are angry at him or her
36.9	Bartering (accepting goods or services) for helping services
36.2	Giving a gift worth $25 or less to a client
34.6	Breaking the law to protect your client's rights
33.6	Selling a product to your client related to the helping relationship
32.5	Pressuring a client to receive needed services
32.1	Reporting a colleague's unethical conduct without first consulting with the colleague
29.3	Counseling clients from a different culture with little or no cross-cultural training
24.4	Based on personal preference, accepting clients who are only male or only female

Table 2.2 | Percentage of NOHS Members Who Believed Situations to Be Ethical (Continued)

% Ethical	Behavior
23.4	Seeing a minor client without parental consent
23	Not having malpractice coverage (on your own or by your agency)
23	Not reporting suspected spousal abuse
21.5	Engaging in a dual helping relationship (a client working with you and another helper) without contacting the other helper
21.1	Becoming sexually involved with a person your client knows well
20.7	Engaging in a professional helping relationship with a family member
19.9	Becoming sexually involved with a former client (five years since helping relationship)
19.9	Kissing a client as a friendly gesture (e.g., in greeting)
19.5	Based on personal preference, accepting clients only from specific cultural groups
18.3	Engaging in a professional helping relationship with a friend
18	Accepting a client's decision to commit suicide
15	Engaging in a dual relationship (e.g., your client is also your child's teacher)
15	Not participating in continuing education (e.g., conferences, workshops, trainings) after obtaining your degree
13.9	Trying to change your client's values
13.1	Not allowing clients to view their records (excluding case notes)
12.7	Accepting a client when you have not had training in their presenting problem
8.9	Giving a gift worth more than $25 to a client
8.6	Telling your client you are attracted to him or her
8.5	Accepting a gift from a client that's worth more than $25
6.5	Keeping client records in an unlocked file cabinet
6.5	Treating homosexuality as a pathology
6.1	Referring a client who is satisfied with his/her homosexuality for reparative therapy
4.9	Lending money to your client
4.9	Attempting to have your client *not have* an abortion even though she wants to
4.5	Terminating the helping relationship without warning
4.1	Counseling while you are emotionally impaired
3.7	Releasing records to a third-party (e.g., another agency) without client consent
3.3	Making grandiose statements about your expertise
2.5	Not reporting suspected elder abuse
2	Recording your client without his/her permission
1.6	Not revealing the limits of confidentiality to your client
1.6	Selling a product to your client that is not related to the helping relationship
1.6	Not informing clients of their legal rights (e.g., HIPPA, FERPA, confidentiality)
1.2	Attempting to have your client *have* an abortion even though she doesn't want to
0.8	Sharing confidential client information with your friends
0.8	Not reporting suspected child abuse
0.4	Becoming sexually involved with a client
0.4	Stating you are credentialed without having a credential
0.4	Sharing confidential client information with your family members
0.4	Counseling while you are impaired by a substance (e.g., drugs or alcohol)
0.4	Attempting to persuade your client to adopt a religious conviction you hold
0	Revealing client records to the spouse of a client without the client's permission

Source: Milliken, T., & Neukrug, E. (2009). Perceptions of ethical behaviors of human service professionals. *Human Service Education*, 29(1), 35–48.

developed by Corey et al. (2011), is an eight-step practical model that consists of: (1) identifying the problem or dilemma, (2) identifying the potential issues involved, (3) reviewing the relevant ethical guidelines, (4) knowing the applicable laws and regulations, (5) obtaining consultation, (6) considering possible and probable courses of action, (7) enumerating the consequences of various decisions, and (8) deciding on the best course of action. Corey's and other similar models can be a great aid to the clinician in the sometimes thorny ethical decision-making process.

Moral Models (Principle and Virtue Ethics Models). While Corey's model emphasizes pragmatism, **moral models** stress moral principles in ethical decision-making and include **principle ethics models** or **virtue ethics models**. For instance, **Kitchener's** (1984, 1986; Urofsky, Engels, & Engebretson, 2008) principle ethics model revolves around six principles to consider in ethical decision-making: *autonomy* has to do with protecting the independence, self-determination, and freedom of choice of clients; *nonmaleficence* is the concept of "do no harm" when working with clients; *beneficence* relates to promoting the good of society, which can be at least partially accomplished by promoting the client's well-being; *justice* refers to providing equal and fair treatment to all clients; *fidelity* is related to maintaining trust (e.g., keeping conversations confidential) and being committed to the client; and *veracity* has to do with being truthful and genuine with the client, within the context of the counseling relationship. On the other hand, rather than focusing on what should be done (principles) some suggest focusing on the helper's character or virtues (Kleist & Bitter, 2009). For instance, Meara, Schmidt, and Day's (1996) suggest that helpers should be *prudent* or careful and tentative in their decision-making, maintain *integrity*, are *respectful*, and are *benevolent*. In addition, virtuous counselors strive to make ideal decisions based on their understanding of their profession and the community. They do this by being self-aware, compassionate, understanding of cultural differences, motivated to do good, and by having a vision concerning decisions that are made.

Developmental Models. Developed by such individuals as **William Perry** (1970) and **Robert Kegan** (1982, 1994), these models attempt to understand how an adult's ways of understanding the world might change over time. Although not specifically developed for ethical decision-making, these models suggest that individuals at "lower" levels of development would respond differently than those who are at "higher" levels (Linstrum, 2005; Neukrug, Lovell, & Parker, 1996). Such models would likely assume that helpers at lower levels of development would want "the answer" to complex questions that might face them, such as those involved in difficult ethical decisions. These helpers often adhere to a rigid view of the truth, and expect, or at the very least, hope that such formal documents as ethical codes hold the answer to complex ethical dilemmas. They are also likely to look at those in positions of authority and power (e.g., supervisors) as being able to quickly tell them the correct answer when faced with thorny ethical dilemmas. These helpers can be said to be making meaning from what Perry calls the stage of **dualism** in that they view the world in terms of black–and–white thinking, concreteness, rigidity, oversimplification, stereotyping, self-protectiveness, and authoritarianism. In contrast, higher-level helpers, sometimes called individuals who are in Perry's stages of **relativism** or **commitment in relativism,** would be more complex thinkers, open to differing opinions, flexible, empathic, sensitive to the context of the ethical dilemma, and nondogmatic (Cottone, 2001; Kohlberg, 1984; McAuliffe & Eriksen, 2010). Although few adults (or human service professionals) reach the highest levels of development (Lovell, 1999), these models suggest that, if afforded the right opportunities, most can. Training programs can offer opportunities to support and challenge students to move toward these higher levels of development.

Summarizing and Integrating the Models. To illustrate various approaches to ethical decision-making, let's examine two human service professionals, Jason, who is at a lower developmental level, and Jawanda, who is at a higher developmental level. Both are faced with the same dilemma—a client of theirs is smoking and selling crack cocaine, and the agency at which they work requires that clients who are selling drugs be reported to an administrator who will then contact the police. Jason examines the ethical code and reads the agency policy guidelines and decides that the "right thing to do" and the only choice he has is to report his client to an administrator. Jawanda, however, views ethical decision making differently. She also reads the agency policy and reviews the ethical guidelines. In addition, she uses a model such as that of Corey et al. (2011) or Kitchener (1984, 1986) in helping her decide what to do. She also tries to be careful, wise, thoughtful, respectful, and caring (virtues). She consults with others to gain other points of view and only then carefully deliberates about what would be best for her client, the agency, society, and herself. After careful consideration, she comes to a conclusion.

The conclusion in this case is really less important than the process—that's why Jawanda's decision is not given. Jawanda has dealt with the situation in a complex and thoughtful manner compared with Jason's somewhat hasty decision. In fact, although both may come to the same conclusion, I would rather work with someone like Jawanda because she shows thoughtfulness and the ability to self-reflect—qualities I would want in a colleague (and a friend!). Thus, we see that ethical decision-making can be, and perhaps should be, a complex process (see Activity 2.1).

Final Thoughts. Ethical guidelines are not legal documents. However, because they reflect the values of our professional associations, we are expected to abide by them. Thus, when a professional violates the codes of ethics, consequences could include removal from a professional association, revocation of his or her credential, or even dismissal from a job. In some instances, states have made part or all of a code of ethics into a legal document. In these cases, stiffer penalties such as fines or even imprisonment could result from an ethical violation. Of course, this depends on the seriousness of the violation. In either case, we hope that when faced with difficult ethical dilemmas you will consider your ethical code as well as some of the models we just discussed and that you come up with a wise decision—whatever that decision is. Throughout this text, we will raise various professional and ethical issues that are related to the NOHS code of ethics.

| **Becky**

A person who is wise at making ethical decisions can integrate the use of one's ethical code with all of the models we have discussed earlier. First, examine NOHS's ethical code (see Appendix A) and see how it might apply. Then, consider how one might use the problem-solving model with the following scenario. Then consider how one might use a principle ethics model and then a virtue ethics model. Finally, consider how a person of higher development could integrate knowledge from the code with the models mentioned earlier in responding to the dilemma.

> As a human service professional for the local department of human services, you have been assisting Becky, a single mother of a four-year-old daughter, for the past few years as she has attempted to remove herself from the welfare rolls,

obtain employment, and secure child care. Today, Becky walks into your office and tells you that she has been HIV positive for the past 8 years and that 2 years ago she developed AIDS.

> Becky has not responded well to her recent new regimen of medication. She is clearly despondent, is very concerned for the well-being of her child, and confides to you that she is considering killing herself. She notes that she has few significant people in her life, realizes that it may only be a matter of time before she dies, and is concerned that in the time she has left she will not be able to adequately care for her daughter. She therefore would like your help in finding a good home for her child and in "getting her affairs in order" before she commits suicide. As a helper, as one of her few confidantes, and as someone who cares, what should you do?

Program Accreditation

A final standard that underscores professionalism is program accreditation. In the case of human service programs, CSHSE is the accrediting body. The CSHSE standards delineate general program characteristics and curriculum areas that must be addressed if a program is to be accredited by the council.

Accreditation is a rigorous process whereby a human services program undergoes an involved self-study, usually makes a number of major changes, and then invites an accreditation team to visit the program to attest to whether or not the program meets the external standards of the accrediting body (Kincaid & Andresen, 2010). After a recommendation from the accreditation team, the CSHSE board votes on whether or not to accredit the program. Benefits of having such a process include the following (Altekruse & Wittmer, 1991; Kincaid & Andresen, 2010; Schmidt, 1999):

- Students who graduate from accredited programs study from a common curriculum are generally more knowledgeable about core issues in the human services and usually participate in fieldwork experiences that are more intensive and longer in duration.
- Program accreditation often becomes the standard by which credentialing bodies determine who is eligible to become certified or licensed.
- Program accreditation offers the impetus for setting and maintaining high standards.

- Program accreditation almost always results in improved programs.
- Administrators and legislators are often more willing to provide money to maintain the high standards of accredited programs as compared to less rigorous nonaccredited programs.
- Those who graduate from accredited programs generally have better job opportunities.
- Accredited programs often attract better faculty.
- Accredited programs often attract better students.

Accreditation of human service programs, which started in 1979, is a relatively new process. Today approximately 40 programs are fully accredited (CSHSE, 2011b). CSHSE accredits associate-, bachelor-, and master-level programs, each of which has its own accreditation standards (see www.cshse.org/standards.html). Although a relatively small number of human service programs are currently accredited, it is clear that progress is quickly being made toward accrediting more programs. As increasing numbers of programs do become accredited, it will become a disadvantage to have graduated from a nonaccredited program. Although a student should not worry if his or her program is currently not accredited, it seems clear that within the next 10–20 years, program accreditation will become increasingly advantageous. If a program values its professional organizations, supports high standards, and wants to develop highly trained students, it should seek program accreditation through CSHSE (DiGiovanni, 2009).

ETHICAL, PROFESSIONAL, AND LEGAL ISSUES: COMPETENCE AND QUALIFICATIONS AS A PROFESSIONAL

As mentioned in Chapter 1, one of the critical characteristics of the effective human service professional is competence, or having a thirst for knowledge and a desire to continue learning throughout one's professional career. Competence is also an important area highlighted in our ethical code. For instance, the Ethical Standards of Human Service Professionals includes the following statements:

> Human service professionals know the limit and scope of their professional knowledge and offer services only within their knowledge and skill base. (See Appendix A, Statement 26)

and

> Human service professionals promote the continuing development of their profession. They encourage membership in professional associations, support research endeavors, foster educational advancement, advocate for appropriate legislative actions, and participate in other related professional activities. (See Appendix A, Statement 30)

I believe that every human service professional should become a member of his or her professional association(s), subscribe to and read the professional journals, attend workshops and participate in other continuing education experiences, and obtain appropriate credentials. Excellence as a human service professional means commitment to educational competence.

THE EFFECTIVE HUMAN SERVICE PROFESSIONAL: PROFESSIONALLY COMMITTED, ETHICALLY ASSURED

The effective human service professional is committed to his or her professional growth and competence. This commitment is not lip service; it is a deeply felt belief that to do one's best in the profession means embracing the field in a professional manner. This human service professional knows the roots of his or her profession and can work in a consultative and mature manner with related professions. This professional knows appropriate ethical conduct because he or she is familiar with the ethical guidelines. Although many ethical decisions are judgment calls, the ethically assured human service professional makes wise decisions because he or she is not only familiar with the ethical codes, but understands ethical decision-making models and has kept abreast of the most recent trends in the field. Finally, the effective human service professional actively supports standards such as program accreditation, credentialing, and Skill Standards as he or she understands that such standards ultimately lead to providing the best possible services to clients.

SUMMARY

In this chapter, we were introduced to the notion of "history as knowledge" and the importance of history in helping us understand the concept of paradigm shifts. We then reviewed some of the antecedents to the human service profession and noted that helpers have been around since the dawn of existence. Moving on to the more recent past, we reviewed the rich history of the fields of psychology, social work, and counseling and examined how each of them has affected the profession we call human services. In particular, we noted that the field of psychology has given us an understanding of the process of therapy and a rich appreciation for testing and research, that the social work field brought us a deep caring for the underprivileged and an awareness of the power of social and family systems, and that the counseling brought us the importance of career as a major life force, a developmental focus in understanding clients, the importance of prevention and education, and a focus on cross-cultural issues and social advocacy.

This examination of the history of closely related professions was followed by a chronology of the more recent events that brought about the actual emergence of the human service field. We noted how the *National Mental Health Act*, and acts and laws that followed in the 1950s

and 1960s, greatly impacted the number of social service agencies in society and the need for more mental health professionals. We pointed out that out of this need came associate-level, then bachelor-level human service programs that trained human service professionals as generalists with interdisciplinary knowledge. We highlighted the fact that this new profession soon had professional organizations, such as NOHS and CSHSE that helped to focus its professional identity.

As a profession matures, standards become increasingly important. Thus, the second part of this chapter reviewed four important standards in the field: Skill Standards, Credentialing, Ethical Standards, and Accreditation. We noted that the recent development of Skill Standards offers us 12 competencies along with a series of skills and tasks that are a natural outgrowth of these competencies. We highlighted the fact that training in these skills can lead to the strengthening of educational programs and can be important in the accreditation and credentialing processes. In reference to credentialing, we distinguished among registration, certification, and licensure and discussed the value of each of these credentials. We also delineated some of the many different types of credentials offered in the human services and by related mental health professions. We highlighted the new credential in the human services: the Human Services—Board Certified Practitioner.

Next in the chapter we examined some of the purposes of ethical guidelines as well as some of their limitations. We pointed out that ethical dilemmas can be difficult and gave the results of one study of human service professionals' perceptions of ethical behaviors. We noted that making ethical decisions is a complex process that optimally should involve a review of ethical guidelines, knowing practical steps to take when facing an ethical dilemma, examining the moral principles and virtues behind making the decision, and making a wise decision. We suggested that those at higher levels of cognitive development make ethical decisions in a manner that differs from the approach taken by those at lower levels. Finally, in discussing program accreditation, we highlighted the advantages of accreditation and noted that CSHSE has developed national accreditation standards for human service programs. We gave a quick review of that process.

As the chapter ended, we highlighted the importance of keeping abreast of changes in the field and the significance of knowing one's limitations as they relate to the ethical issue of competence. Finally, we pointed out that the effective human service professional knows his or her roots, can work side by side with other professionals, is committed to the field, and has a strong sense of ethical correctness.

Experiential Exercises

I. Important Names and Places

Write a brief statement that defines the term or name listed.

1. Paradigm shift
2. Hippocrates
3. Plato
4. Aristotle
5. Augustine
6. Thomas Aquinas
7. Wilhelm Wundt
8. Sir Francis Galton
9. Alfred Binet
10. Sigmund Freud
11. Franz Mesmer
12. G. Stanley Hall
13. American Psychological Association
14. *DSM-IV-TR* (and *DSM-5*)
15. Poor Laws
16. John Minson Galt II
17. Dorothea Dix
18. Charity organization society
19. Friendly visitors
20. Social casework
21. Settlement movement
22. Jane Addams
23. Hull House
24. Mary Richmond
25. Virginia Satir

26. National Association of Social Workers
27. Academy of Certified Social Workers
28. Frank Parsons
29. National Vocational Guidance Association
30. Carl Rogers
31. National Defense Education Act
32. American Personnel and Guidance Association
33. Great Society
34. American Association for Counseling and Development
35. American Counseling Association
36. National Institute of Mental Health
37. *Mental Health Study Act*
38. Primary prevention
39. Block grants
40. Dr. Harold McPheeters
41. Southern Regional Education Board
42. Council for Standards in Human Service Education
43. National Organization for Human Services
44. Skill Standards
45. Ethical standards
46. Ethical decision-making models
47. Credentialing
48. Registration
49. Certification
50. Licensure
51. Program accreditation

II. Identifying Positive Qualities

For each of the great historical figures listed here, generate those characteristics that each of them may have embodied that could be considered vital elements of the helping relationship. Add others of your choosing.

Jesus	Moses	Muhammad
Gandhi	Martin Luther King, Jr.	Eleanor Roosevelt
Joan of Arc	Abraham Lincoln	Rosa Parks
Mother Teresa	Malcolm X	

III. Are We Ready for Another Paradigm Shift?

Do you think the mental health professions are "primed" for another paradigm shift? If yes, what direction do you think it will take? If not, why not?

IV. Visiting an Institution for the Mentally Ill

Make arrangements to visit a modern mental institution. How does the current mental hospital differ from early institutions as discussed in the text? What similarities do you think exist between today's institutions and those in the 1800s?

V. Discussing the Problems of the Poor and Destitute

Have a discussion with a homeless person, visit a shelter for the homeless, and/or visit a storefront walk-in center for the underprivileged. Then, in class, discuss the problems of the poor and destitute. What solutions do you think would work in today's society? How are your solutions similar to or different from the solutions of the COSs and settlement houses of the 1800s?

VI. Skill Standards

Using the competencies identified in Box 2.3, develop a list of five skills that are necessary to implement each competency. Then develop a list of tasks that could be used to develop each skill. Refer to pages 46–48 if you need to review the definitions of competencies, skills, and tasks.

VII. Credentialing: Registration, Certification, and Licensure

What are the advantages of registration, certification, and licensure? Are there any disadvantages? If so, what might they be?

VIII. Comparing Credentialing Processes

Chart 2.1 lists a number of mental health professionals in the columns and three kinds of credentialing along the rows: registration, certification, and licensing. Following is a list of five questions that are represented in each cell in the chart by their corresponding numbers. By matching up the vertical and horizontal columns, respond to the question that the corresponding numbers represent. For example, in the first cell (psychiatrists/registration), across from number "1," you would state whether or not psychiatrists have a credentialing process.

1. Does a credentialing process exist?
2. If a credentialing process does exist, is it regulated by the state legislature, the federal government, or a national professional association?
3. What are the degree requirements for being credentialed?
4. What post-degree experiences, if any, are required for being credentialed?
5. Is a test required to become credentialed?

IX. Ethical Guidelines

Generate a list of ethical issues you would want addressed by a professional association's code of ethics.

1. Bring your list to class and together generate a class list of items you would want addressed by a professional association's code of ethics.
2. As you read the book during the semester, see whether the items on the list you generated in class have been discussed in the ethics section of the chapters.
3. The instructor should have a copy of the code of ethics of APA, ACA, NASW, and the Ethical Standards of Human Service Professionals listed in Appendix A. Examine the different codes and compare them with the list generated in class.
4. Using the ethical and professional vignettes in Exercise XII that follows, compare and contrast how individuals from different developmental levels might make ethical decisions.

Chart 2.1: Comparison of Credentialing Processes Among Select Mental Health Professionals

	Psychiatrist	Psychologist	Mental Health Counselor	School Counselor	Rehab Counselor	Social Worker	Psychiatric-Mental Health Nurse	Psycho-therapist	Human Service Professional
Registration	1.	1.	1.	1.	1.	1.	1.	1.	1.
	2.	2.	2.	2.	2.	2.	2.	2.	2.
	3.	3.	3.	3.	3.	3.	3.	3.	3.
	4.	4.	4.	4.	4.	4.	4.	4.	4.
	5.	5.	5.	5.	5.	5.	5.	5.	5.
Certification	1.	1.	1.	1.	1.	1.	1.	1.	1.
	2.	2.	2.	2.	2.	2.	2.	2.	2.
	3.	3.	3.	3.	3.	3.	3.	3.	3.
	4.	4.	4.	4.	4.	4.	4.	4.	4.
	5.	5.	5.	5.	5.	5.	5.	5.	5.
Licensing	1.	1.	1.	1.	1.	1.	1.	1.	1.
	2.	2.	2.	2.	2.	2.	2.	2.	2.
	3.	3.	3.	3.	3.	3.	3.	3.	3.
	4.	4.	4.	4.	4.	4.	4.	4.	4.
	5.	5.	5.	5.	5.	5.	5.	5.	5.

X. Developing Program Accreditation Standards

In small groups, or as a class, consider the kinds of standards you would require if you were an accreditation body charged with developing program standards for human service programs. Specifically, speak of each of the following.

1. What, if any, admissions requirements would you have?
2. What would you include in the curriculum?
3. How many credits in human services would you require?
4. What would you like to see the faculty-student ratio be in your classes?
5. What philosophy would you like to see permeate the program?
6. How many hours would you require for an internship?
7. What activities would you require in the internship?
8. What kind of competency would you require, if any, for a student to graduate with a major in human services?

XI. Reviewing CSHSE Program Accreditation Standards

Review the CSHSE summary of program accreditation standards that can be found at http://www.cshse.org/standards.html. After you have completed your review, do the following:

1. Summarize and present various aspects of the standards in class.
2. Using the standards as a reference, critically evaluate your human service program.
3. Based on the program accreditation standards and what you developed in Exercise X, make suggestions for changes in your human service program.
4. Critically review the standards. What makes sense? What could be changed?

XII. Ethical and Professional Vignettes

Discuss the following ethical vignettes in class. In your discussion, decide whether the human service professional acted ethically. If you think that he or she acted unethically, what action might you take?

1. A bachelor-level human service professional takes some workshops in how to do Gestalt therapy, an advanced therapeutic approach. He feels assured about his skills and decides to run a Gestalt therapy group. The state in which he works licenses psychologists, social workers, and counselors as therapists. Is it ethical for the human service professional to run such a group? Professional? Legal?
2. An associate-level human service professional who is planning to return to school to obtain his bachelor's and master's degrees tells his colleagues and clients that he is a "master's degree candidate" in human services. If this person is not yet enrolled in a graduate program, is he misrepresenting himself? Might clients be confused by the term *master's degree candidate*? Is this ethical? Professional? Legal?
3. You are working with a client who begins to share bizarre thoughts with you concerning the end of the world. You decide that this individual needs special attention, so you decide to spend extra time with him. Is this appropriate? Ethical? Professional?
4. A client tells a human service professional that she is taking Prozac, an antidepressant, and it isn't having any effect. She asks advice regarding

taking an increased dosage, and the human service professional states, "If the current dosage isn't working, perhaps you should consider taking a higher dosage." Is it appropriate for a human service professional to suggest that a client change dosage levels? Ethical? Professional? Legal?

5. A human service professional who has received specialized training in running parenting workshops on communication skills decides to run a workshop at the local Holiday Inn. She rents a room and advertises in a local newspaper. The advertisement reads, "Learn How to Talk to Your Kid—Rid Your Family of All Communication Problems." Should she do the workshop? Is this ad ethical? Professional? Legal?

6. A bachelor-level human service professional who graduated 10 years ago states that he is "certified"' because the program he graduated from has subsequently obtained accreditation from CSHSE and all students who currently graduate from it are certified. Is this ethical? Professional? Legal? What, if anything, can and should be done?

7. A human service professional is working with a particularly difficult client who presents an ethical dilemma to this professional. In responding to the client, the professional realizes that if he uses the NOHS ethical code, he would have to respond in one way, but if he uses the APA code, he can respond in a different manner, more in harmony with what he would like to do. He decides to go with the APA code. Is this ethical? Professional? Legal?

8. You believe that a human service professional is acting unethically. What should you do? What can be done to this professional if he or she is acting unethically?

9. The American Counseling Association recently revised its ethical code and added the statements that follow relative to end-of-life decisions (ACA, 2005). Considering these statements, revisit Activity 2.1 and discuss whether your views about working with Becky would change based on these guidelines. In addition, do you believe such guidelines should be included in NOHS's code?

Section A.9.b: Counselor Competence, Choice, and Referral

Recognizing the personal, moral, and competence issues related to end-of-life decisions, counselors may choose to work or not work with terminally ill clients who wish to explore their end-of-life options. Counselors provide appropriate referral information to ensure that clients receive the necessary help.

Section A.9.c: Confidentiality

Counselors who provide services to terminally ill individuals who are considering hastening their own deaths have the option of breaking or not breaking confidentiality, depending on applicable laws and the specific circumstances of the situation and after seeking consultation or supervision from appropriate professional and legal parties.

Theoretical Approaches to Human Service Work

CHAPTER **3**

CHAPTER CONTENTS

I have always thought of myself as a kindhearted person. I remember that, even as a young child, I felt a little different from everyone else—a bit more sensitive, a bit more aware of other people's feelings. For instance, if I were playing ball at the park, I would always worry about the feelings of the kid who was picked last. Similarly, I was worried about the feelings of the kids in class who were overweight, or withdrawn, or "nerdy." Later, when I was in college, I still was the "nice guy" trying to do what was just and right and attempting to be the caretaker in the crowd. When shifting my major to psychology, I believed that my caring attitude was in and of itself the sufficient tool I would need to be an effective helper. Therefore, I held an attitude that there was little I could learn that would actually benefit me as a helper. As I went on to graduate school, I continued to think I already had the natural skills that alone would make me an effective helper. Basically, I was going to school to get the degree. I believed this so strongly that no one dared tell me how to interact with a client—I knew it all. Just let me at those clients; I could help them. I didn't need any specific training. After all, wasn't I a caring person? Weren't caring and motivation enough?

Well, I do think that having a caring attitude is one basic ingredient in being an effective helper. However, over the years I have found that often (if not usually) caring alone is not sufficient to be effective at what you do. Although our clients may appreciate our caring, it is often not enough to assist them in the change process. Thus, I now believe that having a solid theoretical background and clearly defined techniques is essential to being an effective counselor.

In this chapter we will explore the importance of counseling theory in the helping relationship. We will first examine the differences, if any, between counseling and psychotherapy. Next, we will examine how a theory is developed and review the theoretical underpinnings of four major conceptual orientations: psychodynamic, behavioral, humanistic, and cognitive. We will then review some cross-theoretical approaches to counseling, including theoretical integration or eclecticism, brief and solution-focused treatment, and gender-aware approaches. The chapter will conclude by reviewing important ethical and professional issues related to supervision, confidentiality, dual relationships, and the importance of continuing to refine one's approach to doing counseling.

COUNSELING OR PSYCHOTHERAPY?

Before we start examining the theoretical underpinnings to doing **counseling** or **psychotherapy**, let's explore the differences, if any, that exist between counseling and psychotherapy. When I ask my students to make associations with the word *counseling,* I usually get responses that include "short-term," "supportive," "conscious," "problem solving," and "present focus." However, when I ask for associations to the word *psychotherapy,* I generally get responses that include "long-term, deep personality change," "secrets unveiled," "unconscious," and "focus on past." In actuality, texts tend to not distinguish counseling from psychotherapy (e.g., see Corey, 2009; Neukrug, 2011). However, how practitioners implement a theory probably has more to do with whether one practices "counseling" or "psychotherapy." For instance, practitioners who see themselves as doing counseling probably have expectations for their clients that fit the previous descriptions of counseling, while those who practice psychotherapy likely have expectations for clients that fit that definition. A rule of thumb may be that as you receive more education and training, you probably will move from more of a counseling role to one of a psychotherapeutic role—your expectations have changed (see Figure 3.1).

Although I would argue that human service professionals do not have the training to do in-depth psychotherapeutic work, there is no question that they counsel clients. Thus, it is crucial that human service professionals understand the basic theory behind doing counseling.

WHY HAVE A THEORY?

In theory-driven science, an unending cycle of discovery and testing creates and evolves theories of ever-increasing scope that can guide counseling practice. (Strong, 1991, p. 204)

Counseling	Psychotherapy
Short-Term	*Long-Term*
Surface Issues	*Deep-Seated Issues*
"Massaging" Personality	*Personality Reconstruction*
Here and Now	*There and Then*
Conscious	*Unconscious*
Moderate Client Revelations	*Deep Client Revelations*
Uncomfortable	*Painful*
Focused Issues	*Life Stories*

Figure 3.1 | The Differences Between Counseling and Psychotherapy

Theory offers us a comprehensive system of doing counseling and assists us in understanding our client, in determining what techniques to apply, and in predicting change. Theories are **heuristic**—they are researchable and testable. Theory comes from practice, is a way of organizing our ideas, and leads to suggested plans of action (Neukrug & Schwitzer, 2006). Without a theory we would be just "doing our own thing," and there would be no rhyme or reason to client interventions (Brammer & MacDonald, 2003). Or, as Hansen, Rossberg, and Cramer (1994) note, "[to] function without theory is to operate without placing events in some order and thus to function meaninglessly" (p. 9). Today, all the current, well-known counseling theories have a long history, have gone through revisions, and have been supported to some degree by research. A counseling theory generally arises from a theorist's view of human nature.

VIEWS OF HUMAN NATURE

Although there are literally hundreds of theories of counseling and psychotherapy (Gabbard, 1995; O'Leary, 2006; List of psychotherapies, 2011), most of them can be placed into four major conceptual orientations: psychodynamic, cognitive-behavioral, existential–humanistic, and postmodern. A theory is placed in one of these orientations because it shares key concepts related to its **view of human nature**. One's view of human nature describes how a person comes to understand the reasons people are motivated to do the things they do. A few of the ingredients that go into the development of one's view of human nature include beliefs about the following:

- The impact of early child-rearing on personality development
- The impact of instincts on personality development (e.g., sex drive, aggressive instincts)
- Whether the individual is born good, bad, or neutral
- Religious beliefs about the nature of the person (e.g., whether we are born with original sin; belief in a hereafter)

- The impact of genetics on personality development
- The impact of social forces on personality development (e.g., poverty, culture, racism)
- Beliefs about the ability of one to change
- Beliefs about one's ability to choose one's circumstances
- Beliefs about whether we are determined by life circumstances (deterministic vs. antideterministic viewpoints)
- Belief in an unconscious

Think about one's view of human nature relative to how you come to understand a person like Charles Manson, a sociopath who, during the 1960s, led a cult of young adults who viciously murdered five people. If you believe people are inherently evil, you would want Manson to learn how to place restraints on his evil nature. You might view his past actions as a product of his evil nature taking over. You might also believe that we all have such an evil side. On the other hand, the individual who believes we are born with innate goodness would see Manson as a person who had lost touch with his innate loving side—perhaps through a series of horribly abusive experiences in childhood. You would therefore want him to get in touch with his caring and loving side, and you would offer him an environment that would allow him to do this. On which side of this philosophical fence are you? (See Box 3.1.)

FOUR CONCEPTUAL ORIENTATIONS AND SELECT THEORIES THAT ACCOMPANY THEM[1,2]

As already noted, there are literally hundreds of counseling theories. For the most part, these theories can be placed in one of four schools or conceptual approaches: **psychodynamic, cognitive–behavioral, existential–humanistic,** and **postmodern.** The following offers an overview of the development and view of human nature of each of the four schools of thought. Each view of human nature is followed by very brief descriptions of a few of the theories from that school. And this is followed by a quick explanation of how that approach may be applied by human service professionals:

Development and View of Human Nature of Conceptual Orientation
↓
Short Descriptions of Select Theories Within Each Orientation
↓
Human Service Applications

Psychodynamic Approaches

It is the latter part of the nineteenth century. A person walks into a physician's office complaining of melancholia and paralysis of the left arm. No apparent physical

---

[1] For flow, many major terms in this section are not in bold but are in the glossary.

[2] Much of the following contains information from: Neukrug, E. (2011). *Counseling theory and practice.* Belmont, CA: Brooks/Cole.

BOX 3.1 | Understanding Your View of Human Nature

For each of the following four statements, circle *all* items that best describe your beliefs. Then using your responses as a guide, develop a paragraph describing your view of human nature. Feel free to add other items.

1. At birth, I believe people are born:
   a. good
   b. bad
   c. neutral
   d. with original sin
   e. restricted by their genetics
   f. with a growth force which allows them to change throughout life
   g. capable of being anything they want to be
   h. with sexual drives that consciously and unconsciously affect their lives
   i. with aggressive drives that consciously and unconsciously affect their lives
   j. with social drives that consciously and unconsciously affect their lives
   k. other attributes? _____

2. Personality development is most influenced by:
   a. genetics
   b. learning
   c. early child-rearing patterns
   d. drives
   e. values that we are taught
   f. environment
   g. relationships with others
   h. biology
   i. instincts
   j. modeling the behavior of others
   k. cultural influences
   l. developmental issues (e.g., puberty)
   m. conscious decisions
   n. the unconscious
   o. language

p. feelings of inferiority
q. primordial images
r. other _____

3. As people grow older, I believe they are:
   a. capable of major changes in their personality
   b. capable of moderate changes in their personality
   c. capable of minor changes in their personality
   d. incapable of change in their personality
   e. determined by their early childhood experiences
   f. determined by their genetics
   g. determined by how they were conditioned and reinforced
   h. determined by unconscious motivations
   i. able to transcend or go beyond early childhood experiences

4. Change is likely to be most facilitated by a focus on:
   a. the conscious mind
   b. the unconscious mind
   c. thoughts
   d. behaviors
   e. feelings
   f. early experiences
   g. the past
   h. the present
   i. the future
   j. the use of medications
   k. unfinished business
   l. repressed memories
   m. biology
   n. language
   o. memories
   p. one's "real" self
   q. other _____

problems are found. What does the physician do? During that time, symptoms such as these were thought to be organic in nature; that is, they were considered physical in origin. If the physical problem could not be immediately discovered, it was because science had not yet found the physical origins of the problems. Then, in the late 1800s, **Sigmund Freud** developed a comprehensive theory that he applied when doing therapy with individuals (Appignanesi & Zarate; 2004; Freud, 1940/2003). Using hypnosis, he discovered some amazing things. For instance, some patients who had lost the use of a limb or were blind were found not to have symptoms while under hypnosis. Freud realized that their illness was not physical but instead had psychological origins (conversion disorder). Freud spent years trying to understand the complex intricacies of the mind. Although he later abandoned the use of hypnosis for other techniques, he felt strongly that there were unconscious factors beyond our everyday awareness that mediated our behavior. In other words, he thought that the reasons we do things are often beyond our understanding and are a function of motivations from the **unconscious**. Freud spent most of his life developing his psychoanalytic theory to explain the causes of human behavior. As the years have gone by, some of Freud's theory has been debunked, other parts have been changed, and still other parts have continued to be seen as important in understanding a person. In addition, a number of theorists have borrowed from Freud's original ideas and moved in innovative directions. Freudians and neo-Freudians are often subsumed under the heading "psychodynamic theorists."

Today, psychodynamic approaches vary considerably but contain some common elements. For instance, they all suggest that an unconscious and a conscious affect the functioning of the person in some deeply personal and dynamic ways. They all look at early child-rearing practices as being important in the development of personality. They all believe that examining the past and the dynamic interaction of the past with conscious and unconscious factors is important in the therapeutic process. Although these approaches have tended to be long term, in recent years some have been adapted and used in relatively brief treatment modality formats. Some of the early psychodynamic approaches are said to be **deterministic,** because personality is seen as "determined" early in life. However, some of the later approaches depart from this. The following offers a very quick overview of three of the more popular psychodynamic approaches: **psychoanalysis, analytical therapy**

Sigmund Freud
(1856–1939)

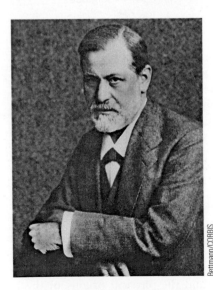

Bettmann/CORBIS

(Jungian therapy), and **individual psychology** (**Adlerian therapy**). In addition, I will briefly describe some recent developments in this area.

Psychoanalysis. Developed by Sigmund Freud, psychoanalysis suggests that **instincts,** such as hunger, thirst, survival, aggression, and sex, are very strong motivators of behavior. The satisfaction of instincts is mostly an unconscious process, and **defense mechanisms** (e.g., rationalizing, repression) are developed to help manage and temper our instincts. Because we are in a constant and mostly unconscious struggle to satisfy our instincts, psychoanalysts believe that happiness is elusive. Early child-rearing practices, which are applied through the oral, anal, and phallic **psychosexual stages** in the first six years of life, are responsible for how we manage our defenses and result in normal or abnormal personality development. Effects of these practices can be observed as we move into adolescence and adulthood (latency and genital psychosexual stages). The fact that early childhood experiences are largely responsible for personality development and that our behaviors are mostly dictated by the unconscious lends a sense of determinism to this approach.

Analytical Psychology. Analytical psychology was developed by **Carl Jung,** who believed that psychological symptoms represent a desire to regain lost parts of self, as well as parts that have never been revealed to consciousness, so that the person can become whole. Analytic therapists believe we are born with two pairs of mental functions of sensation–intuition and thinking–feeling, whose relative strengths are affected by child-rearing. The strengths of each of the mental functions and whether one has an innate tendency to be extraverted (outgoing) or introverted (observer, inward) are called our psychological type. For instance, a person can be 70% sensing, 90% thinking, and 80% introverted. Jung hypothesized that whatever your predominate type is, the complementary type resides in your personal unconscious and longs to be "heard" (in the example just given, the complement is: intuition/feeling/extraverted). Your psychological type affects how you see the world and is the filter through which you develop your consciousness. Analytical therapists also believe that we all inherit the same, immeasurable number of primitive or primordial images called archetypes, which are housed in the collective unconscious (mother archetype, father archetype, the shadow, God archetype). They provide the psyche with its tendency to perceive the world in certain ways that we identify as human and can sometimes interact with repressed material in the personal unconscious and cause complexes.

Individual Psychology. Developed by **Alfred Adler,** individual psychology suggests that early childhood experiences, and the memories of those experiences, result in our character or personality. Believing that we all experience feelings of inferiority as children, Adler suggested that if we learn how to respond to such feelings in healthy ways, we will have a tendency to move toward wholeness, completion, and perfection. However, if a person responds to feelings of inferiority through negative private logic (e.g., "I am not worthwhile"), the result will yield compensatory behaviors (e.g., bullying others to feel worthwhile) that are maladaptive and/or neurotic. Although early experiences influence the development of personality, Adler suggested that education and therapy can be effective in helping a person change. Adler's approach in particular is seen as more optimistic and less deterministic than other psychodynamic approaches, and some have even placed him in the existential–humanistic school, which we will talk about shortly.

Recent Developments/Theories   Although agreeing with many of the basic premises of the psychodynamic view of human nature, some believe that the classic psychodynamic approaches just described have been too lengthy, too deterministic, too impersonal, and/or too focused on the unconscious. Thus, a number of other **"neo-Freudian approaches"** have been developed that still emphasize early child-rearing, the conscious, and the unconscious, but approach counseling in different ways. For instance, **Erik Erikson** developed a theory that looked at how a person develops over the lifetime and focused much more on psychosocial factors (e.g., family, friends, relationships, work; see Chapter 5). Object relation theorists have played down the focus on instincts and played up a focus on the need to be in relationships in building a self. And relational and intersubjectivity perspectives focus much more on how the self is formed in relationship with others and the importance of deep, personal encounters with clients.

The Human Service Professional's Use of the Psychodynamic Approach

Traditionally, the psychodynamic approach has been used mostly in the intensive psychotherapeutic setting. However, some aspects of this approach can be adapted for the human service professional. First, this approach offers us a developmental model by which we can understand the individual. Understanding that clients may be responding to deep-seated motivations that stem from early childhood and are mostly unconscious helps us have empathy and patience when working with very difficult clients. Second, this approach helps us understand deviant behavior. The notion that such behavior is the result of abusive or neglectful early childhood, caretaking may help us understand that deviants, perpetrators, criminals, and abusers are also victims. Only with this knowledge can we begin to have the deeper caring and understanding needed to work with such difficult populations.

Finally, just as our clients might respond to individuals as if they were significant people from their past (called **transference**), mental health professionals who have not resolved their past issues may do the same. Called **countertransference**, this process can have negative effects on relationships with clients because the helper's unresolved issues may cause the helper to respond in unhealthy ways toward his or her clients. It is important for human service professionals to have worked through their own issues to avoid countertransference with their clients (see Bike, Norcross, & Schatz, 2009; Norcross, Bike, & Evans, 2009).

Existential–Humanistic Approaches

At the turn of the twentieth century in Europe, the writings of such existential philosophers as Kierkegaard, Tillich, Sartre, and Camus became particularly well known. American counselors and psychotherapists began to see the value in some of these thinkers' explorations of the struggles of living and how people construct meaning in their lives, eventually embracing some of their concepts and adapting them to the counseling relationship. The new theories that evolved tended to be **antideterministic** and more positive than the earlier psychodynamic approaches and became known as existential–humanistic approaches to counseling. During the 1940s, some of the Americans who were leaders of this revolution included **Carl Rogers** (1902–1987), **Rollo May** (1909–1994), and **Abraham Maslow** (1908–1970). **Maslow's hierarchy** of needs, in particular, became quite popular with its focus on the potential of all people to change and become whole if needs lower on his hierarchy would have the potential to be met (see Figure 3.2).

Today, existential–humanistic approaches embrace a phenomenological perspective by stressing the subjective reality of the client, de-emphasizing the role of the unconscious, and focusing on the importance of consciousness and/or awareness. Deeply opposed to the deterministic tradition of psychoanalysis which de-emphasized the relationship between the helper and client, existential–humanistic therapy is antideterministic and optimistic and stresses the helper's personal qualities and how the helper uses himself or herself in the relationship to effect change. In addition, most existential–humanistic approaches believe in an inborn tendency for individuals to self-actualize, or fulfill their potential, if they are afforded an environment conducive to growth (Maslow, 1968, 1970). Although many modern-day approaches to counseling and psychotherapy have borrowed from the existential–humanistic schools, a few that are particularly based in this tradition include **existential therapy**, which is presented here as an integration of a number of well-known existentially based therapies; the **person-centered counseling** approach of **Carl Rogers**; and **Gestalt therapy**, originally founded by **Fritz Perls**.

Existential Therapy   Developed by **Viktor Frankl, Rollo May,** and others, existential therapy states that we are born into a world that has no inherent meaning or purpose, that we all struggle with the basic questions of what it is to be human,

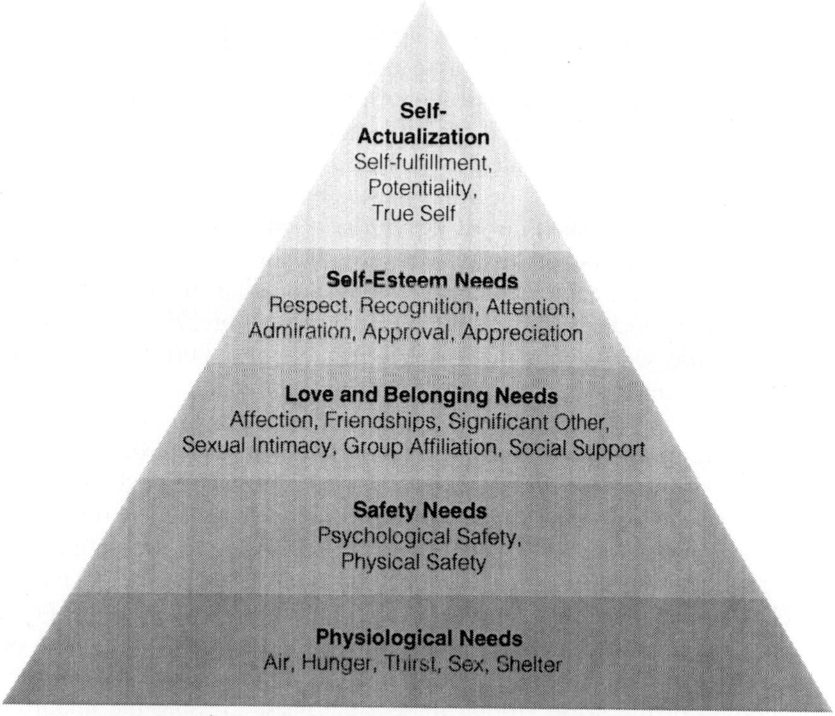

Self-Actualization
Self-fulfillment,
Potentiality,
True Self

Self-Esteem Needs
Respect, Recognition, Attention,
Admiration, Approval, Appreciation

Love and Belonging Needs
Affection, Friendships, Significant Other,
Sexual Intimacy, Group Affiliation, Social Support

Safety Needs
Psychological Safety,
Physical Safety

Physiological Needs
Air, Hunger, Thirst, Sex, Shelter

Figure 3.2 | Maslow's Hierarchy of Needs

and that we alone can create meaning and purpose. Existential therapists believe that we all have the ability to live authentically and experience fully, but sometimes avoid doing so because we fear looking at our existence and our ultimate demise, which is death or nonbeing. In essence, we sometimes create a world void of self-examination in our effort to avoid looking at our existence. Anxiety, feelings of dread, and having struggles are a natural part of living and are important messages about how we live and relate to others, say the existential therapists. If given the opportunity, existential therapists believe that we can choose to find meaningfulness in our lives and, through our choices, experience a limited sense of freedom.

Person-Centered Counseling   Carl Rogers founded this approach, which states that we have an inborn actualizing tendency that lends direction to our lives as we attempt to reach our full potential. However, this tendency is sometimes thwarted as individuals act in ways that they believe significant others want them to act. Rogers suggested that this occurs because of the individual's innate desire to be regarded by significant others and the fact that significant others will sometimes place conditions of worth on a person. This results in the creation of an incongruent self. Anxiety and related symptoms are a signal that the person is acting in an incongruent or nongenuine way and not living fully. Being around people (e.g., helpers) who are congruent (real), empathic, and show unconditional positive regard can help individuals realize their nongenuine ways of being in the world and is the major goal of therapy.

Gestalt Therapy   Founded by Fritz Perls, Gestalt therapy suggests that we are born with the capacity to embrace an infinite number of personality dimensions. With the mind, body, and soul operating in unison, from birth, the individual is in a constant state of need identification and need fulfillment. However, parental dictates, social mores, and peer norms can prevent a person from attaining a need and result in resistances or blockages to the experiencing of his or her needs. Thus, these needs get pushed out of awareness. Gestalt therapy highlights the importance of accessing one's experience in the now because experience = awareness = reality. In other words, experiencing allows an individual to understand his or her resistances and blockages and is the first step toward breaking free from them and living a saner life. Once you realize how you have blocked off your needs, you can then go about meeting them and become whole.

The Human Service Professional's Use of the Existential–Humanistic Approach
Maslow's hierarchy of needs has become an established method of recognizing how to initially understand an individual's struggles. In this model, the human service professional who spends the majority of time attempting to raise an individual's self-esteem when that individual is homeless and cold would be doing the client a disservice (see Figure 3.2). In addition, today, Rogers's personal characteristics of empathy, being nonjudgmental, and being genuine, have become essential qualities for mental health professionals to embrace, regardless of the theoretical orientation of the helper. Along these same lines, stressing the importance of the relationship between the helper and the client has become a key ingredient in the helping

relationship (see section on Characteristics of the Effective Helper in Chapter 1). Finally, the knowledge that clients sometimes have struggles with life and unmet needs that are out of their awareness, enables the human service professional to understand why people respond the way they do.

Cognitive–Behavioral Approaches

Around the turn of the century, the Russian scientist **Ivan Pavlov** (1848–1936) found that a hungry dog that salivated when shown food would learn to salivate to a tone if that tone were repeatedly paired or associated with the food. Eventually the dog would salivate when it heard the tone, regardless of whether food was present. Thus, Pavlov discovered **classical conditioning. John Watson** (1925; Watson & Raynor, 1920) and later **Joseph Wolpe** (1958) would eventually take these concepts and apply them in clinical settings.

During the 1930s, **B. F. Skinner** (1904–1990) showed that animals would learn specific behaviors if the behavior just emitted was reinforced (Nye, 1992, 2000; Skinner, 1938, 1971). His **operant conditioning** procedures demonstrated that **positive reinforcement,** the presentation of a stimulus that yields an increase in behavior, or **negative reinforcement,** the removal of a stimulus that yields an increase in behavior, could successfully change behavior. Skinner also found that **punishment** was not particularly effective in changing behavior (see Box 3.2).

During the 1940s, **Albert Bandura** found that children who viewed a film in which an adult acted aggressively toward a Bobo doll would act out more aggressively than did children who had not seen the film, when all the children were placed in a room together (Bandura, Ross, & Ross, 1963). This third behavioral approach, called **social learning** or **modeling,** showed that we have the capacity to repeat behaviors that we have observed—even at a much later time (Bandura, 1977).

In recent years, cognitive therapists focused on how deeply embedded cognitive structures, or illogical and irrational ways of thinking, can be conditioned in a similar way as behaviors. And, as with behaviors, through **counterconditioning,** old dysfunctional cognitions can be extinguished and new, more functional cognitions can be adopted. Because behavior therapists and cognitive therapists tend to believe there is an intimate, sometimes seamless relationship between cognitions and behaviors, there has been a tendency for these individuals to merge the tenets of both approaches into what has become known as the cognitive–behavioral school. Some of the common assumptions underlying these approaches include the following:

BOX 3.2 | **A Very Bright Pigeon**

I walk into a small store in New York's Chinatown and I see a sign that says "As Seen on the TV Show *That's Incredible*, Play Tic-Tac-Toe with the Pigeon." Being a wealthy man, I place a quarter in the slot, then another quarter, and then another. I can't beat the pigeon. Well I guess operant conditioning really does work, or maybe pigeons are brighter than I thought. On the other hand, maybe I'm not quite as smart as I think.

1. The individual is born capable of developing a multitude of personality characteristics.
2. Significant others and cultural influences play a particularly important role in how the individual is conditioned.
3. Genetics and other biological factors may play a significant role in who we become.
4. Despite the fact that the past plays an important role in how a person is conditioned, long periods of time do not need to be spent on examining the past. Instead, one needs to determine what behaviors and thoughts need to be changed and focus on changing them.
5. Behaviors and cognitions are generally conditioned in very complex and subtle ways.
6. The kinds of behaviors and cognitions that are conditioned play a central role in the development of normal and abnormal behavior.
7. By carefully analyzing how behaviors and cognitions are conditioned, one can understand why an individual exhibits his or her current behavioral and cognitive repertoire.
8. By identifying what behaviors have been conditioned, one can eliminate undesirable behaviors and set goals to acquire more functional ways of behaving and thinking.
9. By actively disputing dysfunctional thinking and through counterconditioning, change is possible in a relatively short amount of time.

This section of the chapter will provide a very brief overview of four cognitive–behavioral approaches: **behavior therapy, rational emotive behavior therapy (REBT), cognitive therapy,** and **reality therapy.**

Behavior Therapy   Behaviorists believe that classical conditioning, operant conditioning, and social learning (or modeling) are all ways that a person can develop a specific personality style. By carefully analyzing how behaviors are conditioned, they suggest that helpers can develop behavioral techniques to eliminate undesirable behaviors and develop new positive behaviors. There are literally dozens of behavioral techniques that use classical conditioning, operant conditioning, and modeling in changing maladaptive behaviors to functional ones, with some of the more popular ones being positive reinforcement, extinction, systematic desensitization, relaxation exercises, modeling, assertiveness training, and the token economy (when tokens can be exchanged for desirable behaviors and later submitted for a reward).

Rational Emotive Behavior Therapy (REBT)   Developed by **Albert Ellis,** REBT suggests that we are born with the potential for rational or irrational thinking, and it is the belief about an event that is responsible for one's reaction to the event, not the event itself. Thus, Ellis said that the <u>A</u>ctivating event precedes the <u>B</u>eliefs about the event, and it is the beliefs that result in the <u>C</u>onsequences or the feelings and behaviors that follow (A → B → C). Ellis said irrational beliefs (iB) result in negative feelings and behaviors and rational beliefs (rB) result in appropriate or good feelings and behaviors. When our lives are run by our irrational beliefs, we end up living a particularly neurotic and unhappy life. Ellis suggested there are three core irrational beliefs that many people buy into (see Box 3.3). The purpose of counseling is to <u>D</u>ispute irrational beliefs by changing our thoughts and by practicing new, healthy behaviors. He came up with many cognitive and behavioral techniques to do this.

Cognitive Therapy   Developed by **Aaron "Tim" Beck,** cognitive therapy suggests that individuals can be born with a predisposition toward certain emotional disorders that reveals itself under stressful conditions. Cognitive therapists also believe that genetics, biological factors, and experiences combine to produce specific core beliefs that are responsible for automatic thoughts (fleeting thoughts about what we perceive and experience), which result in a set of behaviors, feelings, and physiological responses. By understanding one's cognitive processes (e.g., core beliefs, automatic thoughts), one can address and change automatic thoughts and core beliefs that lead to dysfunctional behaviors and distressful feelings. Like Ellis, Beck came up with a number of cognitive and behavioral techniques to change automatic thoughts, core beliefs, and negative ways that one usually responds.

Reality Therapy   Developed by **William Glasser,** reality therapy suggests we are born with five needs: survival, love and belonging, power, freedom, and fun—which can be satisfied only in the present. Reality therapists believe we have a quality world that contains pictures in our mind of the people, things, and beliefs most important to meeting these needs. We make choices based on these pictures, although we can only choose actions and thoughts; feelings and our physiology result from those choices. Sometimes, the choices (actions and thoughts) a person makes as a result of pictures in a person's quality world are ones that result in low self-esteem (e.g., a person's need for power results in the person bullying others). Reality therapists suggest that caring, non-blaming language reflects positive choices and that negative, blaming language reflects poor choices. At any point in one's life, a person can evaluate his or her behaviors, thoughts, feelings, and physiology, and make new choices (e.g., act and think differently and use new, more positive language). Although placed in the cognitive–behavioral school due to its focus on changing behaviors and thoughts, you can see that the concept of "choice" means it can also nicely fit into the existential–humanistic school.

BOX 3.3	**Three Core Irrational Beliefs**

1. I absolutely must under all conditions do important tasks well and be approved by significant others or else I am an inadequate and unlovable person!
2. Other people absolutely must under all conditions treat me fairly and justly or else they are rotten, damnable persons!
3. Conditions under which I live absolutely must always be the way I want them to be, give me almost immediate gratification, and not require me to work too hard to change or improve them; or else it is awful, I can't stand them, and it is impossible for me to be happy at all! (Ellis & MacLaren, 2005, pp. 32–33)

The Human Service Professional's Use of the Cognitive–Behavioral Approach

Unlike the psychodynamic approach, the behavioral approach has been widely applied outside the psychotherapeutic setting. Aside from the preceding examples, behavioral concepts are commonly used in a wide variety of human service settings. For example, reinforcement is used in schools, residential and rehabilitation settings, and day treatment programs, whereas modeling via role-playing is commonly used at employment offices, in educational workshops, and in the training of human service professionals.

Today, finding behavioral techniques incorporated into the human service professional's repertoire of skills is not unusual. In fact, for some disorders, using behavioral techniques has been shown to be so powerful that it would be unethical for a human service professional not to use them (e.g., alleviating phobias, assisting individuals with mental retardation to learn new skills) (O'Donohu, Fisher, & Hayes, 2003). Behavioral techniques are advantageous because, in collaboration with the client, the human service professional can identify client goals, apply specific techniques, and see results within relatively short periods. In residential settings, behavioral techniques are easily understood by clients and help give direction and focus for both staff and clients.

Although human service professionals have not widely adopted the cognitive approach, professionals in most settings can readily use its basic concepts. Helping clients understand the connection between thinking, feeling, and behaving can dramatically affect how they interact in the world. Understanding that our thinking affects our feelings and actions can give clients hope regarding their future. Perhaps one challenge for human service professionals today is to understand and embrace cognitive theory more fully so they can better help clients take responsibility for their thinking, feeling, and acting.

Postmodern Approaches

Postmodern approaches include some of the more recent therapies and are based on the philosophies of **postmodernism** and **social constructionism.** Postmodernists question many of the basic assumptions that are taken for granted as a result of the use of empiricism and the scientific method and suggest there is no one way to understand the world, no foundational set of rules to make sense of who we are, and no one way of understanding a person. These individuals question what "truth is" and can often be found questioning many of the basic tenets of popular therapies which suggest that certain structures cause mental health problems (e.g., id, ego, superego, core beliefs, self-actualization tendency).

Social constructionism has to do with how values are transmitted through language by the social milieu (e.g., family, culture, and society) and suggests that the person is constantly changing with the ebb and flow of the influences of significant others, culture, and society. Social constructionists generally agree that those in positions of power control the type of language that is used in cultures and society. Thus, individuals who are not in power (e.g., nondominant groups such as minorities and women) are at a disadvantage and may be oppressed by the power structure that prevails. Rather than harp on past problems that tend to be embedded in oppressive belief systems, postmodern approaches suggest that clients can find exceptions to their problems, develop creative solutions, and question basic assumptions about their lives. Postmodern therapies tend to be short term, with solution-focused brief therapy being considered a particularly brief approach, sometimes lasting fewer than five sessions. Three postmodern approaches we will examine briefly are **narrative therapy, solution-focused brief therapy,** and **gender-aware therapy.**

Narrative Therapy Narrative therapy, developed by **Michael White,** suggests that reality is a social construction and that each person's reality is organized and maintained through his or her narrative or language discourse. Within this context, values held by those in power are often disseminated through language and become the norms against which individuals compare themselves. Therefore, problems individuals have, including mental disorders, are a function of how people compare themselves to what they have been told are the "norms" of society. Using these arbitrarily created norms, individuals sometimes end up believing their lives are filled with problems which are demonstrated by the problem-saturated stories or narratives they generate and tell others about, including their counselors. By being humble, asking respectful questions, listening to exceptions to the problem-saturated stories, and listening to more subtle positive stories that the client is not quite aware of, narrative therapists can help clients create new, preferred stories that provide a more positive existence for the individual.

Solution-Focused Brief Therapy Steve de Shazer and **Insoo Kim Berg,** two founders of solution-focused brief therapy (SFBT), suggested that problems are the result of language passed down by families, culture, and society, and dialogues between people. Therefore, pathology, for all practical purposes, is not inherently found within the person (inside the person), as is professed by many therapies that describe structures that affect functioning (e.g., id, ego, superego, self-actualizing tendency). Believing there is no objective reality, they suggest there is no reason to spend time looking "inside" the person or spending a lot of time looking at the past. Instead, the focus is on finding solutions and new ways of being. Solution-focused behavior therapists build collaborative relationships and have clients establish preferred goals, so they can quickly move from a problem focus to a solution focus. They argue that change can occur in fewer than six sessions and that extended counseling is often detrimental. One particular technique that has received widespread recognition is the miracle question, which asks the client:

> Suppose that one night, while you were asleep, there was a miracle and this problem was solved. How would you know? What would be different? (de Shazer, 1988, p. 5)

Gender-Aware Approaches Called **feminist therapy** and **men's issues therapy** by some, gender-aware approaches are considered in the postmodern school because they do not assume that problems are inherent, or within the person. Instead, they assume that gender is central to the helping relationship, view problems within a societal context, encourage helpers to actively address gender injustices, encourage the development of a collaborative and equal relationship, acknowledge how language is passed down through culture and affects one's sex-role identity, and respect the client's right to choose the gender roles appropriate for himself or herself regardless of political correctness. Because differences between men and women can be great, gender-aware therapies usually suggest having particular knowledge of women's is-sues and of men's issues so that one can understand how these issues have impacted the client.

The Human Service Professional's Use of the Postmodern Approaches   Post-modern approaches fit neatly into the work of the human service professional. First, human service professionals tend to be more collaborative in their work with clients. That is, they do not believe in the importance of acting in the role of an "authority figure" with the client. The tendency to have an equal relationship with the client supports the notion that one person is not better than another and defuses power dynamics that often happen in counseling relationships. In addition, human service professionals generally understand how societal dynamics and power differentials (poverty, racism, class, gender, etc.) can negatively affect some clients more than others. Finally, human service professionals have always been on the forefront of advocacy and social justice. Postmodern approaches suggest that because power differentials negatively affect some people more than others, it is important that professionals are social justice advocates for those who are disenfranchised.

OTHER THEORETICAL APPROACHES

As noted earlier, there are many, many other approaches to counseling, and what has been discussed in this chapter is just a very brief overview of some of the more popular approaches. However, you may want to look into some of the other approaches that include anything from **eye movement desensitization therapy (EMDR)**, which has cli-ents focus on rapid eye movements or some other rhythmic stimulation (e.g., tapping) while imagining a traumatic or troubling event; to **complementary, alternative,** and **integrative approaches,** which focus on nontraditional ways of healing to treat biolog-ical and mental health problems (e.g., massage, oils, rituals); to **motivational inter-viewing,** which assumes that motivation is the key to change and offers four basic principles to motivate clients: showing empathy, pointing out discrepancies, rolling with resistance, and supporting self-efficacy; to **positive psychology** and **well-being therapy,** which suggest that humans are capable of good and bad but it is important to focus mostly on the positive aspects of the self (see Box 3.4).

Finally, with HMOs overseeing the number of sessions individuals can have with their helpers and with cutbacks in funding for agencies, **brief approaches to counseling** have become popular in recent years. Although solution-focused brief therapy is clearly a form of brief counseling (Rothwell, 2005), brief approaches to counseling can be applied to almost any theoretical orientation (Garfield, 1998), have been shown to be as effective as longer-term counseling, and have been defined as anywhere between 2 and 50 sessions (Carlson & Sperry, 2000; Gingerich &

| BOX 3.4 | **Your Positivity Ratio** |

Want To Know Your Positive to Negative Ratio? Go to: http://www.positivityratio.com/single.php

Eisengart, 2000; MacDonald, 2003). Because human service professionals are generally not doing in-depth therapy, and because they tend to work on highly focused problems, brief treatment approaches have a home with the human service professional.

What is the difference between brief treatment and longer-term approaches? Budman and Gurman (1988) offer some comparisons (see Table 3.1). Finally, Garfield (1998) suggests that all brief treatment approaches pass through four stages: (1) building the relationship and assessing the problem; (2) developing a plan for the client, encouraging homework assignments, and working on the problem; (3) following through on treatment plans and reformulating the treatment plan based on new information and client feedback; and (4) termination, in which the client's feelings concerning progress are assessed, future plans discussed (e.g., follow-up, referral, ways of continuing progress), and closure accomplished.

Do you still want to learn about even other approaches? Google "psychotherapy" or pick up a good counseling theories book, and you'll find many other approaches.

Table 3.1 | Comparison of Long-Term and Short-Term Treatment Approaches

Long-Term Therapist	Short-Term Therapist
1. Seeks change in the basic character.	1. Prefers pragmatism, parsimony, and least radical intervention, and does not believe in notion of "cure."
2. Believes that significant psychological change is unlikely in everyday life.	2. Maintains an adult developmental perspective from which significant psychological change is viewed as inevitable.
3. Sees presenting problems as reflecting more basic pathology.	3. Emphasizes patient's strengths and resources; presenting problems are taken seriously (although not necessarily at face value).
4. Wants to "be there" as patient makes significant changes.	4. Accepts that many changes will occur "after therapy" and will not be observable to the therapist.
5. Sees therapy as having a "timeless" quality and is willing to wait for change.	5. Does not accept the timelessness of some models of therapy.
6. Unconsciously recognizes the fiscal convenience of maintaining long-term patients.	6. Fiscal issues often muted, either by the nature of the therapist's practice or by the organizational structure for reimbursement.
7. Views psychotherapy as almost always being useful.	7. Views psychotherapy as being sometimes useful and sometimes harmful.
8. Sees patient's being in therapy as the most important part of the patient's life.	8. Sees being in the world as more important than being in therapy.

Source: Budman & Gurman, 1988, p. 11.

ECLECTICISM OR INTEGRATIVE APPROACHES TO COUNSELING

Formerly called **eclecticism**, an **integrative approach** to counseling is when mental health professionals draw from a number of different orientations to develop their own theory to working with their clients. Professionals using this approach, however, must not shoot from the hip; instead, they must carefully reflect on their views of human nature and use techniques that fit their ways of viewing the world while meeting the mental health needs of their clients. Unfortunately, my experience has been that many individuals who call themselves eclectic use a hodgepodge of techniques, which may end up being confusing to a client. Today, about one-fourth of helpers state that they are purely eclectic or integrative (Norcross, Bike, & Evans, 2009). Similarly, when human service practitioners and students who had attended counseling were asked the orientation of their counselor, one-fourth stated they their counselor was eclectic (Neukrug, Milliken, & Shoemaker, 2001).

Before you borrow techniques from the differing orientations, you must carefully examine your view of human nature, and throughout this chapter you have had, and will continue to have, an opportunity to do so. Although different models of theoretical integration have been developed (cf. Brooks-Harris, 2008; O'Leary & Murphy, 2006; Stricker & Gold, 2006; O'Leary, 2006), most address some common elements that have led me to view an integrative approach as a developmental process that moves from chaos to coalescence to multiplicity and ends with a commitment to a metatheory (Neukrug, 2012).

Stage 1:   **Chaos:** In this initial stage of developing an eclectic approach, the human service professional has no theory, is sloppy, bases his or her responses on moment-to-moment subjective judgments, and can be harmful to clients. Beginning students who are just starting to understand counseling theory and are attempting to haphazardly combine theories may be at this chaos stage.

Stage 2:   **Coalescence:** As theory is learned, many mental health professionals drift toward adherence to one approach. As they begin to feel comfortable with this approach, they may begin to integrate different techniques from other approaches into their theoretical style.

Stage 3:   **Multiplicity.** During this stage, helpers have thoroughly learned one theory and are beginning to gain a solid knowledge of one or more other theories. They are also now beginning to realize that any of the theories may be equally effective for many clients. This knowledge presents a dilemma for the helper (Spruill & Benshoff, 2000): "What theoretical perspective should I adhere to, and how might I combine, or use at different times, two or more theoretical perspectives so that I could offer the most effective treatment?" Ultimately, this helper is able to feel facile with different approaches and is sometimes willing to integrate other approaches into his or her main approach.

Stage 4:   **Metatheory:** As mental health professionals develop a full appreciation of many theories, they begin to wonder about underlying commonalities and themes among the varying theories. This leads some helpers to develop or take on what some have called a metatheory.

For instance, two mental health professionals with very different integrative approaches may realize that an underlying theme of all clients is how family and social systems affect them (see Chapter 6). Thus, this "systemic understanding" would be seen by these helpers as common to all clients and must be addressed.

If you are just beginning your journey as a human service professional, you might expect to pass through these stages as you begin to sort through the various theoretical approaches and develop your own unique integrative style of counseling.

ETHICAL, PROFESSIONAL, AND LEGAL ISSUES

The Importance of Supervision for the Human Service Professional

To become more effective as a human service professional, it is important to constantly examine your view of human nature, your theoretical approach, and, ultimately, your ability to work successfully with clients. One way of accomplishing this is through the supervisory relationship (Bernard & Goodyear, 2009). The **supervisor** has a number of roles and responsibilities, including ensuring the welfare of the client; making sure that ethical, professional, and legal standards are being upheld; overseeing the clinical and professional development of the **supervisee**; and evaluating the supervisee.

Supervision should start during one's training program and "serve as a unique link between preparation and skilled service" (Cogan & O'Connell, 1982, p. 12). A good supervisor is empathic, flexible, genuine, and open, and is capable of establishing a strong supervisory alliance (Bernard & Goodyear, 2009; Borders & Brown, 2005). In addition, the good supervisor is able to evaluate the supervisee and is comfortable being an authority figure when necessary. Finally, good supervisors know counseling, have good client conceptualization skills, and are good problem solvers.

Unfortunately, all too often I have seen professionals avoid supervision because of fears about their own adequacy. These fears can create an atmosphere of isolation for the human service professional, an isolation that leads to rigidity and an inability to examine varying methods of working with clients. It is important that as professionals we face our own vulnerable spots and look at what we do not do well. A good supervisory relationship can help us look at issues such as when to break confidentiality or when we might be losing our objectivity because of a dual relationship.

Confidentiality and the Helping Relationship

Regardless of the theoretical approach to which one adheres, keeping client information confidential is one of the most important ingredients in building a trusting relationship. However, is **confidentiality** always guaranteed or warranted? For instance, suppose you encounter the following situation:

A 17-year-old client tells you that she is pregnant. Do you need to tell her parents? What if the client was 15 or 12? What if she was drinking while pregnant, or using cocaine, or ... ? What if she tells you she wants an abortion? What if she tells you she is suicidal because of the pregnancy?

Although most of us would agree that confidentiality is an important ingredient in the helping relationship, it might not always be best to keep things confidential. Although all ethical decisions are to some degree judgment calls, we can follow some general guidelines when making a decision to break confidentiality. Generally, you can break confidentiality in these situations:

1. If a client is in danger of harming himself or herself or someone else
2. If a child is a minor and the law states that parents have a right to information about their child
3. If a client asks you to break confidentiality (e.g., your testimony is needed in court)
4. If you are bound by the law to break confidentiality (e.g., a local law requires human service professionals to report the selling of drugs)
5. To reveal information about your client to your supervisor to benefit the client
6. When you have a written agreement from your client to reveal information to specified sources (e.g., other social service agencies that are working with the same client)

Now that we have looked at when it is all right to break confidentiality, let's examine times when it is not usually permissible:

1. When you're frustrated with a client and you talk to a friend or colleague about the case just to "let off steam"
2. When a helping professional requests information about your client and you have not received written permission from your client to disclose such information
3. When a friend asks you to tell him or her something interesting about a client with whom you are working
4. When breaking confidentiality will clearly cause harm to your client and does not fall into one of the categories previously listed

Confidentiality is an ethical guideline, not a legal right. The legal term that ensures the right of professionals not to reveal information about their clients is **privileged communication** (Remley, 2005). In fact, the privilege actually belongs to the client and can be waived only by him or her. Generally, this means that, if called to court, these professionals should not reveal information unless the client allows them to do so. In many states, lawyers, priests, physicians, and licensed therapists have been given privileged communication with their clients, but other mental health professionals, including human service professionals, have not. Thus, they cannot ensure confidentiality in some cases.

The ethical guidelines of all the mental health professions, including those in the human services (see Appendix A), ensure the right to confidentiality, usually with some limitations, as listed earlier. More specifically, the Ethical Standards of Human Service Professionals (NOHS, 1996) states:

> Human service professionals protect the client's right to privacy and confidentiality except when such confidentiality would cause harm to the client or others, when agency guidelines state otherwise, or under other stated conditions (e.g., local, state, or federal

laws). Professionals inform clients of the limits of confidentiality prior to the onset of the relationship. (Appendix A, Statement 3)

Dual or Multiple Relationships and the Human Service Professional

Is it all right to have as a client a friend, relative, or lover? Most professional groups have taken clear stands that dual relationships of these kinds are not ethical (Welfel, 2010). However, could there not be some times when a **dual relationship** (sometimes called **multiple relationships**) might benefit the helping relationship? For instance, what if you have been working with a client on obtaining her GED diploma and she invites you to the graduation ceremony? In this case, would it be reasonable to go? Some would say *yes* (Kaplan, 2006). Although the Ethical Standards of Human Service Professionals (NOHS, 1996) discourages most kinds of dual relationships, they do note that there may be some times when it would be appropriate to cross that line if there are clear benefits to the client:

> Human service professionals are aware that in their relationship with clients power and status are unequal. Therefore they recognize that dual or multiple relationships may increase the risk of harm to, or exploitation of, clients, and may impair their professional judgment. However, in some communities and situations it may not be feasible to avoid social or other nonprofessional contact with clients. Human service professionals support the trust implicit in the helping relationship by avoiding dual relationships that may impair professional judgment, increase the risk of harm to clients or lead to exploitation. (Appendix A, Statement 6)

It is the responsibility of each human service professional to decide whether his or her objectivity and professional judgment are impaired by having a dual relationship with a client, and most importantly, whether the client would be benefited if one were to cross that line.

THE EFFECTIVE HUMAN SERVICE PROFESSIONAL: COMMITTED TO A COUNSELING APPROACH AND WILLING TO CHANGE

Effective human service professionals have reflected on the various approaches to counseling and have made a commitment to an approach. This commitment includes learning more about the approach, reading current research about that approach and other approaches, being open to the supervisory process, and, most important, changing the approach if evidence indicates that it is ineffective. Human service professionals who are committed to this process are willing and eager to explore new theories and to adapt their theories as evidence accrues that a newer approach might be more useful. These are human service professionals who are truly dedicated to growth in the field, in themselves and in their clients.

SUMMARY

This chapter began by contrasting the words *counseling* and *psychotherapy*. We noted that although a text on counseling theories would be indistinguishable from a text on theories of psychotherapy, how a mental health practitioner applies these theories often distinguishes whether he or she is practicing counseling or psychotherapy. We also noted that although human service professionals do not do in-depth counseling or therapy, they do counsel clients, and thus it is crucial that they have a basic understanding of the theory behind what they do. We then discussed the importance of having a theoretical approach drive the way in which one does counseling and that one's theoretical approach is an outgrowth of one's view of human nature.

In reference to views of human nature, we listed a number of ingredients that tend to go into the creation of a view of human nature. We then noted that most theories can be placed into one of four schools or conceptual orientations and that each theory within the specific schools share some common elements in the school's view of human nature. The meat of the chapter examined the view of human nature of four conceptual orientations, very briefly described select theories that accompany them, and highlighted how each conceptual orientation can be used by the human service professional.

For the psychodynamic school, we described Freud's psychoanalysis, Jung's analytical therapy, and Adler's individual psychology, and highlighted some recent theories that have somewhat departed from the original view of nature of the psychodynamic school. For existential–humanistic approaches we discussed Abraham Maslow's hierarchy and highlighted the following approaches to counseling: existential therapy as presented by such individuals as Viktor Frankl and Rollo May, the person-centered counseling approach of Carl Rogers, and Perls's Gestalt therapy. For the cognitive–behavioral approaches, we first highlighted some of the originators of the different kinds of behavior therapy such as Ivan Pavlov who discovered classical conditioning and John Watson and Joseph Wolpe who applied its concepts, B. F. Skinner who researched operant conditioning, and Albert Bandura who taught us about modeling or social learning. Then we offered very brief descriptions of modern-day behavior therapy, Albert Ellis's rational emotive behavior therapy, Aaron Beck's cognitive therapy, and William Glasser's reality therapy. Finally, for the postmodern approaches we discussed Michael White's narrative therapy, Steve de Shazer and Insoo Kim Berg's solution-focused behavior therapy, and gender-aware therapy.

In this chapter we also briefly listed some other popular approaches which you might find interesting, such as eye movement desensitization therapy (EMDR); complementary, alternative, and integrative approaches; motivational interviewing; positive psychology and well-being therapy; and brief therapy. We contrasted some of the differences between the helper who practices long-term counseling and one who practices a brief approach.

In addition to looking at specific theoretical orientations, we briefly reviewed eclecticism, which is now more commonly called an integrative approach to counseling. We noted that such an approach is a developmental process that moves from chaos to coalescence to multiplicity, and ends with a commitment to a metatheory.

As this chapter continued, we examined the ethical and professional issues of supervision, confidentiality, and dual relationships. The supervisory relationship is particularly important because that relationship can help us understand how we interact with our clients, provides feedback when we might be losing objectivity, and can help us make difficult decisions related to breaking confidentiality. For confidentiality, we listed times when it might be important to break confidentiality and times when one should not and also discussed the important right of privilege communication that clients have with some licensed therapists. We noted that dual or multiple relationships can be problematic and stressed that it is the responsibility of each human service professional to decide whether his or her objective and professional judgment would be impaired by such a relationship. We concluded this chapter by noting that the effective human service professional should be committed to a counseling approach yet willing to change as new concepts become known.

Experiential Exercises

I. **Discovering Your Theory and Conceptual Orientation**
    The following offers you a way to determine the counseling and theoretical orientation which is most like your view of human nature. If you prefer, a similar scale that is somewhat more user-friendly can be found at http://www.odu.edu/~eneukrug/therapists/survey.html.

    To discover your theoretical and conceptual orientations, read each of the following items, and using the following scale, write in the spaces provided how strongly you feel about each item (write 1, 2, 3, 4, or 5).

I Don't Believe This   1   2   3   4   5   I Feel Extremely Certain
Statement at All   That This Statement Is True

_____ 1. Instincts (e.g., hunger, thirst, survival, sex, and aggression) are very strong motivators of behavior.

_____ 2. Psychological symptoms represent a desire to regain repressed parts of ourselves as well as parts of self that have never been revealed to consciousness.

_____ 3. Environmental influences on the child can lead to the development of a neurotic character, but through education and therapy, the person can change.

_____ 4. Children learn behaviors through conditioning (e.g., positive reinforcement, punishment).

_____ 5. We are born with the potential for rational or irrational thinking.

_____ 6. We are born with a predisposition toward certain disorders that could reveal itself under stressful conditions.

_____ 7. We are born with five needs: survival, love and belonging, power, freedom, and fun.

_____ 8. We are born into a world that has no inherent meaning or purpose, and we subsequently create our own meaning and purpose.

_____ 9. An inborn actualizing tendency lends direction toward reaching our full potential.

_____ 10. We are born with the capacity to embrace an infinite number of personality dimensions.

_____ 11. Reality is created through interactions or discussions within one's social circle.

_____ 12. Change can occur in fewer than six sessions. Extended therapy is often detrimental.

_____ 13. Deciding how to satisfy instincts (e.g., hunger, thirst, survival, sex, and aggression) occurs mostly unconsciously.

_____ 14. Revealing unconscious material to consciousness allows for an integrated "whole" person.

_____ 15. We all are striving for perfection in our effort to be whole and complete.

_____ 16. Past and present conditioning makes us who we are.

_____ 17. Irrational thinking leads to emotional distress, dysfunctional behaviors, and criticism of self and others.

_____ 18. By understanding one's cognitive processes (thinking), one can manage and change the way one lives.

_____ 19. We all have a quality world containing mental pictures of the people, things, and beliefs most important in meeting our unique needs.

_____ 20. We all struggle with the basic questions of what it is to be human.

_____ 21. Children continually assess whether interactions are positive or negative to their actualizing process, or way of living in the world.

_____ 22. The mind, body, and soul operate in unison; they cannot be separated.

_____ 23. Values held by those in power are disseminated through language and become the norms against which we compare ourselves.

_____ 24. Individuals can find exceptions to their problems and build on those exceptions to find new ways of living in the world.

_____ 25. Our personality is framed at a very young age and is quite difficult to change.

_____ 26. Primordial images that we all have interact with repressed material to create psychological complexes (e.g., mother complex; Peter Pan complex).

_____ 27. Children's experiences by age 5 years, and memories of those experiences, are critical factors in personality development.

_____ 28. Behaviors are generally conditioned and learned in very complex and subtle ways.

_____ 29. Although learning and biological factors influence the development of rational or irrational thinking, it is the individual who sustains his or her type of thinking.

_____ 30. Core beliefs (underlying beliefs that map our world) are the basis for a person's feelings, behaviors, and physiological responses.

_____ 31. We can only choose our actions and thoughts; our feelings and our physiology result from those choices.

_____ 32. We are born alone, will die alone, and except for periodic moments when we encounter another person deeply, we live alone.

_____ 33. The "self" has a need to be regarded positively by significant others.

_____ 34. From birth, the individual is in a constant state of self-regulation through a process of need identification and need fulfillment.

_____ 35. Psychopathology (mental disorders) is a social construction. There is no separate reality that supports its existence.

_____ 36. Although many therapies describe structures that affect functioning (e.g., id, ego, self-actualizing tendency), there is no objective reality proving their existence.

_____ 37. The development of defense mechanisms (repression, denial, projection) are ways of managing instincts.

_____ 38. Archetypes, or inherited unconscious primordial images, provide the psyche with its tendency to perceive the world in certain ways that we identify as human.

_____ 39. As children, how we learn to cope with inevitable feelings of inferiority affects our personality development.

_____ 40. Conditioning (e.g., positive reinforcement, punishment) can lead to a multitude of personality characteristics.

_____ 41. When our cognitive processes result in irrational thinking, we will tend to have self-defeating emotions and exhibit dysfunctional behaviors.

_____ 42. Genetics, biological factors, and experiences combine to produce specific core beliefs that affect how we behave and feel.

_____ 43. At any point in one's life, one can evaluate one's behaviors, thoughts, feelings, and physiology, and make new choices that better meet one's needs.

_____ 44. Meaningfulness, as well as a limited sense of freedom, comes through consciousness and the choices we make.

_____ 45. Because they want to be loved, children will often act in a way in which significant others want them to act instead of acting in a manner that is real or congruent with themselves.

_____ 46. Parental dictates, social mores, and peer norms can prevent a person from attaining satisfaction of a need. This unsatisfied need can affect us in ways of which we are unaware.

_____ 47. Constant discourse and interactions with others within one's social milieu leads to the development of a sense of self.

_____ 48. Language endemic in culture, society, and the individual's social sphere determines the nature of reality.

_____ 49. Because we spend the majority of our time unconsciously struggling to satisfy our unmet needs, happiness is an elusive feeling experienced infrequently.

_____ 50. We are born with the mental functions of sensation–intuition and thinking–feeling, which affect our perceptions. Their relative strengths are affected by how we were raised.

_____ 51. At an early age, we develop a private logic that moves us toward dysfunctional behaviors or toward wholeness.

_____ 52. By carefully analyzing how behaviors are conditioned, one can understand why an individual exhibits his or her current behavioral repertoire.

_____ 53. It is not events that cause negative emotions, but the belief about the events.

_____ 54. We all have automatic thoughts (fleeting thoughts about what we are perceiving and experiencing) that result in a set of behaviors, feelings, and physiological responses.

_____ 55. When language shows caring and the taking of responsibility, good choices are made. When language is blaming, critical, and judgmental, poor choices are made.

_____ 56. We sometimes avoid living authentically and experiencing life fully because we are afraid to look squarely at how we are making meaning in our lives.

_____ 57. Anxiety, and related symptoms, can be conceptualized as a signal to the individual that he or she is acting in a nongenuine way and not living fully.

_____ 58. Breaking free from defenses (e.g., repression) allows one to fully experience the present and live a saner life.

_____ 59. Reality is a social construction, and each person's reality is organized and maintained through his or her narrative and discourse with others.

_____ 60. Pathology, in all practical purposes, does not exist and is not inherently found within the person.

_____ 61. Early child-rearing practices are largely responsible for our personality development.

_____ 62. People are born with a tendency to be either extraverted (e.g., being outgoing) or introverted (e.g., being an observer, looking inward).

_____ 63. Child experiences, and the memories of them, impact each of our unique abilities and characteristics integral to the development of our character or personality.

_____ 64. By identifying what behaviors have been conditioned, one can eliminate undesirable behaviors and set goals to acquire more functional ways of acting.

_____ 65. The depth at which and length of time for which one experiences a self-defeating emotion are related to one's beliefs about an event, not to the event directly.

_____ 66. Automatic thoughts (fleeting thoughts about what we are perceiving) reinforce core beliefs we have about the world.

_____ 67. Needs can be satisfied only in the present, so focusing on how past needs were not met is useless.

_____ 68. People can gain a personally meaningful and authentic existence by making new choices that involve facing life's struggles honestly and directly.

_____ 69. Being around people who are real, empathic, and show positive regard results in the individual's becoming more real.

_____ 70. The ultimate way of living involves allowing oneself access to all of what is available to one's experience. Essentially, Now = Awareness = Reality.

_____ 71. Problems individuals have are a function of their problem-saturated stories or narratives. However, new preferred stories can be generated.

_____ 72. Problems are the result of language passed down by families, culture, and society, and dialogues between people.

SCORING

Scoring I: Place the numbers you chose across from the respective item. In each column, add up your score for each theory and divide the total by 30. That will give you the percentage score for that approach. Place your percentage in the parentheses. For the "psychodynamic score," add the total scores from each of the bottom rows and place it in the far right column. Divide that score by 90, and that will give you the percentage score for psychodynamic therapy. Place that percentage in the parentheses next to *psychodynamic*.

	Psychoanalysis ( )	Analytical ( )	Individual Psychology ( )	Score for Psychodynamic ( )
	1 _____	2 _____	3 _____	
	13 _____	14 _____	15 _____	
	25 _____	26 _____	27 _____	
	37 _____	38 _____	39 _____	
	49 _____	50 _____	51 _____	
	61 _____	62 _____	63 _____	
TOTAL:	_____	_____	_____	_____

Scoring II: Place the numbers you chose across from the respective item. In each column, add up your score for each theory and divide the total by 30. That will give you the percentage score for that approach. Place your percentage in the parentheses. For the "existential–humanistic score," add the total scores from each of the bottom rows and place it in the far right column. Divide that score by 90, and that will give you the percentage score for existential–humanistic therapy. Place that percentage in the parentheses next to *existential–humanistic*.

	Existential ( )	Person-Centered ( )	Gestalt ( )	Score for Existential–Humanistic ( )
	8 _____	9 _____	10 _____	
	20 _____	21 _____	22 _____	
	32 _____	33 _____	34 _____	
	44 _____	45 _____	46 _____	
	56 _____	57 _____	58 _____	
	68 _____	69 _____	70 _____	
TOTAL:	_____	_____	_____	_____

Scoring III: Place the numbers you chose across from the respective item. In each column, add up your score for each theory and divide the total by 30. That will give you the percentage score for that approach. Place your percentage in the parentheses. For the "cognitive–behavioral score," add the total scores from each of the bottom rows and place it in the far right column. Divide that score by 120, and that will give you the percentage score for cognitive–behavioral therapy. Place that percentage in the parentheses next to *cognitive–behavioral*.

	Cognitive–Reality Behavioral ( )	REBT ( )	Behavioral ( )	Therapy ( )	Score for Cognitive–Behavioral ( )
	4 _____	5 _____	6 _____	7 _____	
	16 _____	17 _____	18 _____	19 _____	
	28 _____	29 _____	30 _____	31 _____	
	40 _____	41 _____	42 _____	43 _____	
	52 _____	53 _____	54 _____	55 _____	
	64 _____	65 _____	66 _____	67 _____	
TOTAL:	_____	_____	_____	_____	_____

Scoring IV: Place the numbers you chose across from the respective item. In each column, add up your score for each theory and divide the total by 30. That will give you the percentage score for that approach. Place your percentage in the parentheses. For the "postmodern score," add the total scores from each of the bottom rows and place it in the far right column. Divide that score by 60, and that will give you the percentage score for postmodern therapy. Place that percentage in the parentheses next to *postmodern*.

	Narrative ( )	Solution-Focused ( )	Score for Postmodern ( )
	11 _____	12 _____	
	23 _____	24 _____	
	35 _____	36 _____	
	47 _____	48 _____	
	59 _____	60 _____	
	71 _____	72 _____	
TOTAL:	_____	_____	_____

II. Understanding Your View of Human Nature

Now that you've read this chapter, go and redo the exercise in Box 3.1. Compare the paragraph you wrote then with the one you wrote now. Any differences? Discuss your paragraph(s) with others in class.

III. Applying Differing Theoretical Orientations

Read the description of each of the following clients and think about how each theoretical orientation listed in this chapter would describe the origins of this person's current situation. Then discuss how you might apply each orientation.

The story of Jill. Jill is a 32-year-old married mother of two children, ages 7 and 2. She states that before getting married 6 years ago, she drank heavily, smoked pot, and "hung out with bikers and slept with a lot of guys." She has settled down since then but recently has started hanging out with her neighbor Steven, is drinking again, and is thinking about having an affair with Steven. She says that she loves her husband, but he has not been paying attention to her lately. She is angry at him but reports that she and her husband rarely talk about their feelings. Although she maintained average grades in school, she never completed high school and would like to obtain her GED. She reports having frequent anxiety attacks and rarely leaves her house other than to go to her part-time job in a factory.

Jill, the second child in a family of four, states that her father was verbally abusive, drank a lot, and generally didn't pay attention to her. Since he stopped drinking a few years ago, however, he has become closer to her. She reports her childhood as being chaotic because she never knew whether her father would blow up at her or at other members of her family when he was drunk. No one in her family has ever received a high school diploma.

The story of Harley. Harley was recently released from the state mental hospital where he spent most of his adolescence. Harley has a history of being psychotic; that is, he has periodically been out of touch with reality. His parents abandoned him when he was 9 years old, and he has lived in foster homes and at state hospitals since that time. He just turned 18 years old. Harley is currently taking antipsychotic and antianxiety medications and is in the day treatment program at the local community mental health center. At day treatment, he spends the day attending support groups, doing vocational skills training, and socializing. He has little memory of his childhood, but what he can remember is very painful. For instance, he does have vague memories of verbal and sexual abuse, and he thinks there were older siblings in his home. Harley's lifelong dream is to own a motorcycle, and he seems to talk about a motorcycle as if it were his lover. Confidentially, he reports having had sexual feelings toward a motorcycle.

Harley has few friends and has an impulsive temper; that is, he periodically just blows up. Although he generally does not act out physically toward people, on rare occasions he has been known to attack someone in an impulsive rage. His medication seems to help him with his outbursts.

IV. The Human Service Professional's Implementation of Varying Theoretical Approaches

Describe how a human service professional in each of the following occupations might apply the theoretical orientations discussed in this chapter.

1. A human service professional who helps at a shelter for the homeless
2. A human service professional who helps the mentally retarded at a residential home
3. A human service professional who helps the mentally ill at a day treatment program in a mental health center
4. A human service professional assisting poor women at a problem-pregnancy counseling center
5. A human service professional who helps the poor at an unemployment office

V. Have one person role-play a supervisor and one person role-play a human service professional, and then discuss the case of Harley or Jill in Exercise III.

1. What theoretical approach do you think would work best with your client? Discuss with your "supervisor" what you think you might want to do to assist your client.
2. Did the "supervisor" offer a supervisory environment that was conducive to your talking about the client? What supervisory qualities were helpful? Unhelpful?

VI. Eclecticism or Integrative Approaches to Helping

1. Using Exercises I and II as a resource, make a list of items that reflect your view of human nature.
2. Based on this list, begin to develop your own theory of counseling.
3. What "techniques" are natural outgrowths of your theory?
4. Do you think your theory will change over time?

VII. Ethical and Professional Issues: Supervision
1. Make a list of the qualities you would want in a supervisor.
2. How does your list differ from the qualities noted in the book?

VIII. Ethical and Professional Vignettes: Confidentiality and Dual Relationships
1. Refer to Harley and Jill in Exercise III to discuss the following vignettes.
    a. While you are helping Jill find study classes for the GED exam, she reveals that sometimes when she's drinking she takes the belt out and "whacks my kids good—they just won't shut up." Do you break confidentiality and tell Child Protective Services?
    b. While driving to work one day, your car breaks down. Harley sees you and says, "I'm good with mechanical things, let me help for a small fee—besides, I could use a little money for buying my bike." You want to get your car fixed, and you want Harley to have his bike. Do you let him help you?
    c. One day Jill tells you she is pregnant by Steven. She's going to have an abortion. Your state has a law requiring women to tell their spouses if they're to have an abortion. She refuses. What do you do?
    d. Jill's husband shows up at your office demanding information about his wife. You tell him things are confidential. He tells you that he'll sue you and the rest of this "fleabag" operation. What do you do?
    e. You've been encouraging Jill for months to get involved in more social activities and to get out of the house more. One day Jill shows up at the same art class you are taking. What do you do?
    f. Jill tells you that from time to time, usually when she's drinking, she gets severely depressed and thinks about killing herself. You ask her if she has a plan, and she says, "Well, sometimes I think about just doing it with that gun my husband has." One day she calls you; she's been drinking, and she tells you she's depressed. She hangs up saying, "I don't know what I might do." What do you do?
    g. Harley stops taking his medication, stops by your office, and seems pretty angry. He says, "That cheating Harley dealer, he's trying to rip me off. He told me I could have that bike at a discount and went back on his word." You try to talk with Harley, but he storms out of your office saying, "I'm going to get that man!" What do you do?
2. Other ethical vignettes
    a. Your supervisor tells you that he is going to have to report your client to social services for possible child abuse. You believe that reporting your client is breaking confidentiality and will have a deleterious effect on your relationship with your client. Is what he's doing ethical? Professional? Legal?
    b. A colleague of yours who works with female clients who have been abused encourages all of her clients to leave their husbands and states that this is the "right thing to do" from a feminist perspective. Does she have a point? Is what she's doing ethical? Professional? Legal?
    c. A fellow student of yours tells you that being eclectic is the way to go because then you can pretty much pull any techniques you like from

the different theories and combine them into your own approach. When working in an internship, you discover that this student is counseling clients without a solid theoretical base—just using techniques she likes. What is your responsibility to this student? To the clients? What is your ethical obligation?

d. After obtaining your first job, you discover that many of your human service colleagues have forgotten the theories they have learned in school and do not feel obligated to participate in continuing education. What is your responsibility in this situation? What is your ethical obligation?

e. You discover that a colleague of yours is seeing clients for extended periods to "pad" his contact hours. With many of these clients, a brief treatment mode could have been used, but your colleague has continued to see them for extended periods of time regardless of this fact. What is your responsibility to the clients? To your colleague? To the agency? To your profession? What should you do?

The Helping Interview: Skills, Process, and Case Management

CHAPTER CONTENTS

The first time I did counseling, I was a volunteer at the drug crisis clinic at my college. I had no training, but somehow I instinctively knew that it was probably best to listen a lot and be kind. Having been a psychology major, I never had a course in counseling theories or counseling methods. I knew little about the "correct" way to respond to a drop-in at the center. I hope I did more good than harm as I tried to help students who had overdosed or were "bumming" from doing hallucinogens.

Immediately following receipt of a bachelor's degree, I went on to obtain my master's degree in counseling. I then spent a few months painstakingly looking for employment. I obtained my first real job at "The Rap House." Funded by a government agency, this storefront drop-in and crisis center was the place where many of the homeless alcoholics could stop in, get a cup of coffee, and, if need be, talk to a helper or get a referral to a detox center. These were my first clients in a professional setting.

Now that I had a graduate degree, I at least had some training in appropriate ways to respond to a client. At that time, my theoretical approach was humanistically based, and I felt it was good if people could express their feelings and let things out. Although my counseling approach had become somewhat focused, my old untrained self, which sometimes would get very advice oriented, periodically raised its ugly head.

From these experiences, I have come to learn that one is not born with an ability to counsel. Helping skills can be learned and the more training you have, the more effective you will be (Armstrong, 2010). However, one need not have an advanced degree to become a fairly effective helper (Barz, 2001). What is important is learning the skills and practicing them. Much like riding a bicycle or skateboard for the first time, learning helping skills feels awkward at first. However, you will find that the more you practice, the more natural and at ease you'll feel. In my own life, I now approach the learning and refinement of my skills as a never-ending process. One never "gets there"; instead, we hope to get better as we learn new and more effective ways of working with our clients. Some of us are lucky because we had good modeling from our parents or other significant people, and thus we have a head start in learning skills. Unfortunately, I have found that most of us have not been so blessed, so practicing tried-and-true techniques becomes extremely important.

More than any other area in the human services, I have found that learning skills is the most sensitive and awkward area for many students. This part of the curriculum is where students often feel that they are putting themselves "out there," showing their capabilities to their peers. Unfortunately, because students often feel so vulnerable in front of their peers, I find many protect themselves and partially shut out this important learning experience. If you are apprehensive, that's normal. However, if you find that this fear prevents you from taking an active role in learning these important skills, then reflect on what you are doing and see whether you can take a more open approach.

In this chapter, we will examine the importance of creating a favorable atmosphere for the helping relationship and examine techniques that over the years have been shown to be effective in working with a wide range of clients. We will also examine the typical stages clients pass through during the helping relationship and the kinds of skills that are generally used during each of these stages. In addition to responding effectively to your clients and knowing the predictable stages of the interview, good case management is critical to successful work with clients and will be examined in this chapter. Case management involves attendance to a myriad of sometimes mundane tasks important to maintaining the optimal functioning of clients (e.g., diagnosis, paperwork, and follow-up), and we will take a brief look at some of these tasks. This chapter will conclude with an examination of ethical, professional, and legal issues related to the helping relationship.

CREATING THE HELPING ENVIRONMENT

In creating an environment that is conducive to a facilitative helping relationship, the helping professional needs to pay attention to a number of areas. First, the helper must assure a comfortable office environment. Second, the helper needs to embody the personal characteristics necessary to foster a positive helping relationship. Finally, the helper needs to know how to attend nonverbally to the client. Let's take a look at each of these areas.

Office Environment

I'm sure you've had the experience of walking into someone's office and finding it cold and inhospitable. The arrangement of one's office can be crucial to eliciting positive attitudes from people and should give a message to our clients that they are welcome (Bedi, 2006; Pressly & Heesacker, 2001). Although not all human service professionals have their own offices, wherever we meet our clients we should attempt to make the environment as conducive as possible to a positive working relationship. If we are lucky enough to have an office, simple things like nonglare lighting, comfortable seating, and not having obstructions (e.g., large desks) between ourselves and our clients can be helpful in creating a comfortable helping environment. You may want to review Exercise I at the end of this chapter to determine how you might arrange your office.

Personal Characteristics of the Helper

Whether the human service professional is found doing one-to-one counseling within an office or chatting with clients in a group home, the personal characteristics he or she brings can destroy or foster a helping relationship. Many common attitudes that would be destructive to a helping relationship which need little explanation include being critical, disapproving, disbelieving, scolding, threatening, discounting, ridiculing, punishing, and rejecting (Benjamin, 2001; Glasser & Glasser, 2007; Van Nuys, 2007). Clearly these attitudes and behaviors, as well as others of a similar nature, are to be avoided. In contrast, many of the attitudes which can foster a positive helping relationship and which the human service professional should embrace were noted in Chapter 1. They included **relationship building; empathy; genuineness, acceptance, cognitive complexity; wellness;** and **competence** and **cross-cultural sensitivity.** These characteristics allow our clients to feel a sense of safety and trust with us and each of them help facilitate a positive helping relationship.

If you find a client who is particularly nasty or angry, first examine your attitudes to see how you bring yourself to the session. If you are not embodying the characteristics of the effective helper, perhaps your attitude is feeding the client's anger.

Importance of Nonverbal Behavior

Don't *say* things. What you are stands over you the while, and thunders so that I cannot hear what you *say* to the contrary. (Emerson, 1880, p. 80)

Sometimes condensed to "What you do speaks so loud that I cannot hear what you say," the previous quote says volumes about the importance of **nonverbal behavior.** Supporting the quote, in 1971 **Albert Mehrabian** published his classic research which suggested that when talking about feelings and attitudes, words accounted for 7% of what was being communicated while voice intonation accounted for 38% and body language for about 55%. Years later, it continues to be clear that nonverbal behavior is a major aspect of how we communicate to others (Guerrero & Floyd, 2006; Planalp & Knie, 2002).

How we present ourselves nonverbally can greatly add or detract from our overall relationship with our clients. For instance, **posture, eye contact,** or a **tone of voice** that says "don't open up to me" will obviously affect our clients differently from behaviors through which the helper nonverbally conveys, "I'm open to hearing what you have to say." **Personal space** is an additional nonverbal factor that affects the counseling relationship (Guerrero & Floyd, 2006; Zur, 2007). Mediated at least somewhat by culture, age, and gender, individuals vary greatly in their degree of comfort with personal space. Therefore, the human service professional must allow for enough personal space so that the client feels comfortable, yet not so much that the client feels distant from the helper. When necessary, the helper should take the lead in respecting the client's need for personal space.

Touch is a final aspect of nonverbal behavior (Ferch, 2000; Zur, 2007). Touching at important moments is quite natural. For instance, when someone is expressing deep pain, it is not unusual for us to hold a hand or embrace a person while he or she sobs. Or, during a helping interview, one might find it natural to place a hand on a shoulder or give a hug. However, in today's litigious society, touch has become a particularly delicate subject, and it is important for each of us to be sensitive to our clients' boundaries, our own boundaries, and limits to touch set by our professional code of ethics. Some have become so touchy over this issue, that a therapist in Massachusetts, branded "the hugging therapist," was fired from his job at a mental health agency because he hugged his clients too much. Brammer and MacDonald (2003) suggest that physical contact with a client should be based on (1) the helper's assessment of the needs of the helpee; (2) the helper's awareness of his or her own needs; (3) what is most likely to be helpful within the counseling relationship; and (4) risks that may be involved as a function of agency policy, customs, personal ethics, and the law.

Even though many nonverbal behaviors seem to be universal, there do seem to be some cross-cultural differences (Matsumoto, 2006; Pease & Pease, 2006). With this in mind, helpers who have been traditionally taught to lean forward, have good eye contact, speak in a voice that meets the client's affect, and rarely touch the client are now being asked to be acutely sensitive to client responses to nonverbal behaviors. Some clients will expect to be looked at, while others will be offended by eye contact; some clients will expect you to lean forward, while others will experience this as an intrusion; and some clients will expect you to touch them, while others will see this as offensive. In respect to nonverbal behavior, effective helpers keep in mind what works for the many while remaining sensitive to what works for the few.

COUNSELING TECHNIQUES

A number of helping skills have traditionally been shown to be important in building a positive counseling relationship, and here you will have the chance to examine them. They include listening; empathy; silence; encouragement and affirmations; modeling; self-disclosure; the use of questions; information giving, advice giving, and offering alternatives; confrontation; and collaboration.

Listening Skills

> First there is the hearing with the ear, which we all know; and the hearing with the non-ear, which is a state like that of a tranquil pond, a lake that is completely quiet and when you drop a stone into it, it makes little waves that disappear. I think that [insight] is the hearing with the non-ear, a state where there is absolute quietness of the mind; and when the question is put into the mind, the response is the wave, the little wave. (Krishnamurti, cited in Jayakar, 1996/1986, p. 328)

Assuming we have created an environment conducive to a positive client/helper relationship, we are now ready to assess the client situation. Usually, our first step is to understand the issues our clients bring with them. This means being able to hear our clients—good listening. Effective listening helps to build trust, convinces the client you understand him or her, encourages the client to reflect on what he or she has just said, ensures that you are on track with your understanding of the client, and can facilitate information-gathering from your client (Neukrug & Schwitzer, 2006).

Finally, whenever I teach **listening skills**, I like to stress that good listening involves not talking. Although obvious, I have found that too many people confuse listening with advice giving. It's almost as if we have learned that if someone is in distress or has a problem, we should tell them what to do. Although advice giving has its place (we will talk more about this later), my experience has been that, more often than not, most people want to be heard rather than to receive advice (see Box 4.1).

Hindrances to Listening   Even when we know how to listen, our own prejudices, biases, and unfinished business can prevent us from fully hearing another person.

BOX 4.1 | **Listen to Me**

When I ask you to listen to me and you start giving me advice, you have not done what I asked.

When I ask you to listen to me and you begin to tell me why I shouldn't feel that way, you are trampling on my feelings.

When I ask you to listen to me and you feel you have to do something to solve my problem, you have failed me, strange as that may seem.

Listen: All that I ask is that you listen, not talk or do—just hear me.

When you do something for me that I can and need to do for myself, you contribute to my fear and inadequacy.

But when you accept as a simple fact that I do feel what I feel, no matter how irrational, then I can quit trying to convince you and get about this business of understanding what's behind these feelings.

So, please listen and just hear me.

And, if you want to talk, wait a minute for your turn—and I'll listen to you.

(Author Unknown)

Thus, knowing ourselves is the first step we can take toward hearing another (see Activity 4.1). Once we have examined our own issues, we are ready to listen, and a few pointers can go a long way in doing this effectively (Egan, 2010; Ivey, Ivey, & Zalaquett, 2010):

1. *Calm yourself down.* Before meeting with your client, calm yourself down—meditate, pray, jog, or blow out air, but calm your inner self.
2. *Stop talking and don't interrupt.* You cannot listen while you are talking.
3. *Show interest.* With your body language and tone of voice, show the person you are interested in what he or she is saying.
4. *Don't jump to conclusions.* Take in all of what the person says and don't assume you understand the person better than he or she understands himself or herself.
5. *Actively listen.* Focus on the client and pay attention. Many people do not realize that listening is an active process that takes deep concentration.
6. *Concentrate on feelings.* Listen to, identify, and acknowledge the person's feelings to him or her.
7. *Concentrate on content.* Listen to, identify, and acknowledge what the person is saying.
8. *Maintain appropriate eye contact.* Be willing to look directly at your client, but also be sensitive to how eye contact might make some clients feel uncomfortable.
9. *Have an open body posture.* Show, by your body language, that you are inviting the client to talk (e.g., do not sit there with your arms crossed).
10. *Be sensitive to personal space.* Obtain a sense of the optimal distance needed between you and your client for effective communication.
11. *Don't ask questions.* Don't ask questions except if they are used to clarify content (e.g., Can you repeat that, I didn't hear exactly what you said?).

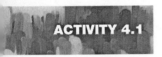 **ACTIVITY 4.1** | # Hindrances to Effective Listening

In class, break into triads (groups of three). Within your group, number yourselves 1, 2, and 3. With the three topics listed later (or other topics of the instructor's choice), have the instructor assign one of the topics to persons 1 and 2. Number 1, you be "pro" the situation, and, number 2, you be "con" the situation. Now, one of you start debating the situation while the other listens. When the first person is finished, the second person should repeat verbatim what he or she heard (do not do reflective listening—just repeat verbatim). Then, debate back and forth, taking turns listening and repeating verbatim until the instructor tells you to stop. Number 3, you are an objective helper, to give feedback if needed. As the objective person, don't forget also to give feedback concerning each person's body language. When you have finished this first situation, have numbers 2 and 3 do the second situation, and then numbers 3 and 1 do the third situation. Each time, the third person will be the objective helper.

When you have finished, the instructor will ask for feedback concerning what things prevented you from hearing the other person. Make a list on the board, and in particular make sure you discuss some of the following items: preoccupation, defensiveness, emotional blocks, and distractions. Also, remember to give feedback on the appropriateness of each person's nonverbal behaviors.

Situations: Abortion, torturing suspected terrorists to gain information, capital punishment

Empathy: A Special Kind of Listening

Highlighted as one of the eight personal qualities of the effective helper, **empathy** is also one of the most important counseling skills. Many of the early Greek philosophers noted the importance of listening to another person from a deep inner perspective (Gompertz, 1960). In the twentieth century, Lipps (1960) is given credit for coining the word *empathy* from the German word *Einfühlung*, "to feel within." However, the person who had the most impact on our modern-day understanding and usage of empathy was **Carl Rogers (1959):**

> The state of empathy, or being empathic, is to perceive the internal frame of reference of another with accuracy and with the emotional components and meanings which pertain thereto as if one were the person, but without ever losing the "as if" condition. (pp. 210–211)

Since Rogers' original definition of empathy, others have attempted to operationalize the concept. This means that they have taken Rogers's definition and developed a method to measure one's ability to make empathic responses. For instance, **Robert Carkhuff (1969)** developed a five-point scale to measure empathy (see Figure 4.1). He notes that Level 1 and Level 2 responses in some ways detract from what the person is saying (e.g., advice giving, not accurately reflecting feeling, not including content), with a Level 1 response being way off the mark and a Level 2 only slightly off. For instance, suppose a client said, "I've had it with my dad; he never does anything with me. He's always working, drinking, or playing with my little sister." A Level 1 response might be, "Well, why don't you do something to change the situation, like tell him what an idiot he is?" (giving advice and being judgmental). A Level 2 response might be, "You seem to think your dad spends too much time with your sister" (does not reflect feeling and misses some important content).

On the other hand, a Level 3 response accurately reflects the affect and meaning of what the helpee has said. Using the same example, you might say, "Well, it sounds as if you're pretty upset at your dad for not spending time with you." Level 4 and Level 5 responses reflect feelings and meaning beyond what the person is outwardly saying and add to the meaning of the person's outward expression. For instance, in the example, a Level 4 response might be, "It sounds like you're pretty hurt because your father seems to ignore you" (expresses new feeling, hurt, which the client did not outwardly state). Level 5 responses are usually made in long-term therapeutic relationships by expert therapists. They express a deep understanding of the pain the client feels as well as recognizing the complexity of the situation.

Usually, in the training of helpers, it is suggested that they attempt to make Level 3 responses because such responses have been shown to be effective for clients (Carkhuff, 2009). Using the Carkhuff (1969) operational definition of empathy, an enormous body of evidence indicates that making good empathic responses

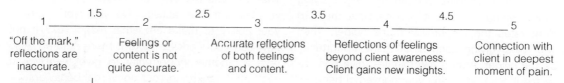

Figure 4.1 | The Carkhuff Scale

(Level 3 or above) can be taught in a relatively short amount of time and that such responses by both paraprofessionals and professionals are beneficial to clients (Carkhuff, 2009; Neukrug, 1980, 1987; Schaefle, Smaby, Maddux, & Cates, 2005).

Over the years, good empathic responses sometimes have been confused with active listening or reflection of feeling. Although Rogers was instrumental in encouraging the use of empathy, he warned against a mechanistic and wooden response to clients:

> Although I am partially responsible for the use of this term [reflection of feelings] to describe a certain type of therapist response, I have, over the years, become very unhappy with it. A major reason is that "reflection of feelings" has not been infrequently taught as a technique, and sometimes a very wooden technique at that. Such training has very little to do with an effective therapeutic relationship. (Rogers, 1986, p. 375)

As Rogers implied, although it is important to learn this new skill of empathy, sometimes making such responses will feel stilted and mechanistic. With practice, your responses to clients will become naturally empathic. Activity 4.2 gives you an opportunity to practice this important skill of empathy.

Silence

When   is   empty   space   facilitative,   and
when   does   it   become   a   bit   much?

Silence is a powerful tool that can be used advantageously by the helper for the growth of the client (Linda, Miller, & Johnson, 2000; Sommers-Flanagan & Sommers-Flanagan, 2009). Silence allows the client to reflect on what he or she has been saying and allows the helper to process the session and to formulate his or her next response. Silence says to the client that communication does not always have to be filled with words, and it gives the client the opportunity to look at how words can sometimes be used to divert a person from his or her feelings. Silence is powerful. It will sometimes raise anxiety within the client, anxiety that on one hand could push the client to talk further about a particular topic and on the other hand could cause a client to drop out of the helping relationship.

A former professor of mine used to suggest waiting 30 seconds before making a response. Thirty seconds during a helping relationship is a VEEEEEEEEEERY LOOOOONG TIIIIIIIIIIME. There have been times when I've had a student

---

ACTIVITY 4.2   **Making Empathic Responses**

In class, break up into triads. Two students role-play a helping relationship, with the helper trying to make Carkhuff Level 3 responses, while the third student rates the responses of the helper. Then switch roles, giving each student the opportunity to be the helper. After a few minutes, give one another feedback concerning your nonverbal behavior and the ability to make Carkhuff Level 3 responses. Then discuss the level of comfort (or discomfort) you felt with this activity. Do you feel natural in your ability to make empathic responses? If not, how can you work to make it more natural? Also, here is another opportunity to give feedback to each other regarding your nonverbal behaviors.

role-play a client, and I've waited 30 seconds before responding. Trust me, this is a VERY LONG TIME. I would have difficulty waiting this long during a helping relationship. However, others may feel comfortable with this amount of silence. For instance, my former professor could do this. During these 30 seconds you could SEE him moving in his chair, SEE him thinking about the last client statement, and SEE him thinking about what he was to say next. This worked for him. Silence is powerful.

Finally, the value of silence on the part of the helper or client may be somewhat culturally determined. For instance, some research has found that the typical pause time varies for different cultures. Therefore, one's natural inclination to talk—to respond to another—will vary as a function of culture (Tafoya, 1996; Zur 2007). As a human service professional, you may want to consider your pause time to discover your comfort level with silence. When working with clients you might consider a client's pause time. In fact, Tafoya notes that Native Americans have at times been labeled reticent to talk and resistant in the helping relationship when in fact they have long pause times. If they had been treated by Native American helpers, they most likely would not have been labeled in this fashion.

Encouragement and Affirmation

> The need for supporting core self-esteem doesn't end in childhood. Adults still need "unconditional" love from family, friends, life partners, animals, perhaps even an all-forgiving deity. Love that says: "no matter how the world may judge you, I love you for yourself." (Steinem, 1992, p. 66)

Many of the clients with whom you will be working are coming in with hurts from the past that continue to infiltrate their lives and cause low self-esteem. These hurts create depression and anger that sometimes seem to have lost their origins. Such feelings can create negativity and sometimes an "attitude" toward the world that can make these individuals some of our more difficult clients. In fact, sometimes our inclination may be to tell these clients to "cut it out" or "pick yourself up off your duff." However, this is the last thing they need. In fact, such clients have generally been so abused and put down throughout their lives that unconsciously they may be expecting to be treated this way by everyone, even the human service professional. Carrying around this attitude in life rarely, if ever, brings them what they really need—affirmation of self and an attitude that says "you can do it."

Human service professionals must be able to see beyond the hurts, the depression, the anger, and the attitude. They need to believe that clients have potential—that they can "do it." Human service professionals can express this positive attitude toward clients through **encouragement** and **affirmation**. Affirming a client is reinforcing a client's existing way of being, whereas encouragement is reinforcing a client's ability to perform a task. For instance, affirming a client by saying "good job," "I know you are lovable and capable," or "You are a good person inside" helps the client feel supported and worthwhile. Similarly, encouraging a client by saying "I know you can do this" or "I'm confident of your ability to change" can help build a client's sense of self-worth. Ultimately, clients need to internalize, or believe that they possess these feelings on their own. Although too many affirmations or too much encouragement can lead to client dependency issues, encouragement and

Gloria Steinem believes that our need for high self-esteem continues throughout adulthood. Fulfilling that need starts with our ability to love ourselves.

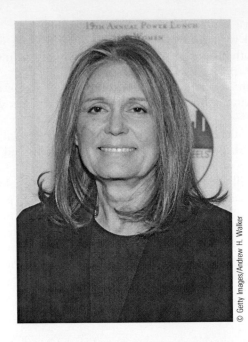

© Getty Images/Andrew H. Walker

affirmation done appropriately can be important tools in helping clients integrate a more positive attitude about life (Orlinsky, Ronnestad, & Willutzki, 2004).

Modeling

I once was asked to talk to a large family reunion about the importance of education. School always came easy for me, but I knew that this was not the case for most of this family. For them, finishing high school was difficult, and going on to college was rarely considered. Instead of specifically talking about education, I decided to talk about something that had always been very difficult for me—being athletic. So, I talked about how I trained for years as a runner, preparing myself over and over to do the one big run—the New York marathon. I told them this was one of the finest accomplishments of my life and how triumphant I felt when I finally did it. And, I told them how that moment in time is indelibly pictured in my mind and has given me a major self-esteem boost. Then, I talked more generally about doing something important yet difficult in life—something like finishing one's education. I noted that like running a marathon, finishing one's education takes perseverance and leaves one with something to be proud of. It's no easy task, but in the "long run," you feel better about yourself. This, example, and the analogy that it had for education, I thought, would be a good model for them. I think it was!

We are constantly **modeling** behavior for our clients, sometimes in intentional ways, as in the previous example, and sometimes in very subtle ways (Brammer & MacDonald, 2003). Because our clients look up to us, and sometimes even idealize us, the ways in which we model behaviors can have a powerful effect and dramatically influence our clients' change process (Cooper, Heron, & Heward, 2007; Naugle & Maher, 2003).

When modeling occurs in very subtle ways, clients learn new behaviors simply as a by-product of being in a helping relationship with us. If we are empathic, then they may learn how to listen to loved ones more effectively. If we are assertive, they may learn how to positively confront someone in their lives. And, if we can show them that we can resolve conflict, then they may learn new ways of dealing with conflict in their lives.

When modeling occurs in an intentional manner, the helper deliberately assists the client in establishing new behaviors. For instance, a former client of mine wanted to become more assertive with his peers. Thus, he described certain situations with his peers in which he was passive. I then modeled ways in which he could have been assertive. After watching me as a model, he practiced similar behaviors in the office, then at home, and finally with his peers. Now, he didn't miraculously become assertive, but with time and patience, he slowly changed some behaviors that he did not feel good about.

Self-Disclosure

A former student once shared with me that her psychiatrist had recently committed suicide. She told me that for months prior to his suicide, during her sessions, *he* was increasingly revealing more about himself and listening to her less. She now was feeling guilty about his death, thinking that she should have been attending to his needs. What a terrible legacy to leave her! We are helpers, caregivers. We are not in this business to take—to have our needs met. Keeping a check on when and why we are self-disclosing is extremely important.

Self-disclosure has been broadly defined as anything that a helper may reveal "verbally, nonverbally, on purpose, by accident, wittingly, or unwittingly ..." (Bloomgarden & Mennuti, 2009, p. 8). Although self-disclosure, as in the previous case, can have the potential for harm, it can also be an important tool to help clients open up, as research has shown that when one person is open in a relationship, the other person is more likely to be open (Bloomgarden & Mennuti, 2009; Farber, 2006; Maroda, 2009). Self-disclosure needs to be done sparingly, at the right time, and as a means for promoting client growth rather than satisfying the counselor's needs (Zur, 2009). A general rule of thumb that I use is: "If it feels good to self-disclose, don't." If it feels good, you're probably meeting more of your needs than the needs of your client. Hill and Knox (2002) suggest a number of guidelines for when to use self-disclosure:

1. Disclose infrequently.
2. The least appropriate disclosure is about sexual issues.
3. The most appropriate disclosure is about professional issues.
4. Disclosure is best used to normalize situations, validate reality, build the relationship, or offer alternatives.
5. Avoid disclosures for one's own needs or disclosures that are intrusive, blur boundaries, interfere with the flow, or confuse the client.
6. The best disclosures are ones in which the information given by the helper somehow matches that given by the client.
7. Some clients respond better to disclosures than others—know your client.

Finally, I agree with Kahn (2001), who states:

> I try not to make a fetish out of not talking about myself. If a client, on the way out the door, asks in a friendly and casual way, "Where are you going on your vacation?" I tell where I'm going. If the client were then to probe, however ("Who are you going with? Are you married?") I would be likely to respond, "Ah … maybe we'd better talk about that next time." (p. 150)

The Use of Questions

Generally, **questions** can be helpful in uncovering patterns, gathering information quickly, inducing self-exploration, challenging the client to change, and moving a client along quickly to preferred goals (Benjamin, 2001; Sommers-Flanagan & Sommers-Flanagan, 2009). However, their overuse can create an authoritarian atmosphere in which the client feels humiliated and dependent as he or she expects the counselor to come up with a solution for him or her. In addition, a question may not be as helpful as an empathic response in allowing a client to delve deeper into self (Neukrug, 2002; Neukrug & Schwitzer, 2006; Rogers, 1942). In fact, sometimes, helpers rely on questions rather than make an empathic response because it feels easier to ask a question. For instance, suppose the client said the following:

CLIENT: You know, I'm a bit disturbed that my parents never taught me how to be more in charge of my life.

A human service professional could respond by saying something like this:

HSP: Do you feel angry at your parents for not teaching you how to take charge?

However, probably a more effective response would be:

HSP: I get a sense that you're angry at your parents for not teaching you how to take charge.

In this previous case, the empathic response is more focused and allows the client to expand on the topic—if he or she so wishes to. However, sometimes it may be important to ask questions. For example **closed questions** might be more useful than **open questions** when you need to gather specific information like medical or employment history, **tentative questions** are helpful when you want a client to ponder a subject, and **solution-focused questions** are important if you want to help a client focus on **preferred goals.** Let's take a look at each of these and finish with a short discussion on the use of **Why questions.**

Open Versus Closed Questions   Open questions are stated in a manner that allows clients to respond in a variety of ways, whereas closed questions tend to limit client responses. If you are going to ask a question, an open question is generally more effective than a closed question in terms of facilitating client self-exploration, but a closed question is more effective in gathering information quickly. For instance, an open question such as "How did your parents treat you when you were growing up?" allows for a wide variety of responses by the client, thus allowing the client to direct the flow of the session. On the other hand, a closed question, such as, "Were your parents strict with you?" elicits a yes or no response from the client and is useful when one is under a time crunch and is hoping to garner information quickly.

Tentative Questions   Benjamin (2001) notes that almost any question can be made more facilitative if it is asked tentatively. For instance, rather than asking "Were your parents strict with you while growing up?" one could ask, "I'm wondering how strict your parents were with you while you were growing up." Or, one can even say, "I would guess you had some feelings about how your parents brought you up." This kind of tentative question is much more akin to an empathic response and is more facilitative when trying to build a relationship with a client and for client self-exploration. Closed questions are easy to ask—there's little need for practice. However, tentative questions and empathic responses take practice. Thus, I often suggest that students spend more time practicing making tentative questions and empathic responses rather than closed questions.

Solution-Focused Questions   If you find yourself in a setting where brief treatment is being used and reaching goals quickly is desired, you might want to consider the kinds of questions that follow. Based on the work of solution-focused theorists, as noted in Chapter 3, we find the following kinds of questions (Neukrug, 2011).

Preferred goals questions: These are questions that are generally asked near the very beginning of the helping relationship to assess what the goals or hope of counseling would be. For instance, one might ask, "How will you know that coming to counseling has been worthwhile for you?"

Evaluative questions: These questions help clients distinguish behaviors that have led to preferred goals from those that have not (e.g., Has that new behavior worked for you?)

Coping questions: Coping questions focus on past behaviors that have been successful in dealing with problems (e.g., So, you've had this problem in the past, how did you tend to cope with it then?)

Exception-seeking questions: These questions help clients examine when they haven't had the problem in their lives, so that they can explore how they previously lived a problem-free life (e.g., So, what was going on in your life when you were not feeling this way?).

Solution-oriented questions: Future oriented, these questions offer clients the opportunity to develop new, positive ways of reaching their preferred goals (e.g., What kinds of things do you think you can do to help reach your preferred goals?).

"Why" Questions   Generally, asking a "why" question is not recommended. Although asking *why* seems to make sense, people often feel interrogated and put on guard when asked why they felt or did something. Usually "what" or "how" questions are more palatable for clients. For instance, compare the following "why" and "what" questions:

HSP: Why did you feel depressed and angry at your parents' divorce?

In this case, it is almost as if the interviewer is challenging the helpee about how he or she felt. The following question is similar, but instead of starting with "why," I've started it with "what."

HSP: What was it about your parents' divorce that made you feel depressed and angry?

In this case, the helpee is not being put on the defensive.

Although much more can be said about the different uses of questions in the interviewing process, suffice it to say that one should always be careful whenever questions are being used. Keeping this in mind, consider the following if you are to ask a question (Benjamin, 2001; Neukrug & Schwitzer, 2006):

- Are you aware you are about to ask a question?
- Have you weighed carefully the desirability of asking a question?
- Have you examined your tendency to use questions and why you use them at all?
- Have you considered alternatives to asking questions?
- Will the question(s) you are about to ask inhibit the flow of the interview?

Offering Alternatives, Information Giving, and Advice Giving

Have you ever been in a situation where you've had someone try to give you advice or information and you felt like telling that person to mind his or her own business? Unfortunately, I have seen this happen all too often. **Offering alternatives, information giving, and advice giving** are three ways of facilitating client movement, all of which assume there is information the helper holds that he or she can give to the client to foster positive change. However, they all also hold the potential of damaging the helping relationship (Benjamin, 2001). From least potential to harm to most potential for harm, the following are brief definitions of these three types of skills.

Offering alternatives is a response that suggests to the client that there may be a number of ways to tackle the problem and has the helper offer options from which the client can choose. This type of response has the least potential for harm because it does not presume there is one solution to the problem. It does not set up the helper as the final expert, and to some degree, allows the client to pursue various options while maintaining a sense that he or she is directing the session. For example, the helper might say:

"You know, there are many kinds of birth control. For instance, you can ..."

Information giving is a response that offers the client valuable "objective" information which will facilitate client understanding and client growth. This kind of a response sets up the helper as the expert, thereby increasing the potential for the client to become dependent on the relationship. Unfortunately, more often than not, the client already knows the information given and sometimes the information is given in a judgmental fashion, as if the client *should* follow through with some task that underlies the information given. For example, the helper might say:

"You know, Planned Parenthood offers birth control counseling."

Advice giving suggests to the client that the helper is the expert and that he or she may hold the solution to the problem. This type of response is generally value-laden, carries with it the potential for developing a dependent relationship, and may mimic control issues from the client's family of origin (e.g., parents giving advice). For example, the helper might say:

"You know, you really need to practice birth control if you're not going to get pregnant."

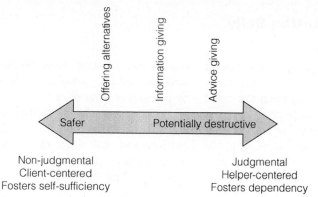

Figure 4.2 | Damaging Effects of Offering Alternatives, Information Giving, and Advice Giving

Offering alternatives, information giving, and advice giving are similar in the sense that they all move the focus of the session from the client to the helper. With each having the potential for being destructive to the helping relationship, their effectiveness as a helping tool must always been considered relative to their potential benefits (Orlinsky et al., 2004) (see Figure 4.2). When counseling is optimal, the timing of this kind of response should be such that the client is a step ahead of the advice that would have been offered. Thus, the client in essence is gaining so much from counseling that he or she is coming up with solutions prior to the counselor suggesting them.

Confrontation: Support with Challenge

When hearing the word **confrontation,** many people think of someone yelling at another or telling another person how to live his or her life. Along these lines, I have found that once in a while, a client "hooks me," and I start to argue with him or her about how to live life. This is rarely if ever helpful to the client and is almost always the result of some unfinished business of my own. In fact, trying to get another person to change if he or she is not ready is nearly impossible. Confrontation that is facilitative is usually very different from this, and revolves around giving feedback without being judgmental, critical, or aggressive (Egan, 2010; Evans, Hearn, & Uhlemann, 2011; Polcin, 2006). To do this, it is first important to spend time trying to understand the life circumstances of the client, often by using good listening and empathy skills. This is then followed by challenging the client, which may include making a **high-level empathic response, suggesting alternatives,** and **pointing out discrepancies.**

Making a high-level empathic response, such as a Level 4 response can be very effective in helping a client see hidden parts of himself or herself. Such responses reflect feelings that you sense from the person, feelings of which the client is not quite aware. Therefore, when you tell the client that you hear some deeper feelings underlying what he or she is saying, and if you have that base of caring, the client might be more receptive to this kind of feedback.

BOX 4.2	Confronting Sally

One time I worked with a client who was making almost $60,000 a year, was in an abusive relationship, had no major bills, and insisted that she could not leave the relationship because she could not afford to live on $60,000. Clearly, her verbal statement that she could not leave the relationship did not match the reality that one could live on this amount (certainly, most of us would be happy to live on this amount). After building a relationship using empathy, I gently challenged this perception by pointing out the discrepancy between what she earned and her statement that she did not earn enough to live on her own. This allowed her to examine the real reasons she was not leaving—reasons that had more to do with low self-esteem and fears of being alone.

Suggesting alternatives challenges the client to look at new ways of viewing the world. Like the case of higher-level empathy, such a confrontation should be done only if there is a base of caring; otherwise, the client may respond defensively.

Pointing out discrepancies highlights an incongruence in the client's life, such as between the client's values and behaviors (e.g., client talks about the importance of honesty in all aspects of life and then states he is collecting unemployment insurance despite the fact that he is working) or between the client's feelings and his or her behaviors (e.g., man who says he loves his wife deeply and then tells the helper about the affair he is having) (Hackney & Cormier, 2009; Hill, 2009). Be aware that if you point out a discrepancy before building a relationship, the client may walk out on you. For instance, I have seen clients who drink heavily, perhaps the equivalent of five or more beers a night, yet state they do not have a drinking problem. I have learned that unless I have established a relationship with these clients, they typically will not be able to examine the discrepancy between how much they drink and their statement about not having a drinking problem.

Whether you use higher-level empathic responses, the offering of alternatives, or pointing out discrepancies, using confrontation can be a very powerful technique in the helping relationship (see Box 4.2).

Collaboration

The last important skill that helpers should know is that of **collaboration.** Collaboration involves showing that you respect the client's opinion by eliciting feedback from the client about perceived progress in the helping relationship, by hearing criticism about your skills, and by being willing to adjust the direction of the helping relationship, if need be (Sommers-Flanagan & Sommers-Flanagan, 2009). Generally, collaboration includes the following:

1. The use of one's basic skills (e.g., listening, empathy) to offer a summary of what has been discussed thus far.
2. Asking the client, through the use of questions, how he or she feels about the helping relationship thus far.
3. Asking the client, through the use of questions, about the direction he or she would like to take in the helping relationship.

| BOX 4.3 | What Skills Would You Use? |

You work at a problem-pregnancy clinic and a 17-year-old woman comes in seeking information about birth control. She has been sexually active for two years, has not used any birth control, and knows little about sexually transmitted diseases (STDs). When she comes into your office, you affirm her decision to come to the clinic. You then listen carefully and try to understand her situation. After you spend some time listening, you tell her about the various types of birth control, suggest that she may not want to have unprotected sex, and give her information about AIDS and other STDs. You also suggest that she might want to consider being tested for STDs. You then ask her if she has any thoughts about what she would like to do. She thinks a while and then says that she will try to use condoms but also thinks it might be smart if she is on the Pill.

She thinks she would like to be tested for STDs but would like more information on the testing process. After you explain the testing process to her, she agrees to come back to the clinic for the tests. You then thank her for coming in and schedule another appointment. In this short scenario, one can easily see how a human service professional can be affirming, empathic, an information giver, an advice giver, a person who offers alternatives, and a problem solver. What do you think would be most effective for this 17-year-old? How might you work with her fears of having an STD? Are there other techniques that we have talked about that might be helpful for this young woman?

4. Sharing with the client one's own thoughts about which areas might be important to focus upon.
5. Having an honest discussion concerning any discrepancies between numbers 3 and 4, which leads to a mutual decision about the helpfulness of the helping relationship thus far and the direction to take in the future.

Collaboration can occur throughout the helping relationship and is often most useful at transitional points, such as when you are transitioning to a new stage in the counseling relationship.

Using Helping Skills Wisely

The proper use of helping skills occurs when a helper feels at ease with the use of a variety of skills and is able to reach into his or her bag of skills and choose those that will be most facilitative for client growth. An effective helper is intentional in his or her delivery of helping skills and prior to making responses can quickly and deliberately choose the most effective skills and tools (Neukrug & Schwitzer, 2006). Read Box 4.3 and consider what skills you might use with the client presented.

THE STAGES OF THE HELPING RELATIONSHIP

The application of the helping skills we just examined can vary considerably as a function of the helper's job role, setting, and theoretical orientation. Despite these differences, there are many commonalities within the helping relationship. For instance, all helpers have to address technical issues unique to the first session (e.g., meeting times, length of session, payment issues, and frequency of sessions).

All helpers will face issues of trust. All helpers will need to identify client concerns, develop goals, and assist the client in working on identified goals. And all helpers will have to deal with termination. These commonalities will be displayed in a series of stages of the helping relationship through which all clients will pass (Neukrug & Schwitzer, 2006). Progress through these stages can vary dramatically as a function of setting, and helpers should recognize the stages through which their clients are passing. They include the rapport and trust building stage, problem identification stage, deepening understanding and goal-setting stage, work stage, and closure stage.

Stage 1: Rapport and Trust Building

Clients come to the helper with one major agenda: "Can I trust my helper enough to discuss with him or her what I need to discuss?" The helper, on the other hand, is dealing with a number of issues that are crucial to the development of an effective working relationship. For instance, the helper is concerned about using basic skills to build trust in the relationship, assuring that the physical environment feels safe, and informing the client about the counseling process (Brammer & MacDonald, 2003; Hackney & Cormier, 2009). Recently the use of a written **professional disclosure statement** to cover many of these issues, as listed here, has become increasingly popular (Remley & Herlihy, 2010):

1. Limits of confidentiality
2. Length of the interview
3. Purpose of the interview
4. Your credentials
5. Limits of the relationship
6. Your theoretical orientation
7. Legal issues of concern to you and your client
8. Fees for services
9. Agency rules that might affect your client (e.g., reporting a client's use of illegal drugs)

After providing the professional disclosure statement to the client, it is important to obtain **informed consent** from the client. Informed consent indicates that the client has been given this information and agrees to participate in the helping relationship. Although such consent can be obtained verbally, it is better to have clients sign a statement noting that they gave their informed consent.

During the first stage, the development of a comfortable, trusting, and facilitative relationship can be accomplished through the use of listening skills, empathic understanding, cultural sensitivity, and a fair amount of good social skills (Hackney & Cormier, 2009). As this stage continues, the helper will begin to identify and delineate the issues presented by the client.

Stage 2: Problem Identification

The building of a trusting relationship and the ability to do an assessment of client problems are signs that you are moving into the second stage where you and your client will validate your initial identification of the problem(s). Perhaps the reason that the client initially provided for coming in for counseling was masking other issues. Or additional issues may arise as you explore the client's situation—perhaps even issues of which the client was not fully aware. In either case, during these sessions you validate your original assessment and make appropriate changes as necessary. During this stage the use of questions is often important as the helper attempts to clearly focus on the problems the client wishes to work on. It is also at this stage that client and helper begin to work collaboratively in the sense that the helper is "checking in" with the client so that the client agrees with the identification of the problem(s).

Stage 3: Deepening Understanding and Goal Setting

Although your basic helping skills are still important, the fact that trust has been built in the earlier stages means that other skills can now be added—skills that will allow you to understand your client in deeper ways. For instance, the client will now allow you to confront him or her, ask probing questions, and give advanced empathic responses. You can increasingly push the envelope and move into the inner world of the client. However, it is always crucial to maintain sensitivity to your client's needs and to maintain a supportive and nurturing base. Move too fast and the client will rebuff your attempts to expose his or her inner world. Move at the right pace and the counseling relationship will deepen, and you might consider using advanced skills based on your expertise and the client's issues. The result of your continued probing and analysis of the situation should be anything from an informal verbal agreement concerning goals to a collaboratively written contract that is signed by both the client and helper.

Stage 4: Work

During the fourth stage, the client is beginning to work on the issues that were identified in Stage 3 and agreed upon between the helper and client. The helper will use his or her helping skills to facilitate progress, and, if necessary, the helper and client may want to revisit and in a collaborative manner, reevaluate some of the goals set. During this stage it is not uncommon to find the helper using a variety of skills. For instance, the helper may use empathy, to assure deep understanding and self-reflection; modeling, to offer new kinds of behaviors with which to experiment; self-disclosure, to bond with the client and offer hope for change; questions, to assure one is on track with client issues; confrontation, to gently encourage the client to continue working; and affirmations and encouragement, to reinforce client behavior. The client in this stage is taking responsibility for and actively working on his or her identified issues and themes and is generally building higher self-esteem as he or she accomplishes identified goals.

Stage 5: Closure

As the client accomplishes some or most of his or her goals, clients and helpers will logically think about ending the helping relationship. Because the helping relationship is one of the few intimate relationships that is time-limited, clients and helpers will inevitably have to work through their feelings of loss about the ending of the relationship (Murdin, 2000). Termination should be a gradual process in which the client and helper have time to deal with the loss involved and discuss whether or not stated goals have been met. Successful termination is more likely if (1) clients discuss termination early, (2) goals are clear so clients know when counseling is near completion, (3) the helper respects the client's desire to terminate yet feels free to discuss feelings that termination may be too soon, (4) the relationship remains professional (e.g., does not move into a friendship), (5) clients know they can return, (6) clients are able to review the success they had in counseling, and (7) clients can discuss feelings of loss around termination (Hill, 2009; Sommers-Flanagan & Sommers-Flanagan, 2009). During this stage, a number of skills will be used. For instance, helpers will use empathy to summarize client accomplishments. In addition, they will affirm clients for reaching their goals and encourage clients to continue on track, even after the helping relationship has ended. Finally, some helpers feel comfortable during this stage with a small amount of self-disclosure as they share their good feelings about their client's accomplishments and their sad feelings about saying good-bye.

CASE MANAGEMENT

Managing a caseload of clients can be tedious and time-consuming and involves a myriad of activities collectively called **case management.** Although definitions of case management have varied, generally, case management has been viewed as the overall process that is involved in maintaining the optimal functioning of clients (Neukrug, 2002; Neukrug & Schwitzer, 2006; Woodside & McClam, 2006). Thus, case management involves such things as: (1) treatment planning; (2) diagnosis; (3) monitoring the use of psychotropic drugs; (4) case report writing; (5) managing and documenting client contact hours; (6) monitoring, evaluating, and documenting progress toward client goals; (7) making referrals; (8) follow-up; and (9) time management. The following is a quick overview of the case management process. However, you are encouraged to look at the literature for a more in-depth understanding of this important process.

Treatment Planning

Treatment planning involves the accurate assessment of client needs that results in the formation of client goals (Jongsma & Peterson, 2003; Seligman, 2004). As the helper utilizes a greater number of ways to assess the client, the ability to develop accurate goals is increased. Thus, ideally, assessment involves a myriad of information-gathering activities that can include (1) the clinical interview, (2) personality testing, (3) ability testing, and (4) the use of informal assessment instruments such as observation, reviews of records, and personal documents (Neukrug & Fawcett, 2010).

The actual development of client goals should be a relatively easy process if the helper has completed a thorough assessment of the client. Goal setting should be a collaborative process and goals need to be attainable. Progress toward goals should be monitored and the pace adjusted, if necessary.

Diagnosis

A **diagnosis** is a natural outgrowth of the assessment process that can occur in many ways. For instance, one can make an informal diagnosis to be used in goal setting, a rehabilitation diagnosis for physical problems, a vocational diagnosis for career planning, a medical diagnosis, and a mental health diagnosis, such as those made from the ***Diagnostic and Statistical Manual IV-Text Revision*** (***DSM-IV-TR***, American Psychiatric Association [APA], 2000; note: ***DSM-5*** is scheduled to be published in 2013). The *DSM* deserves special attention because it has become the most widespread and accepted diagnostic classification system of emotional disorders and has become increasingly important for a number of reasons, including the following:

- enhancing communication among professionals,
- increasing accuracy of diagnosis,
- determining treatment plans, and
- providing information for insurance companies that need a diagnosis if they are to pay for treatment (Neukrug & Schwitzer, 2006, Neukrug, 2012).

A *DSM-IV-TR* diagnosis includes five axes, although many clinicians will not use all of the axes every time they make a diagnosis. Axis I describes "Clinical Disorders and Other Conditions That May Be a Focus of Clinical Attention." Axis II delineates "Personality Disorders and Mental Retardation." Axis III explains "General Medical Conditions." Axis IV describes "Psychosocial and Environmental Problems," and Axis V offers a "Global Assessment of Functioning Scale," which helps identify the client's current level of functioning and can be used to assess whether progress is being made (see Box 4.4). However, you may find when reading this book

BOX 4.4 | Global Assessment of Functioning Scale

The **"GAF" scale**, which can be found in its entirety in *DSM-IV-TR* (APA, 2000), helps clinicians assess the level of functioning of a client by rating the client from 1 to 100. Review the summarized and shortened version of the GAF scale, and assign scores to role-played clients or descriptions of clients.

- 91–100: Optimal level of functioning; exhibits no signs of mental distress and deals with life in appropriate and effective ways
- 81–90: Minimal symptoms
- 71–80: Transient symptoms related to stressors in life
- 61–70: Mild symptoms, but generally good functioning
- 51–60: Moderate symptoms that are affecting social and occupational functioning
- 41–50: Serious symptoms that affect many aspects of life, such as suicidal thoughts or being obsessive-compulsive
- 31–40: Serious impairment in judgment and mood that affects many areas of life (e.g., ongoing abuse, problems with reality testing)
- 21–30: Very serious impairment, such as being delusional and/or hallucinating; problems functioning in many areas of life
- 11–20: Serious danger of harming self or others and/or having problems caring for self and communicating
- 1–10: Likelihood that client will harm self or another and an inability to care for self

that *DSM-5* has been published and some dramatic changes may be found (e.g., collapsing of Axis I and Axis II).

Although the *DSM* has its critics, including some who believe it is dehumanizing, leads to labeling, and does not fully take into account societal factors that impact on a diagnosis, it has become the most widespread and accepted diagnostic classification system of mental disorders (Eriksen & Kress, 2005, 2006, 2008; Halstead, 2007; Kress, Eriksen, Rayle, & Ford, 2005; Madsen & Leech, 2007; Seligman, 2004). Whole courses are taught on the *DSM* and you are encouraged to learn more about it.

Psychotropic Medications

Today, a host of **psychotropic medications** can be used as an adjunct to counseling in the treatment of many disorders (National Institute of Mental Health, 2010; Preston, O'Neal, & Talaga, 2010; Videbeck, 2011). For such treatment, medications are often classified into five groups: **anti-psychotics, mood-stabilizing drugs, anti-depressants, anti-anxiety agents,** and **stimulants.** Today, it is common for helpers to consult or refer to a physician, generally a psychiatrist, who can assess the client and prescribe appropriate psychotropic medications. Therefore, it is important for human service professionals to have a basic working knowledge of psychopharmacology, more than what can be offered in this text.

Finally, it is important to recognize that psychopharmacology has come a long way since the 1950s when the first modern-day psychotropic medications were introduced. Increasingly, medications used for a wide array of disorders are more effective and have fewer side effects than in the past. As the mechanism for psychological disorders becomes increasingly understood, new and even more effective medications can be developed to target the underlying physiological mechanism causing some disorders.

Case Report Writing

A client's record consists of a complete file of the individual's concerns, progress during treatment, final disposition, and other pertinent information. Although ethics codes and recent laws suggest clients can have access to most of their records, their purpose is usually to aid the helper. For instance, good case records can do the following (Neukrug, 2002; Neukrug & Schwitzer, 2006; Prieto & Scheel, 2002):

1. Be used in court to show that adequate client care took place
2. Assist helpers in conceptualizing client problems and making diagnoses
3. Help determine whether clients have made progress
4. Be useful when obtaining supervision
5. Assist the helper in remembering what the client said
6. Be part of the process through which insurance companies and government agencies approve the treatment being given to clients
7. Be a determining factor, in this age of accountability, regarding whether or not an agency will receive funding

Depending on the agency, many kinds of **case report writing** may be required, such as daily case notes, intake summaries, quarterly summaries, termination summaries, and reports that aid in educational and vocational planning, to name just a few.

Today case notes are often written on the computer, although you may find yourself using the tried-and-true fashion of writing them out, which can help organize one's thoughts about a client (Cameron & turtle-song, 2002; Prieto & Scheel, 2002). One approach to writing case notes that has gained popularity over the years is called the **SOAP format,** which stands for Subjective, Objective, Assessment, and Plan. Table 4.1 shows how such notes are used.

More involved summaries than those found in SOAP notes often include demographic information (e.g., DOB, address, phone, e-mail address, date of interview), reason for report, family background, other pertinent background information (e.g., health information, vocational history, history of adjustment issues/emotional

Table 4.1 | SOAP Case Notes

	Subjective-Description	Subjective-Examples	Subjective-Pointers
S	• What the client tells you (feelings, concerns, plans, goals, thoughts) • How the client experiences the world • Client's orientation to time, place, and person	• Client reports... • Client shares... • Client describes... • Client indicates...	• Avoid quotations • Full names of others are generally not needed • Be concise • Limit adjectives
	Objective-Description	**Objective-Examples**	**Objective-Pointers**
O	• Factual: What the helper personally observes and/or witnesses • Quantifiable: What was seen, heard, smelled, counted, or measured (may include outside written materials)	• Appeared _____ as evidenced by... • Test results indicate... • Client's hair uncombed; clothes unkempt	• Avoid words like client "appeared" or "seemed" when not supported by objective examples • Avoid labels, personal judgments, or opinionated statements
	Assessment-Description	**Assessment-Examples**	**Assessment-Pointers**
A	• Summarizes the helper's clinical thinking • Includes diagnoses or clinical impressions and reasons for behavior	• Behavior/attitude consistent with individuals who... • *DSM* diagnosis • Rule out...	• May note themes, or recurring issues • Remain professional • Remember that others may view assessment
	Plan-Description	**Plan-Examples**	**Plan-Pointers**
P	• Describes parameters of treatment • Includes action plan; interventions; progress; prognosis; treatment direction for next session	• Counselor established rapport, challenged, etc. • Client progress is indicated by... • Next session, counselor will... • Client and counselor will continue to...	• Give supporting reasons for progress • "Progress is fair due to client's inconsistent attendance at sessions"

Source: Adapted from Cameron, S., & turtle-song, I. (2002). Learning to write case notes using the SOAP format. *Journal of Counseling & Development, 80*(3), 286–292.

problems/mental illness), mental status, assessment results, diagnosis, summary, conclusions, and recommendations.

Managing and Documenting Client Contact Hours

Human service professionals are increasingly being asked to find ways to meet with all their clients on a consistent and ongoing basis. For accountability, it is essential that human service professionals find a credible way of doing this. This sometimes means using some creative activities, such as running special groups (e.g., medication review groups), and working additional evening hours to meet with clients who cannot meet during the day.

In addition to providing a record of how the helper manages to meet with all of his or her clients, the **documentation** of these contact hours has become crucial because reimbursement by insurance companies, as well as local, state, and federal funding agencies, is often based on the clear documentation of contact hours. Thus, most agencies today have some mechanism for documenting these hours. Often, this is done on a simple grid, but increasingly, documentation can be completed using computer software specifically developed for this purpose.

Monitoring, Evaluating, and Documenting Progress Toward Client Goals

The documentation of progress toward goals is increasingly being reviewed by funding agencies, and today such agencies will often not renew funding if documentation and progress are not shown. The simplest way to document progress toward goals is to make a note in the client's chart. Innovative human service professionals can also create charts and graphs to visually document client progress. Finally, the GAF scale of *DSM-IV-TR* has been used as one measurement of progress toward goals and treatment success (see Box 4.4).

Making Referrals

There are many reasons to refer a client to another professional. For instance, a client may be referred as a part of the treatment plan, because the professional is leaving the agency, because the professional feels incompetent to work with the client, or because the client has reached his or her goals and is ready to move on to another type of helping relationship. In any case, the manner in which the **referral** is made is crucial, and in this process the human service professional should do all of the following:

1. Discuss the reason for making the referral with the client and obtain his or her approval.
2. Obtain, in writing, permission to discuss the client with another professional, even if one is simply sharing the client's name with another professional.
3. Monitor the client's progress with the other professional.
4. Ensure that confidentiality of client information is maintained in the referral process.

Follow-Up

Follow-up, another important function of case management, can be accomplished in many ways. Some helpers follow up with a phone call, e-mail, or letter, while others may do an elaborate survey of clients. Follow-up can be done a few days to a few weeks after the relationship has ended and serves many purposes (Neukrug, 2002; Neukrug & Schwitzer, 2006):

1. Functions as a check to see if clients would like to return to the helping relationship or would like to follow up with a different helper
2. Allows the helper to assess if change has been maintained
3. Gives the helper the opportunity to look at which techniques have been most successful
4. Offers an opportunity to reinforce past change
5. Offers a mechanism whereby the helper can evaluate services provided

Time Management

With ever-increasing case loads and demands placed on the helper, **time management,** the last aspect of case management, has become crucial if the helper is to avoid burnout (Woodside & McClam, 2006). Time management strategies serve a number of purposes. They are useful in planning activities and can help a human service professional ensure that all clients are seen within a reasonable period of time. They also help professionals remember meetings, appointment times, and other obligations. Today, there are a number of time management systems. Although this text will not delve into these different systems, suffice it to say that addressing time management concerns is paramount in today's world.

ETHICAL, PROFESSIONAL, AND LEGAL ISSUES: PRIMARY OBLIGATION

Client, Agency, or Society?

Think about the following scenario:

> In building your relationship with a 17-year-old client, you discover that she is using crack cocaine, is possibly selling drugs to friends, and is involved in gang violence including looting. Your agency has a policy to report any illegal acts to the "proper authorities."

What is your responsibility to this client? What are the limits of confidentiality with her? If you are primarily responsible to your client, what are the implications of being required to report her actions to the proper authorities? If you do not report her actions to the proper authorities as you are supposed to do, what implications might this have for your employment? What responsibility do you have to protect society from the illegal activities in which she is involved? What liability concerns do you have if you do not report the illegal acts in which she is participating? These are some of the tough ethical, professional, and legal questions human service professionals sometimes have to face.

If this were a dualistic world, there would be an easy answer to these tough dilemmas. The world is fortunately (unfortunately?) more complex than this.

| BOX 4.5 | The Tarasoff Case |

The case of *Tarasoff et al. v. Regents of University of California* (1976) set a precedent for the responsibility that mental health professionals have for maintaining confidentiality and acting to prevent a client from harming self or others, often called "duty to warn." This case involved a client who was seeing a psychologist at the University of California–Berkeley health services. The client told the psychologist that he intended to kill Tatiana Tarasoff, whom he had formed a crush on despite her not being romantically interested in him. After the psychologist consulted with his supervisor, the supervisor suggested that he call the campus police. Campus security subsequently questioned the client and released him. The client refused to see the psychologist any longer, and two months later, he killed Ms. Tarasoff. The parents of Ms. Tarasoff sued and won, with the California Supreme Court stating that the psychologist did not do all that he could have done to protect Tatiana Tarasoff.

Although state laws vary on how to handle confidentiality, this case generally is seen as signifying to mental health professionals that it is their responsibility to protect the public if serious threats are made.

Although most ethical guidelines, including the **Ethical Standards of Human Service Professionals** (National Organization of Human Services, 1996; see Appendix A), imply that the mental health professional has a primary responsibility to the client, we all must acknowledge legal and moral responsibility toward others. Therefore, ethical guidelines usually include a statement that requires the mental health professional to take responsible action if a client's behavior is perceived as potentially harmful to the client or others. For instance, the Ethical Standards of Human Service Professionals has such a statement and suggests that the human service professional seek consultation or supervision if a client's actions might harm self or others (see Box 4.5). The same standards also require that the human service professional follow agency guidelines, whenever reasonable, as well as local, state, and federal laws. With these guidelines in mind, it is prudent to be clear about the limitations of the helping relationship before starting your work with clients. Probably the best way to do this is by using a professional disclosure statement.

Confidentiality of Records and Clients' Rights to View Their Records

Clients generally have a legal right to view their records, and increasingly they have been exercising these rights in schools and agencies (Remley & Herlihy, 2010). Along these same lines, it has generally been assumed that parents have the right to view records of their children (Attorney C. Borstein, personal communication, April 1, 2011).

In terms of federal law, the *Freedom of Information Act of 1974* allows individuals to have access to any records maintained by a federal agency that contain personal information about the individual, and every state has passed similar laws governing state agencies (U.S. Department of Justice, 2004). Similarly, the *Family Educational Rights and Privacy Act (FERPA)* assures parents the right to access their children's educational records (U.S. Department of Education, 2011), although FERPA generally excludes counseling notes from the category of educational records. Finally, the *Health Insurance Portability and Accountability Act*

(HIPAA) ensures the privacy of client records and limits sharing of such information (Zuckerman, 2008). In general, HIPAA restricts the amount of information that can be shared without client consent and allows clients to have access to their records, except for process notes used in counseling (U.S. Department of Health and Human Services, n.d.).

In a more practical vein, rarely does a client ask to view his or her records. However, if one of my clients were to make such a request, I would first explore why he or she wanted to see the records. Next, I would talk with the client about what is written in the records. If this was not satisfactory to the client, I would suggest that I might write a summary of the records. However, if a client continued to steadfastly state a desire to view his or her records, I would comply with this request.

Generally, clients should have the expectation that information they share with their helper will be kept confidential. However, there are some exceptions to this rule, such as (1) if a helper shares client information with a supervisor as a means of assisting the helper in his or her work with the client, (2) if the court subpoenas a helper's records, or (3) if a client gives permission, in writing, to share information with others. You should also remember that human service professionals do not have the legal protection afforded to licensed professionals through **privileged communication** (see Chapter 3). Privileged communication is the client's legal right to not have information shared with third-party sources, especially the court. Thus, if a client asks that a human service professional not share information requested from the court (e.g., case notes), the practitioner will probably have to go against the client's wishes. In fact, there is a fair chance that a human service professional who does not share requested information with the courts will be found in contempt of court.

Security of Case Notes

Due to the importance of client records, and because federal law requires it, records should be kept in a secure place and should be accessible only to a limited few who have permission to view such records. Written client records need to be kept in secured places such as locked file cabinets. Computer records should be kept on nonaccessible computer disks or thumb drives and be password-protected. Clerical help needs to understand the importance of confidentiality when working with records. In fact, some agencies have clerical staff sign statements acknowledging that they understand the importance of protecting the confidentiality of records.

THE EFFECTIVE HUMAN SERVICE PROFESSIONAL: LOOKING FOR FEEDBACK FROM OTHERS

Developmentally mature human service professionals are open to hearing both positive and negative feedback about their helping skills. They want to "stretch" and are willing to take a critical look at how they interact with clients. They want to try out new approaches to working with clients and are willing to feel vulnerable in the learning process. Finally, such professionals actively seek out supervision and consultation from experts in the field and view the learning of helping skills as a process in which one continually grows and adjusts his or her approach to meet the needs of clients.

SUMMARY

In this chapter we presented an overview of the basic helping skills used for working effectively with clients. We first noted that creating an environment that is conducive to the helping relationship involves paying attention to the physical comfort of the surroundings (the office environment), embodying positive personality characteristics of the human service professional, and using nonverbal behaviors appropriately, including posture, eye contact, tone of voice, personal space, and touch.

Next, we outlined the foundations of good helping skills. We discussed the importance of effective listening; the use of empathy, as measured by the Carkhuff scale; the importance of silence; the effective use of encouragement and affirmation; and knowing how to use modeling and self-disclosure into the helping relationship. We then examined how and when one might use questions and specifically discussed open versus closed questions, tentative questions, solution-focused questions, and the use of "why" questions. From there we moved on to compare offering alternatives, information giving, and advice giving, and we noted that offering alternatives has the least potential for harm. We next discussed confrontation and noted that the gentlest and probably most effective type of confrontation is a higher-level empathic response such that the client feels supported while perceiving new feelings. We also suggested that offering alternatives and pointing out discrepancies are two other means of confronting the client. We concluded this section by highlighting the importance of having a collaborative relationship with one's client—one which includes eliciting feedback, hearing criticism about skills, and being willing to adjust the direction of the helping relationship.

We next discussed the stages of the interview and noted that a number of stages are typically passed through in the helping relationship, including rapport and trust building, problem identification, deepening understanding and goal setting, work, and closure. We highlighted the kinds of skills generally used in each of these stages, and we noted some special issues involved in various stages such as the importance of giving a professional disclosure statement and receiving informed consent from clients.

As this chapter continued, we explained that case management is a broad term that includes such things as (1) treatment planning, (2) diagnosis, (3) monitoring the use of psychotropic drugs, (4) case report writing, (5) managing and documenting client contact hours, (6) monitoring, evaluating, and documenting progress toward client goals, (7) making referrals, (8) follow-up, and (9) time management. We briefly reviewed these important areas of managing cases, and we highlighted the importance of examining these areas in more detail to be effective in the case management process.

As we neared the end of the chapter, we discussed ethical, professional, and legal issues related to the helping relationship. For instance, we discussed the importance of knowing whether the human service professional is responsible to the client, agency, or society, especially when dealing with issues related to "duty to warn" such as in the Tarasoff case. We talked about the importance of protecting the confidentiality of records and noted a number of laws that protect client confidentiality and allow clients to access their records. These include the Freedom of Information Act (FERPA) and *Health Insurance Portability and Accountability Act (HIPAA)*. We also highlighted the difference between confidentiality and privileged communication, and we discussed the importance of keeping client records secure. Finally, we noted that the effective human service professionals are those who see their helping skills as continually in process; that is, mature human service professionals are always willing to adapt their skills to become better helpers.

Experiential Exercises

I.   Arranging Your Office

The instructor will distribute a number of magazines, some scissors, glue, and a large piece of paper. From the magazines, cut out pieces of furniture and office accessories that you like and paste your furniture and accessories on the piece of paper. Compare your office to that of other students. What makes your office more or less conducive to the counseling relationship? Come up with a justification for your office arrangement based on your counseling style.

II.   Listening Quiz

Take the listening quiz that follows. Place an X in the appropriate space to represent how you *generally* respond to someone when you are listening. Then, go through the quiz again, this time placing an O to represent how you think you *should* listen to another. (See answers at the end of this chapter.)

Usually	Sometimes	Rarely	
_____	_____	_____	1. I try to determine what should be talked about during the interview.
_____	_____	_____	2. When listening to someone, I prepare myself physically by sitting in a way that I can make sure that I hear what is being said.
_____	_____	_____	3. I try to be "in charge" and lead the conversation.
_____	_____	_____	4. I usually clear my mind and take on a nonjudgmental attitude when listening to another.
_____	_____	_____	5. When listening to another, I try to tell the other my opinion of what he or she is doing.
_____	_____	_____	6. I try to decide from the other's *appearance* whether or not what he or she is saying is worthwhile.
_____	_____	_____	7. I attempt to ask questions if I need further clarification.
_____	_____	_____	8. I try to judge from the person's opening statement whether or not I know what is going to be said.
_____	_____	_____	9. I try to listen intently to feelings.
_____	_____	_____	10. I try to listen intently to content.
_____	_____	_____	11. I try to tell the other person what is "right" about what he or she is saying.
_____	_____	_____	12. I try to "analyze" the situation and give interpretations.
_____	_____	_____	13. I try to use *my* experiences to best understand the other person's feelings.
_____	_____	_____	14. I try to convince the other person of the "correct" way to view the situation.
_____	_____	_____	15. I try to have the last word.

After finishing the listening quiz, as a small group or as a class, define the term *listening*. After you have defined the word *listening*, see if the answers you gave on your quiz reflect this definition. To assist you in your group definition, use the definition of *to listen* from the *Oxford English Dictionary*, which means (1) to hear attentively, (2) to give ear to, and (3) to pay attention to.

III. Affirmation and Encouragement

Make a list of times in your life when you have been affirmed or encouraged. What did that do to improve your self-esteem?

IV. Making Empathic Responses

A good empathic response accurately reflects to the client the feelings and the meaning of what the client has said (Carkhuff's Level 3 response). For the following situations, write the feeling in the spaces provided, followed by the meaning of what the client has said. Follow this by writing another statement that again reflects the feelings and meaning of the client, but this time in your own words. In small groups in class, share some of your responses and get feedback from others about the accuracy of what you wrote. For example, suppose a female client makes the following statement to a human service professional:

CLIENT: I don't know what's wrong with my husband. Since he lost his job, he just sits around all day and does nothing, doesn't look for a job, doesn't cook, just does nothing. He seems worthless.

Next is an example of a feeling word *(angry)* followed by the client's meaning ("husband doesn't do anything all day long") in response to the preceding client statement:

HSP: You feel angry because your husband doesn't do anything all day long.

The following is an example of a response to the same client, but this time in one's own words, again reflecting feeling and meaning:

HSP: I guess I hear you're disappointed and upset at your husband for not taking charge of his life.

Now, respond to the following scenarios:

1. Teenager to human service professional:

CLIENT: Why should I use condoms? I'm not going to get AIDS or nothing like that. Only fags get AIDS. Don't you agree?

HSP: You feel _____ because _____

HSP: _____

2. Abused wife to human service professional:

CLIENT: I don't know why I keep going back to him. He just keeps beating on me. But afterward, he always tells me he loves me. I think he loves me, but he just drinks too much sometimes.

HSP: You feel _____ because _____

HSP: _____

3. Pregnant teenager to human service professional:

CLIENT: I want this baby; I don't care what my parents say about an abortion. I can bring this baby up by myself. I'll quit school and get a job and bring the baby to work with me.

HSP: You feel _____ because _____

HSP: _____

_____

4. Disabled enlisted person to human service professional:

CLIENT: Even though I lost my leg, I have lots to live for. I have a good family, and I know I'm employable. I just hope I can get through rehab quickly.

HSP: You feel _____ because _____

HSP: _____

_____

_____

5. Older person to human service professional:

CLIENT: Since I moved to this retirement home, I have nothing to live for. I can't drive anymore, and I know nobody here.

HSP: You feel _____ because _____

HSP: _____

_____

6. Person of color to human service professional:

CLIENT: I think I'm getting the shaft from my realtor. I keep telling her I want to move to this one community, and she says she can't find anything for sale there. I don't believe it!

HSP: You feel _____ because _____

HSP: _____

_____

7. Pro-life client to human service professional

CLIENT: I refuse to let any more babies die. I'll do anything to close down those murdering abortion clinics.

HSP: You feel _____ because _____

HSP: _____

_____

8. Pro-choice client to human service professional:

CLIENT: I believe a woman has a right to choose what to do with her body, and I'm sick and tired of these pro-lifers interfering with other people's right to choose!

HSP: You feel _____ because _____

HSP: _____

_____

9. Estranged husband to human service professional:

CLIENT: So I wasn't faithful to my wife. So what? I loved her. She didn't have to leave me. I still was good to her despite my failings. I miss her so much!

HSP: You feel _____ because _____

HSP: _____

_____

10. Estranged wife to human service professional:

CLIENT: I loved my husband, but I couldn't put up with his unfaithfulness any longer. He just couldn't give me the love I needed in a relationship. I'm sorry he is so depressed now, but I can't go back to him.

HSP: You feel _____ because _____

HSP: _____

_____

V. An Interview with a Client

The following is an interview between a client and a human service professional who is employed at an employee assistance program for a large business. Go through the interview and identify the type of response being made by the helper (empathy, advice giving, information giving, offering alternatives, confrontation, self-disclosure, modeling, open questions, closed questions, affirmation or encouragement, collaboration, referral, and/or summarizing). Each response may have more than one answer. Check the end of this chapter for the answers.

1. **Client/employee:** I woke up this morning feeling depressed. My life is out of sorts, and I'm not sure why. Do you think this is something that will pass?

   HSP: So, it seems as if your depression just came out of nowhere, and you're not sure what's causing it.

2. **Client:** Well, yeah. I guess I haven't been real happy at work lately. I've been at this same job for 20 years, and it seems like I never get promoted. All my friends get promoted, and I just make my little yearly salary increases but never move up. Maybe I'm just no good.

   HSP: Well, I hear how you're not feeling real good about yourself and it seems to be at least partly related to the fact that things haven't worked out at your job as you thought they might.

3. **Client:** That's true. You know, maybe I should take some courses and that would help me do better at work. What do you think?

   HSP: I'm not sure. But it seems as if you've had some ideas about how to change your life.

4. **Client:** Yeah, I've thought about going back to school, quitting my job, looking for another job, and even just storming into my boss's office and telling her what I think.

   HSP: What do you think about all these different options?

5. **Client:** Well, I guess I have thought about at least talking to my boss and asking her what she thinks I might do. That would be at least a beginning.

   HSP: Do you feel good or bad about your relationship with your boss?

6. **Client:** Well, I don't know if it's either. Perhaps more neutral. I don't really know her real well. She is not approachable, but on the other hand, maybe I'm not either.

   HSP: So on one hand it might be difficult to talk with her, but on the other hand, you also see that maybe you haven't made it easy for her to approach you.

7. **Client:** Kind of. Maybe I need to talk with her to see what the different options are for me.

   HSP: When you say "options," I'm unclear what you mean. Can you explain that to me?

8. **Client:** Well, I guess I mean whether I should take a course for credit, do some in-house workshops, or maybe something else ... like, like talk to my supervisor more and get feedback from her, or become more active in the employees' association, or something.

   HSP: Well, it seems as if you have a lot of ideas that you can approach your boss with.

9. **Client:** Yeah, I guess I do. I hope I can do it. You know, I get pretty nervous talking to her.

   HSP: I know you can do it if you want to. I know you're capable of lots!

10. **Client:** Yes! I can do it. But you know, this fear I feel with her, that's something I feel with a lot of people in positions of authority. Like, take my church. You know, I've been on this fund-raising committee now for a number of years, and I've had a lot of ideas, but I never tell them to the chair because I think he's going to put me down.

    HSP: So, you see this as a pattern in your life; that is, this fear you have of expressing yourself with people in positions of authority.

11. **Client:** Yeah, I think it goes back to the fact that my parents, particularly my father, were really strict and always told me how to live my life. I get so scared sometimes around authority figures that I just don't know what to say or do.

    HSP: Well, you're bringing up some really important issues for yourself. What are your thoughts about seeking out counseling for this?

12. **Client:** It had crossed my mind. Especially because I believe this issue is something that prevents me from getting ahead in my life. What do you think?

    HSP: I know of some good helpers, and I know of an assertiveness training group. I think considering some counseling might be really good for you. But, I'd like to know, what are your thoughts on that?

13. **Client:** Yes, I think so.

    HSP: I admire your wanting to work on this issue. Here, let me give you the names of some helpers and a couple of groups. [HSP gives the names.]

14. **Client:** I really appreciate this. Sometimes I think I'm never going to get through this problem I have. I guess I think that change is really not possible.

    HSP: You know, I had some problems once in my life that were really difficult for me, and I saw a therapist. It really helped me get through it, and I feel much better about me now.

15. **Client:** Really?

    HSP: Yeah, it was really helpful. I know you can move on in your life in a positive way and feel good about you. You have all the ingredients in you to make this work.

16. **Client:** I hope so. I think this is a really good start. Can I talk about one other thing?
    HSP: Sure.

17. **Client:** I notice that on some nights, not all nights, mind you, I seem to drink a lot. I wake up in the morning feeling terrible. I wonder if this affects my work performance. I've been thinking about maybe trying out an AA meeting. What do you think?

    HSP: I hear your concern about your drinking and the fact that you have been giving some serious thought to doing something about it.

18. **Client:** To be honest, sometimes I really think I go overboard with my drinking.
    HSP: Well, it sounds to me as if you might have a problem with alcohol and perhaps you should do something about it.

19. **Client:** Do you know of any AA meetings?

HSP: Yep, let me give you a list I have right here. You know AA meetings usually last a couple of hours and one's anonymity is ensured. I have heard that people who go to AA meetings are usually accepting of one another.

20. **Client:** Well, you've been helpful. I appreciate all of what you've done for me.

HSP: Well, thanks. I hear that you are ready to do some important things for yourself. For instance, today you talked about some concerns you were having at work relative to getting promoted, as well as how this might relate to both issues with authority figures and your drinking. You've gotten some referrals from me, and it sounds as if you're seriously thinking about following up on them. I think that it's great that you're so motivated, and I know you can make great strides. Maybe next week you can touch base with me to let me know what you've done to follow up. What do you think about all we've done today and some of the ideas we came up with?

VI. **Writing Case Notes**

Using the interview in Exercise V, and following the guidelines in this chapter, write case notes that include the following information:

1. Reason for referral
2. Summary of contact with client
3. Recommendations for client

VII. **Writing Case Reports**

Meet with someone in class and have each student role-play a problem situation. Then write a two- to three-page case report that addresses the following categories:

1. Client information

    Name

    Address

    E-mail address

    Date of birth

    Date of interview

2. Reason for interview
3. Background information about the client that is relevant to the interview (e.g., family background, educational background, work background)
4. Assessment of client problem
5. Summary and recommendations
6. Signature with credentials

VIII. **Ethical and Professional Vignettes**

For the following vignettes, write some possible solutions and be prepared to discuss them in class.

Case Note Security

1. A client who is coming to your agency demands to see her case notes. In them, you have noted that you suspect she may be lying about her Social Security eligibility and that you also suspect she might be paranoid. What do you do?

2. A client you have been seeing at a crisis center comes in and asks to see all records pertaining to him. These include crisis logs that have information in them about other clients, as well as case notes you have made concerning his contacts. What do you do?

Confidentiality and Primary Obligation: Client, Agency, or Society?

3. You're working for social services, and in the course of a conversation with a client, you discover that she has been using heroin. An agency dictate states that any client suspected of using illegal drugs must be immediately referred to rehabilitation, and if he or she refuses, you can no longer see the client at your agency. You explain this to her, she gets angry, walks out, and states she'll "blow this place up." What do you do?

4. In your conversation with a client at the homeless shelter, you discover that he is drinking and taking Quaaludes in amounts that you believe could kill him. You mention this to him, but he tells you to mind your own business. What do you do?

5. In the course of working with a client, she expresses her concern about her grandmother who, she states, lives by herself, is depressed, has stopped eating, and has lost a considerable amount of weight. You contact the grandmother, but she refuses services. What do you do?

6. While you are talking with a 15-year-old male client, he informs you that on a recent vacation he was sexually molested by an uncle. He asks you not to tell his parents. What do you do?

7. A 15-year-old client tells you he is having sexual relations with his 14-year-old step-sister. What do you do?

8. An adult client informs you that he wants to kill his ex-girlfriend and her new boyfriend. He denies that he actually will act on these feelings but says that he just "thinks about it a lot." What do you do?

Answers to Exercises

Exercise II: Usually: 2, 4, 9, 10; Sometimes: 7, 13; Seldom: 1, 3, 5, 6, 8, 11, 12, 14, 15

Exercise V: 1. empathy; 2. empathy; 3. empathy; 4. open question; 5. closed question; 6. empathy; 7. open question; 8. empathy, affirmation; 9. encouragement; 10. empathy; 11. empathy, open question, referral; 12. offering alternatives, advice giving, collaboration, referral; 13. referral, affirmation; 14. modeling, self-disclosure; 15. affirmation, encouragement; 16. not ratable; 17. empathy; 18. confrontation; 19. referrals, information giving; 20. summarizing, affirmation, encouragement, collaboration.

Development of the Person

CHAPTER CONTENTS

With each passage from one stage of human growth to the next we, too, must shed a protective structure. We are left exposed and vulnerable—but also yeasty and embryonic again, capable of stretching in ways we hadn't known before. These sheddings may take several years or more. Coming out of each passage, though, we enter a longer and more stable period in which we can expect relative tranquility and a sense of equilibrium regained. (Sheehy, 1976, p. 29)

In my senior year in college, I was staying with my girlfriend, and in the middle of the night I began to have what I now would call a panic attack. I walked the campus the rest of the night trying to calm myself down. I thought I had lost it. The next day I went to the college counseling service and saw a psychologist who reassured me that I was not "crazy." I was soon referred to a group at the center for what became my first therapeutic experience.

Subsequently, I participated in different groups and in individual counseling. Through these experiences, I have had the opportunity to examine some of my life events that have dramatically affected my development. Some of these experiences, such as a childhood heart disorder and the death of my father, might be considered situational, in that they were unexpected events in my life that had a dramatic effect on me. Other experiences, however, such as developing a sense of my own values or belief system, dealing with puberty, struggling with issues of intimacy as in the previous example, making decisions about entering the world of work, and dealing with mid-life issues, are all related to developmental milestones which we all face at around the same times in our lives.

This chapter will examine the developmental process, from birth through death. Whether it is physical changes, psychological growth, cognitive development, or moral development, theories have been developed to explain the natural progression of the person over the life span. These theories can help the human service professional understand some of the reasons why people act the way they do, and they provide a knowledge base that helpers can use when easing people through these natural transitions.

DEFINING DEVELOPMENT

The development of a person is complex and occurs on many levels. Although developmental models differ, they tend to share a number of common elements. For instance, most see development as having the following qualities (Crandell, Crandell, & Vander Zanden, 2008; Roberts, Brown, Johnson, & Reinke, 2005; Santrock, 2008, 2009):

1. *Continual:* It starts at birth, and we continue to develop until we die.
2. *Orderly, sequential, and builds upon itself:* Models that describe human growth have a predictable pattern of development from earlier to later stages in which the latter stages build on what has already been experienced and integrated into our lives.
3. *A change process:* By its very nature, development means that we are constantly changing, moving on to different life phases and stages. Our core remains the same, but like a piece of clay we can be molded, sometimes torn apart and then put back together, but we are always clay. Each piece has a different shape, and it can come in different colors, different weights, and different consistencies, but it is all clay.
4. *Painful yet growth producing:* Because development implies giving up past ways of behaving or perceiving the world, it is painful because we have to let go of something that is familiar. On the other hand, it is growth producing, as we move on to newer ways of being in the world that will, by their very nature, help us adapt more easily to the world.
5. *Hopeful:* Developmental theories are optimistic—they see the potential in people and have as their basis the idea that if nurtured and allowed to develop

naturally, the individual will blossom, much like a seed that turns into a flower. And if the individual can understand the stages of growth, he or she can optimize movement to higher stages of development.

6. *Preventive and wellness-oriented:* The nature of developmental theory lends itself toward prevention and a wellness model of mental health. By knowing the expected transitions an individual will be facing, helpers can develop workshops and educational seminars that can assist individuals in understanding their natural progression from one developmental level to another. It also offers helpers a framework from which to develop strategies to assist the client who may want to revisit unfinished developmental tasks.

Developmental counseling offers the human service professional a unique perspective when working with clients. The developmentally astute helper knows the (1) characteristics that are commonly displayed by clients at different developmental stages, (2) types of social issues and personal problems often experienced by clients as they pass through specific developmental stages, (3) reasons why such problems occur, and (4) techniques that might work with clients who have similar developmental concerns. Clearly, knowledge of human development can go far in assisting the human service professional in his or her work with clients.

Many theories of human development have been described over the years, and a text such as this can cover only some of the more popular ones. In this chapter we will focus on some of the more prevalent theories of child development, cognitive and moral development, personality development, and life span development.

PHYSICAL DEVELOPMENT OF THE GROWING CHILD

As the child develops, major physiological changes take place (see Rice, 2001; Santrock, 2008, 2009). Although the rate of children's physical development is fairly consistent, the scope of a specific child's development is based on the genetic predisposition of the child in interaction with the environment. For instance, although most children will be ready to learn multiplication in third grade, the rate and depth of learning will vary based on genetics and environment. Along these lines, a brilliant child is at a major disadvantage if he or she is brought up in a home that has lead paint and lead in the water or in an environment that does not nurture the child's innate intelligence. On the other hand, a child who is less able can shine if placed in a stimulating and nurturing environment.

The importance of a nurturing environment can be seen through the success of the **Head Start Program**. This federally funded program, which was started in the 1970s, places disadvantaged preschool children in intellectually stimulating and nurturing environments before they enter public school. On average, these children have done noticeably better academically and socially than have children of similar backgrounds who have not received such opportunities (Puma et al., 2010).

Because most children will develop at fairly predictable rates, if a child specialist is aware of the expected physiological timetable normed for children, he or she can determine whether a child is on target for his or her development (Brooks-Gunn, 2004; Stearns, Allal, & Mace, 2008). Sometimes, lagging behind in physical development can be a first indication of a physiological, emotional, or intellectual impairment. For instance, a friend of mine has a daughter who could not crawl at age 1. Because most children are beginning to walk at this time, my friend was concerned that this might be an indication of a developmental disability. In this case, the child had a rare but harmless form of hypertrophy of the muscles and was walking within a few months of being tested. If tests had revealed a developmental disability, however, early diagnosis could have been crucial for optimizing the skills that the child did possess.

Typically, child specialists will examine age-appropriate milestones in such areas as motor development, cognitive ability, speech development, sensory development, intelligence, moral development, memory, and physical development in determining what may be considered normal compared with what could be a deviation from the norm (Schneider & Bullock, 2009). A course on human growth and development will help familiarize human service professionals with many of these expected developmental milestones.

THE DEVELOPMENT OF KNOWING: COGNITIVE AND MORAL CHANGES

Jean Piaget and Cognitive Development

Probably the person who most helped us understand the intellectual or cognitive development of children is **Jean Piaget** (Flavell, 1963). Piaget stated that as the child grows, he or she takes new information into an already existing view of the world. Known as **assimilation,** this process refers to incorporating new information within the framework that the child already has for understanding the world. For instance, when my daughter Emma was 3 years old, she asked me for some M&M's. I gave her two, and she told me she wanted five more. So I then gave her five more of the miniature M&M's (which are equivalent to about two regular-size ones). She was very pleased, not realizing that five of the small ones were not the same as five of the larger ones. Emma had not yet learned the concept of conservation, or the "notion that liquids and solids can be transformed in shape without changing their volume or mass" (Mussen, Conger, & Kagan, 1969, p. 452). As children grow older, they clearly understand this difference in mass. As they learn the concept behind this, they **accommodate** to this way of knowing. In other words, they change their previous way of understanding the world and adopt a new method. Piaget stated that in accommodating to the world, certain **schemata** or new **cognitive structures** (new ways of thinking) are formed that allow an individual to adapt and change his or her view of the world. The processes of assimilation, forming new schemata, and eventual accommodation occur throughout the life span.

Through his research on child cognitive development, Piaget determined that as children grow they pass through predictable periods, which he called the **sensorimotor, preoperational, concrete-operational,** and **formal-operational** stages. During the sensorimotor stage, from birth through 2 years, the infant responds to physical and sensory experiences. Because the child hasn't acquired full language ability, he or she cannot maintain mental images and responds only to the here and now of experience. Thus, trying to have a logical and reasoned conversation with a child at this age would make little sense because he or she cannot yet make rational sense out of the world. For instance, imagine a parent saying to a two-year-old child who has just reached out for candy at a checkout counter, "Let's sit down and talk about this when we get home so you'll understand why you shouldn't take candy without asking." Unfortunately, some parents try to make children understand this kind of logic. Can you consider other options to a reasoned approach that can change this child's behavior without using anger or punishment?

As the child moves into the preoperational stage (ages 2–7 years), he or she is developing language ability and can maintain mental images. This way of being in the world is intuitive, meaning that the child responds to what seems immediately obvious rather than having the ability to think logically. When a child in this stage sees a tall glass of water, he or she assumes that it has more volume than a smaller but wider glass of water (or the piece of toast cut in two is more than the one piece of toast). Because children at this age have not yet adopted logical thinking, trying to explain such logical principles would be difficult, if not impossible (unless the child is on the verge of entering the concrete-operational stage). Imagine trying to explain to 3-year-old Emma why five small M&M's are the same as two large M&M's. She just wouldn't get it!

From ages 7 through 11, the child enters the concrete-operational stage in which he or she can begin to "figure things out" through a series of logical tasks. Children in this stage often are very adamant about their logical way of viewing the world. For instance, when helping a friend's son figure out a math addition problem, I suggested to him a new way of doing it. However, because my method did not follow his "logical" way, he became very angry and told me I was wrong, even though the answer was the same. I was wrong because I didn't do it the way he learned, and he did not yet have the flexibility to examine other ways of problem-solving. Children in this stage will have difficulty with metaphors or proverbs because they have not developed the capacity to think abstractly. However, when children move into Piaget's final formal-operational stage (ages 11–16) they

When Emma was 3, she did not realize that five small M&M's are not more than two large M&M's, thus supporting Piaget's theory on conservation.

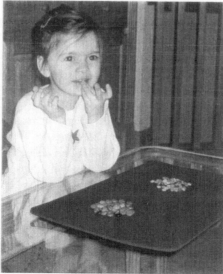

Kristina Williams-Neukrug

begin to think abstractly and apply more complex levels of knowing to their under-standing of the world. A child in this stage can understand how objects might have symbolic meaning (e.g., the Liberty Bell is more than just a bell), test hypothe-ses, understand proverbs, and consider more than one aspect of a problem at one time.

Piaget's research on child development has greatly helped us understand how children learn and the limitations of their abilities based on their age and develop-mental stage. Such knowledge has greatly affected styles of teaching, ways to parent effectively, and methods of counseling children.

Kohlberg's Theory of Moral Development

By having children respond to **moral dilemmas** (problems of a moral nature that have no clear-cut answer), **Lawrence Kohlberg** (1963, 1981, 1984) discovered that moral understanding and reasoning develop in a predictable pattern. He identified three levels of development, each containing two stages.

The first level, **preconventional** (roughly ages 2–9 years), is based on the notion that children make moral decisions out of fear of being punished or out of desire for reward. In Stage 1 of this level, moral decision-making is based on perceived power that others hold over them and the desire to avoid punishment from these in-dividuals in authority. In Stage 2, decisions are made with an egocentric/hedonistic desire to satisfy one's own needs and in hopes of gaining personal rewards. Imagine a 6-year-old wanting to watch her favorite DVD. A parent might say, "No, you can't watch that now, but after dinner we'll make special time to do whatever you want." A child might initially say, "Sure, Mom" (not wanting to get punished for doing the wrong thing), but then, when Mom is not watching, secretly put the DVD in the DVD player.

In Kohlberg's **conventional level** (ages 9–18), moral decisions are initially based on social conformity and a desire to gain approval from others (Stage 3), whereas later, the accent is on adhering to rule-governed behavior—carrying out one's duty to society to avoid guilt and dishonor (Stage 4). In this level, children are motivated less by punishment or reward and more by a wish to avoid displeasing others and out of a sense of right and wrong as defined by rules of law and order. In Stage 3 of this level, the child responds to what he or she believes significant others would view as morally correct, in hopes of avoiding their disapproval and of gaining their acceptance. Most children will reach Stage 3 by age 13 (Gerrig & Zimbardo, 2010). For example, when my daughter Hannah was 9 years old she had a strong need to be approved by my wife and me, so she acted in a manner that she felt would not disappoint us. When she did "go against the rules," she often felt guilty because she believed that she had not lived up to our expectations. However, when Hannah turned 11, approval from her parents took a back seat in her moral deci-sion-making, and a rigid adherence to societal rules of law and order took hold (Stage 4). She began to live by the adage, "It is important to follow the law if we are going to have a moral society that functions adequately."

Kohlberg noted that many individuals never reach the final **postconventional** level of moral development. If postconventional thinking comes at all, it comes only at or after age 13. It is based on acceptance of a social contract that is related to democratically recognized universal truths (Stage 5) or on individual conscience based perceived universal principles and moral values (Stage 6). In Stage 5, the first stage of the postconventional level, the individual now believes that laws can be examined, interpreted, discussed, and changed. Although an individual in this stage would generally be law-abiding, this individual is no longer rigidly adhering to the law, as was the case of the Stage 4 individual. Instead, this individual would reflect on a law to consider whether it makes sense at all times and might attempt to change the law at times when it does not seem justified (e.g., perhaps stealing would be allowed if the parent of a starving child stole food for the child).

In Stage 6, the final stage of the postconventional level, moral decisions are based on a sense of universal truths, personal conscience, individual decision-making, and respect for human rights and dignity (Rice, 2001). Here an individual would consider moral truths in his or her decision-making process and, after deep reflection, might choose to break a law, deciding that such an action is taken out of respect for the dignity of people and for the betterment of society. For instance, during the civil rights movement of the 1960s, some individuals broke laws to advance the cause of civil rights for all people (see Box 5.1).

Gilligan's Theory of Women's Moral Development

In 1982, **Carol Gilligan** wrote *In a Different Voice,* a book that questioned some of Kohlberg's assumptions. Gilligan, who had worked with Kohlberg, points out that most of his research had been done on a small group of boys. She proposes that moral reasoning for females might be based on a different way of knowing or understanding the world. Gilligan notes that Kohlberg's theory stresses the notion that high-stage individuals make choices autonomously, whereas her research

---

| **BOX 5.1** | **The Heinz Dilemma** |

Kohlberg gave dilemmas, such as the one here, to adolescent boys to help him understand the moral development of children (well, at least boys—see Gilligan in the next section). After reading the dilemma and reflecting back on Kohlberg's stages, devise responses that a "typical" person might make as a function of the stage he or she is in. Do you think responses will vary as a function of gender? What about as a function of ethnicity?

In Europe, a woman was near death from a special kind of cancer. There was one drug that the doctors thought might save her. It was a form of radium that a druggist in the same town had recently discovered.

The drug was expensive to make, but the druggist was charging ten times what the drug cost him to make. He paid $200 for the radium and charged $2,000 for a small dose of the drug. The sick woman's husband, Heinz, went to everyone he knew to borrow the money, but he could only get together about $1,000 which is half of what it cost. He told the druggist that his wife was dying and asked him to sell it cheaper or let him pay later. But the druggist said: "No, I discovered the drug and I'm going to make money from it." So Heinz got desperate and broke into the man's store to steal the drug for his wife. Should the husband have done that? (Kohlberg, 1963, p. 19)

Carol Gilligan
states that
women's moral
development is dif-
ferent from men's
in that women tend
to stress interde-
pendence rather
than autonomy.

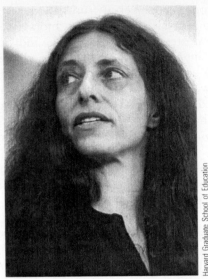

Harvard Graduate School of Education

seems to indicate that women value connectedness and interdependence and view the relationship as primary when making moral decisions. In describing the differences between men and women, Gilligan observes the responses of one of Kohlberg's subjects and compares him with a woman she interviewed:

> Thus while Kohlberg's subject worries about people interfering with each other's rights, this woman worries about "the possibility of omission, of your not helping others when you could help them." (1982, p. 21)

Gilligan states that in the development of moral reasoning, women will emphasize a **standard of care** as they move toward self-realization. She believes that women tend to be more concerned about the effect their choices have on others, whereas men are more concerned about a sense of justice being maintained (Gerrig & Zimbardo, 2010). Noting these male and female differences, Gilligan states:

> Given the differences in women's conceptions of self and morality, women bring to the life cycle a different point of view and order human experience in terms of different priorities. (1982, p. 22)

More specifically, the Level 1 preconventional girl is not dissimilar to Kohlberg's Level 1 boy, in that her moral reasoning is narcissistic—she reasons from a survival, self-protective perspective. For Gilligan, the Level 2 conventional female shows a concern for others and feels responsible for others compared with Kohlberg's Level 2 person who is concerned about pleasing others or following the rules. Gilligan's Level 3 postconventional woman is a complex thinker who recognizes the interdependent nature of humans and who knows that every action a person takes affects others in deeply personal ways. Gilligan also found that because adolescent girls tend to be more concerned with the feelings of others, they will often lose their "voice" as they defer in decision-making. However, as women age and grow, their voice, or strong sense of self, will often return as they realize they can be concerned about others and also have a perspective on the world that they will stand up for (see Gilligan's novel, *Kyra*, 2008).

In thinking about the examples given to clarify Kohlberg's theory, you might consider how a woman's decisions might differ from a man's if her decision-making process takes into account how a person's decisions affect others, based on her awareness of the interconnectedness of people (reflect on the Heinz dilemma again, in Box 5.1, this time from Gilligan's perspective). Gilligan has added a unique perspective to the concept of moral development and may be bringing to the forefront major differences in how men and women approach moral reasoning. Understanding such differences is crucial in helping us comprehend why the different sexes make certain choices. Table 5.1 compares Kohlberg and Gilligan and shows how their theories are both related to Piaget's stages.

Table 5.1 | A Comparison of Piaget to Kohlberg and Gilligan

Piaget's Stages	Piaget	Kohlberg/ Gilligan Levels	Kohlberg	Gilligan
Sensorimotor	Responds to physical and sensory experience.			
Preoperational	Intuitive responding. Maintenance of mental images. No logical thinking.	Preconventional	1. Punishment/ reward. 2. Satisfy needs to gain reward (you get from me, I get from you).	Concern for survival.
Concrete-operational	No complex thinking. Uses logical thinking sequencing, categorizing, to figure things out.	Conventional	1. Social conformity/ approval of others. 2. Rules and laws to maintain order.	Caring for others. Sacrifice of self for others. Responsible to others.
Formal-operational	Abstract thinking. Complex ways of knowing.	Postconventional	1. Social contract/ democratically arrived at, rules that can be changed through a logical process. 2. Individual conscience.	Decision-making from an interdependent perspective. All that we choose affects everyone else.

Note: Kohlberg's levels are each divided into two stages as shown.

Knowledge of Child Development: Applications for the Human Service Professional

Although the human service professional is not necessarily an expert in child development, knowledge of such development can help him or her understand whether the child is developing within a normal range. If the human service professional can recognize physical problems or delays in social, cognitive, or moral reasoning, then appropriate referrals can be made to medical, psychological, or educational sources that can assist the child in his or her development. Early identification of such problems can greatly help to ameliorate these concerns.

PERSONALITY DEVELOPMENT

How are our personalities formed? This question has intrigued philosophers for centuries. In the last 100 years, psychologists have attempted to answer this question through a number of theories that seek to explain the personality development of the individual. Paralleling the counseling theories discussed in Chapter 3, theories of personality development are based on views of human nature of the major counseling theories and describe a system for the developing person.

Although many theories of personality development have been developed over the years, we will examine Freud's theory of psychosexual development, learning theorists' views on development, and Rogers's humanistic understanding of growth and development. These represent three of the more prevalent views concerning personality development of the individual. This section will also feature a new take on personality development and the creation of reality—postmodernism and social constructionism. As you will see, this approach questions all reality that has come before it.

Freud's Psychosexual Model of Development

Sigmund Freud viewed individual personality as forming within the first five or six years of life. As noted in Chapter 3, he believed that the person is born with sexual and aggressive **instincts** that are regulated as a function of parenting received in early childhood. Freud stated that the child is born all **id.** Ruled by the **pleasure principle,** the id embodies all of our instincts and attempts to blindly satisfy our needs. As the child develops, the type of parenting he or she receives greatly affects the formation of the **ego,** where we see the beginning of consciousness. Ruled by the **reality principle,** the ego attempts to deal with reality of everyday life. As the ego is developing, the formation of the **superego** begins to develop. The superego represents the formation of the child's morality and values and is greatly affected by the values of parents and society (Freud, 1940/2003). Freud collectively called id, ego, and superego the **structures of personality** (Neukrug, 2011) and believed the individual passes through five **psychosexual stages of development,** each of which affects the expression of the id, and formation of the ego, superego, and consciousness (see Figure 5.1).

Stating that sexual satisfaction and resulting psychosexual development is centered on **erogenous zones,** Freud presented a unique view of the developing

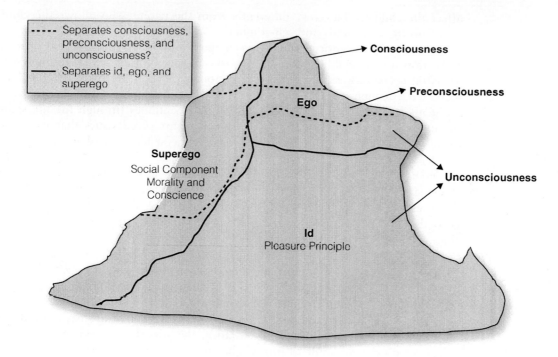

Figure 5.1 | The Relationship of the Id, Ego, Superego, Consciousness, Preconsciousness and Unconsciousness

individual. During the **oral stage,** the first stage of psychosexual development, the infant receives pleasure through feeding. The major developmental task of this stage, which occurs between birth and age 1, is how the child becomes attached to the mother (or the major caretaker). Therefore, the relationship between caretaker and infant is extremely important. Clearly, a child who goes hungry or is physically abused will have difficulty successfully passing through this stage. Invariably, Freud stated, this child would develop trust problems as an adult.

Freud stated that during the **anal stage,** the child receives pleasure from bowel movements. During this stage, which occurs between ages 1 and 3 years, the child becomes physiologically ready to be toilet trained. How parents assist with the child's newfound ability to control his or her bodily functions greatly affects the child's ability to be independent, feel powerful, and express negative feelings. Think about the parent who demands the child "sit on the potty" versus the parent who encourages and supports the child's newfound control of his or her bodily functions. These two types of parenting will affect the child's sense of autonomy very differently.

During the **phallic stage,** which occurs between ages 3 and 5 years, the child becomes aware of his or her genitals as well as of the genitals of the opposite sex. Now the child receives pleasure from self-stimulation. How parents respond to a child in this stage can greatly affect the child's attitudes and values. The parent who consistently tells his or her child that it is sinful to touch the genitals will affect the child's values very differently from the parent who allows the child to touch his or her genitals and self-stimulate.

The **latency stage,** occurring between age 5 and puberty, is a period of relative relaxation for the child, in which he or she replaces earlier sexual feelings with a focus on socialization. Here, the child becomes more aware of peers and devotes increased attention to peer-related activities. Freud's final stage of development is the **genital stage,** which begins at puberty and continues through the life span of the individual. Here, we see the emergence of unresolved issues that were raised in the first three stages of development, as well as a focusing of sexual energy on social activities with peers and on love relationships.

Freud believed that becoming **fixated,** or having problems with maturation and showing dysfunctional patterns resulting from incomplete development during a stage, is the result of inadequate parenting or caretaking. These dysfunctional ways of being generally occur unconsciously, that is, outside of our awareness. For instance, the child who is sexually abused at age 5 might have repressed these memories, yet Freud would say that the abuse would continue to affect the child's behaviors in unconscious ways. Therefore, it is not uncommon to see an adult who was sexually abused find ways to avoid dealing with his or her sexuality (e.g., becoming obese, becoming a workaholic, or, in an extreme case, taking on multiple personalities).

Typically, to avoid anxiety that unresolved issues might arouse, the individual develops **defense mechanisms.** For instance, the sexually abused child might develop defenses as an adult to protect the ego that became so fragile as a result of the abuse. Although there are many defense mechanisms, some of the more common ones are *repression*, pushing out of awareness threatening or painful memories; *denial*, distorting reality to deny perceived threats to the person; *projection*, viewing others as having unacceptable qualities that the individual himself or herself actually has; *rationalization*, explaining away a bruised or hurt ego; and *regression*, reverting to behavior from an earlier stage of development that is a less demanding way of responding to anxiety (e.g., sucking one's thumb).

With volumes having been written on Freud's theory, the previous text represents just a small fraction of his ideas about personality development. Freud's psychoanalytic model of personality development has added much to our understanding of the complexity of the individual and has helped to explain why people behave in so many different ways. His stage theory and the concepts of the structures of personality, the unconscious, and defense mechanisms represented the first comprehensive approach to understanding the development of personality.

Learning Theory

B. F. Skinner and other **learning theorists** hold the belief that each individual is born a **blank slate,** or **tabula rasa,** and that personality development is based on the types of conditioning that happen throughout one's lifetime (Bandura, Ross, & Ross, 1963; Skinner, 1971). Drastically differing with Freud's notion of instincts, Skinner believed that "the most important causes of behavior are environmental and it only confuses matters to talk about inner drives" (Nye, 2000, p. 80).

As noted in Chapter 3, learning theorists believe that one adopts behaviors through **operant conditioning, classical conditioning,** or **modeling (social learning).**

Learning theorists do not view personality development as a function of developmental stages as in the psychoanalytic model. Although behaviorists do not deny that a person's genetics or biology can affect behavior, they emphasize how positive or negative reinforcement (as suggested by operating conditioning), social learning (i.e., modeling), and the pairing of an unconditioned stimulus with a conditioned stimulus (i.e., classical conditioning) affect our personality development.

Operant conditioning is generally considered to be the most common type of conditioning and occurs when behavior that is emitted is reinforced, thus increasing the probability of that response occurring again. Through years of rigorous research, Skinner and others delineated many principles of operant conditioning, each of which is crucial to the shaping of behaviors and the development of personality. A small portion of these include the following:

1. *Positive reinforcement:* Any stimulus that, when presented following a response, increases the likelihood of that response.
2. *Negative reinforcement:* Any stimulus that, when removed following a response, increases the likelihood of that response.
3. *Punishment:* Applying an aversive stimulus to decrease a specific behavior. Punishment is often an ineffective method of changing behavior as it may lead to undesirable side effects (e.g., counteraggression).
4. *Schedules of reinforcement:* The numerous ways in which a stimulus can be arranged to reinforce behavior; based on elapsed time and frequency of responses.
5. *Discrimination:* The ability of a person to respond selectively to one stimulus but not respond to a similar stimulus.
6. *Generalization:* The tendency for stimuli that are similar to a conditioned stimulus to take on the power of the conditioned stimulus.
7. *Extinction:* The ceasing of a behavior because it is not reinforced.
8. *Spontaneous recovery:* The tendency for responses to recur after a brief period of time after they have been extinguished.

Learning theorists believe that personality development is generally shaped by the significant people in one's life. This is because those individuals are most readily available to apply these principles, although such application is rarely, if ever, done in a purposeful or deliberate manner. Skinner and other learning theorists believe that reinforcement from significant others often occurs very subtly and in ways that we do not immediately recognize (Nye, 2000; Skinner, 1971; Wolpe, 1969). Therefore, changes in voice intonation, subtle glances, or body language could subliminally affect one's personality development. Learning theorists note that if a situation is examined closely enough, one could attain an understanding of the types of reinforcement contingencies, or modeling, that were instrumental in shaping behavior.

Because reinforcement contingencies are so powerful, behaviors are generalized to other situations. This is why an individual's behavior will be relatively consistent from situation to situation. Extinguishing behaviors that have been continually reinforced is difficult, and a major task of helpers who work with individuals exhibiting maladaptive behaviors is to use counterconditioning (conditioning new adaptive behaviors) so the individual can learn more effective ways of living in the world.

Recently, many learning theorists have included a cognitive framework within their conceptualization of development. **Albert Ellis** (Ellis & Harper, 1997), **Michael Meichenbaum** (1977), and **Aaron Beck** (J. Beck, 1995, 2005) believe that not only do behaviors of individuals become reinforced, but so do the ways in which people think. Therefore, thinking can dramatically affect behavior, and behavior can dramatically affect thinking in complex ways. **Cognitive-behaviorists** have challenged the beliefs of the original behavioral purists and have changed the manner in which most learning theorists conceptualize the development of the individual.

Because development is seen as a result of reinforcement contingencies, learning theorists believe that change can occur at any point in the life cycle. Therefore, one can identify dysfunctional behaviors and irrational thinking, determine the reinforcements that continue the dysfunctional ways of living in the world, and devise a method of reinforcing new behaviors and different cognitions.

Summarizing some of the major factors that can lead to healthy or abnormal development, modern-day learning theorists hold the following beliefs:

1. The individual is born capable of developing a multitude of personality characteristics.
2. Behaviors and cognitions are continually reinforced by significant others and by cultural influences in our environment.
3. Reinforcement of behaviors and cognitions is generally very complex and can occur in very subtle ways.
4. Abnormal development is largely the result of the kinds of behaviors and cognitions that have been reinforced (other factors such as genetics may also affect development).
5. By carefully analyzing how behaviors and cognitions are reinforced, one can understand why an individual exhibits his or her current behavioral and cognitive repertoire.
6. Through the application of principles of learning, old dysfunctional behaviors and cognitions can be extinguished and new healthy behaviors and cognitions can be learned.

Learning theory offers a unique, objective, straightforward method of understanding personality development. In addition, it has had a great impact on our ability to change maladaptive behaviors (see Chapter 3). We owe much to Skinner and his colleagues for adding this important dimension to our understanding of personality development.

Humanistic Theory

As noted in previous chapters, **Carl Rogers** greatly affected our understanding of the person. His thoughts on personality development starkly contrast with the views of Freud and Skinner. Although representing just one of the many **humanistic approaches** to understanding personality development, Rogers's ideas embody many of the key concepts put forth by the humanistic theorists.

Rogers believed that individuals are born good and have a natural tendency to actualize and obtain fulfillment if placed in a nurturing environment that includes **empathy, congruence,** and **unconditional positive regard** (see Chapters 1 and 3). In contrast with Freud, Rogers did not emphasize the importance of instincts, the unconscious, or developmental stages in the formation of personality. In contrast with Skinner, Rogers did not place much value on reinforcement contingencies as a factor in personality development. Instead, he viewed the relationship between the child and his or her major caretakers as the most significant factor in personality development (Rogers, 1951, 1957, 1980).

Rogers believed that we all have a need to be regarded or loved by others. He stated that significant people in our lives often set up **conditions of worth,** or ways we should act so we can receive their love. Therefore, as children we will sometimes act in ways that please others to obtain a sense of acceptance—even if the pleasing self is not their real self. At this point, the child has learned that if he or she practices **incongruity,** or not being real, he or she will receive acceptance (see Box 5.2). This nongenuine way of living then becomes our way of relating to the world and prevents us from becoming **self-actualized**—becoming our true selves. Often this incongruity occurs as the result of our **introjection** (swallowing whole) of the values of others without ever giving ourselves the opportunity to reflect and decide whether we truly adhere to these values. This is when our **self-actualizing tendency** is squashed. The helper who works with an individual who is incongruent attempts to set up an environment in which the client feels safe enough to get in touch with his or her true self. Only when one realizes his or her true self can one become self-actualized, as noted by **Abraham Maslow's** hierarchy of needs (see Chapter 3).

The humanistic approach downplays, and in many cases challenges, the concept of abnormality. Instead, so-called abnormal behavior is seen as an attempt by

| BOX 5.2 | **The Story of Ellen West** |

This story, so eloquently told by Rogers (1961), describes the history of a famous psychotherapy client (a client Rogers knew about but never saw himself). Rogers described the estrangement of this person from her feelings—how she felt obligated to follow her father's wishes and not marry the man she loved, how she disengaged herself from her feelings by overeating, how a few years later she again fell in love but instead married a distant cousin according to her parents' wishes. Following this marriage, she became anorexic, taking 60 laxative pills a day, again as an apparent attempt to divorce herself from her feelings. She saw numerous doctors, who gave her differing diagnoses, treated her dispassionately, and generally denied her humanness. Eventually, disenchanted with her life, Ellen West committed suicide.

This story, Rogers noted, gives a poignant view of what it is like to lose touch with self—to be incongruent. Because Ellen West felt she needed to gain the conditional love of her parents, she gave up the most valuable part of self—her real self. Losing touch with self led to a life filled with self-hate and a sense of being out of touch. Eventually, therapists viewed her as being mentally ill, which Rogers implied might have added to her feelings of estrangement and her eventual suicide.

dispassionate clinicians to objectify and isolate the client. If we call the individual "abnormal," we take away his or her humanness and no longer need to deal with this person as a human being. In fact, humanists would say, abnormal behavior can be seen as a healthy response to an unhealthy situation. In this case, responding to conditions of worth is natural as the person attempts to survive in a world where significant individuals in the person's life are attempting to have the person act in a certain manner. What is abnormal, say the humanists, is the attempt to call something abnormal that is actually natural.

The humanistic approach to personality development represents a departure from the **deterministic** views of Freud (i.e., we are determined by instincts and child-rearing) and the **reductionistic** ideas of the learning theorists (i.e., reducing personality down to reinforcement contingencies). The humanist's stress on the importance of significant relationships has added an important dimension to our understanding of personality development.

Postmodernism and Social Constructionism

In recent years, there has been a challenge to the traditional psychodynamic, humanistic, and learning theory perspective of personality development. In fact, **postmodernists** and **social constructionists**, such as **Michael White** and **David Epston**, turn the concept of abnormality on its head. From their perspective, abnormal behavior is simply a **social construction**—a construct that has been developed by certain individuals within the helping professions who have tended to be in power (e.g., psychiatrists) and have subtly, but forcefully, pushed their viewpoint onto the rest of the mental health field. They also believe that through dialogue and by introducing new knowledge, people can build new constructions of their sense of self. In fact, these individuals tend to believe the following four premises (Freedman & Combs, 1996):

1. Realities are socially constructed.
2. Realities are constituted through language.
3. Realities are organized and maintained through narrative.
4. There are no essential truths.

If this is the case, what do you think causes differences in personality development? Is it just the result of dialogues we have with significant people in our lives? Are these dialogues somewhat a function of the language used in our families, in our culture, and in society? Have we all constructed for ourselves our own realities? (see Box 5.3).

Knowledge of Personality Development: Applications for the Human Service Professional

When we initially meet clients, we are sometimes bewildered by their actions. Why does a rapist rape? Why does a parent abuse his or her child? Why does an adult who seemingly has everything live in a state of depression? Why does an able-bodied, intelligent person end up on the streets as a homeless person? Understanding the personality development of the individual can give us insight into the

BOX 5.3	**Color Therapy**

Imagine there was a counseling approach that stated color preference was an indication of mental health, and the closer a person's favorite color was to "red," the healthier he or she was. Those who liked red most were very healthy, those who liked orange were pretty healthy, those who liked yellow were somewhat healthy, and so forth down the spectrum to green, then blue, and then those who liked violet were really unhealthy. Now imagine that this approach became so popular that it was accepted throughout the land and most people "know" that color preference is related to mental health.

Now, imagine a client sees a counselor who is a "Color Counselor." Naturally, one of his first questions is to ask the client what her favorite color is. She says "blue." Well, immediately, the counselor assumes the client is not mentally healthy. After all, blue is way down the list toward violet. So, the counselor begins to treat her and tries to change her favorite color. He even has a systematic way of having her work up the hierarchy toward red. If she practices the system every day, she will eventually get closer to red, says the counselor. After a few months, she has worked her way up to green, and the counselor says he thinks that she might want to consider taking some medication, for medication will help her experience the red more often. And, the counselor tells her that after a few years of

experiencing more red, she can try to reduce her medication because maybe she can begin to like red on her own.

Frustrated that she is not making progress fast enough, the client decides to see a new counselor. The new counselor is clearly nonconventional and does not even believe in Color Therapy. She asks the client to tell her what her problem is. The client states "Well, everyone says that liking blue is bad, and so I must be mentally ill. What do you think?" This counselor replies by saying, "How about we don't focus on the color right now. Instead, let me ask you: What do you want your life to look like? Where do you want to take counseling? What do you want as your end goal? And, what would make you happier?"

With counselor number one, there is an external reality based on preconceived notions about colors. This reality has been bought into by many, and a whole system of working with clients has been developed. And, almost everyone "knows" and believes in this approach. The second counselor, however, does not have these preconceived ideas, and indeed even questions the moral authority that asserts that this reality exists. This counselor does not believe there are any internal structures that mediate mental health based on color. This helper is the postmodern, social constructionist helper!

client's world. Such insights into the developing world of the person as offered to us by psychoanalysts, learning theorists, humanists, and postmodernists can enhance our ability to empathize with our clients, help us in treatment planning for our clients, and give us the knowledge base to make appropriate referrals. If we did not have this basic understanding of personality development, we could be left without a clue to the makeup of the person or how to work with the individual (see Box 5.4).

LIFE SPAN DEVELOPMENT THEORIES

Some developmental models suggest that the individual continues to grow through a series of life stages, with development not suddenly ending as one enters adulthood. One of the more prevalent life span development theories has been

BOX 5.4 | A Psychotic Relative

When I was about ten years old, I had a favorite relative named Joyce with whom I loved to play. Suddenly, she no longer came to visit. I heard rumors that Joyce's father, David, had had a "nervous breakdown" and that his wife had divorced him. The families became estranged at that point. David, who was college educated, never seemed the same after his nervous breakdown. He rarely bathed, wore dilapidated clothes, and often would come up with delusional and grandiose ideas about life. When I was older, I realized that David had been psychotic. He had lost touch with reality, was paranoid, and had been hospitalized in a large, urban psychiatric hospital. After being released from the hospital, he would often stay in sleazy apartments and at times was homeless. What had happened to David? Recently, when I asked my mother about David, she stated that he had at times seemed different, even before the hospitalization.

I often wonder about David's personality development. What kinds of early childhood development affected his personality? What kind of parenting did he receive? Were there genetic or biological factors that affected his mental health? Unfortunately, much of David's life is shrouded in mystery. Perhaps with early intervention and knowledge of personality development, the tragedy that befell him and his family might have been averted.

Erik Erikson's stages of psychosocial development. More recently, **Robert Kegan's subject/object theory** has gained some prominence. In Chapter 1, we viewed the adult stages of Kegan's model; here, we will look at the whole model, from birth through adulthood.

Erik Erikson's Stages of Psychosocial Development

Although Erikson started out studying Freud's psychoanalytic approach, he later developed a model that rejected many of Freud's tenets. Contrary to Freud, Erikson believed that the individual is not determined by instincts, early childhood development, and the unconscious. Instead, he suggested that **psychosocial forces** (i.e., forces outside of ourselves that affect our psyche) affect personality development over the life span. As opposed to Freud's deterministic philosophy, Erikson had faith in the ability of the individual to overcome many of his or her problems and believed that healthy ego development and a positive identity is contingent on the individual's ability to master specific age-related developmental tasks as highlighted by a particular **virtue** or **strength** associated with each stage (see Table 5.2). On the other hand, if the individual cannot cope with the developmental tasks, then he or she will develop a low self-image and bruised ego and carry dysfunctional behaviors into the next levels of development. Erikson's eight life span stages offer a means of helping us understand the typical developmental tasks of the individual (Erikson, 1968, 1998) (see Box 5.5).

Robert Kegan's Constructive Model of Development

Kegan (1982, 1994) believes that our understanding of the world is based on the ways in which we construct reality as we pass through life. His **subject/object**

Table 5.2 | Erikson's Psychosocial Stages of Development

Stage	Name of Stage with Ages	Virtue of Stage	Description of Stage
1	Trust vs. mistrust (birth–1)	Hope	In this stage the infant is building a sense of trust or mistrust that can be facilitated by significant others' ability to provide a sense of psychological safety to the infant.
2	Autonomy vs. shame and doubt (1–2)	Will	Here, the toddler explores the environment and is beginning to gain control over his or her body. Significant others can either promote or inhibit the child's newfound abilities and facilitate the development of autonomy or shame and doubt.
3	Initiative vs. guilt (3–5)	Purpose	As physical and intellectual growth continues and exploration of the environment increases, a sense of initiative or guilt can be developed by significant others who are either encouraging or discouraging of the child's physical and intellectual curiosity.
4	Industry vs. inferiority (6–11)	Competence	An increased sense of what the child is good at, especially relative to his or her peers, can either be reinforced or be negated by significant others (e.g., parents, teachers, peers) leading to feeling worthwhile, or discouraged by others, which leads to feeling inferior.
5	Identity vs. role confusion (adolescence)	Fidelity	Positive role models and experiences can lead to increased understanding of temperament, values, interests, and abilities that define one's sense of self. Negative role models and limited experiences will lead to role confusion.
6	Intimacy vs. isolation (early adulthood)	Love	A good sense of self and self-understanding leads to the ability to form intimate relationships that are highlighted by mutually supporting relationships that encourage individuality with interdependency. Otherwise, the young adult feels isolated.
7	Generativity vs. stagnation (middle adulthood)	Caring	Healthy development in this stage is highlighted by concern for others and for future generations. This individual is able to maintain a productive and responsible lifestyle and can find meaning through work, volunteerism, parenting, and/or community activities. Otherwise, the adult feels stagnant.
8	Ego integrity vs. despair (later life)	Wisdom	The older adult who examines his or her life either feels a sense of fulfillment or despair. Successfully mastering the developmental tasks from the preceding stages will lead to a sense of integrity for the individual.

BOX 5.5 | The Case of Miles

I once saw a 32-year-old client who was having trouble with intimacy. Miles was engaged to be married, despite the fact that he had rarely dated, had very poor interpersonal skills, and was quite fearful of having a sexual relationship. He was a virgin when he eventually married, and he soon found that he could not maintain an erection and have intercourse with his wife. Although he was dealing directly with Erikson's intimacy versus isolation stage, it became evident that he had never successfully passed through earlier stages. He had been verbally abused as a child, which had resulted in a fearful attitude and difficulty building trust. His fears gave him an inferiority complex, which made him want to hide from people. He therefore was unable to interact successfully with his peers and generally felt lost in the world. He had never discovered what he was good at, what he liked, or what he valued. Clearly, he had a very poor identity formation. His problems with intimacy seemed closely related to not having successfully completed earlier stages of development.

As Miles and I worked on his concerns related to intimacy, we also spent much time examining issues related to earlier stages of development. As he reflected on his life and as he worked through his issues, he eventually was able to have a closer, more intimate relationship with his wife. This ultimately also led to their having a satisfactory sexual relationship.

---

theory states that individuals pass through specific developmental stages that reflect a meaning-making system. Movement from a lower to a higher stage necessitates a letting go of the earlier stage. This is not done easily, and Kegan (1982) suggests that movement occurs most successfully if there is challenge to one's existing view of the world within a supportive environment.

Being born into the **incorporative stage,** Kegan states that the self-absorbed infant is all reflexive and has no sense of self as separate from the outside world. However, as very young children begin to experience the world, reflexes are no longer the primary focus; instead children attempt to have their needs met through attainment of objects outside of self: "In disembedding herself from her reflexes the two-year-old comes to have reflexes rather than be them, and the new self is embedded in that which coordinates the reflexes, namely, the 'perceptions' and the 'impulses'" (Kegan, 1982, p. 85). In this **impulsive stage,** children have limited control over their actions and act spontaneously to have needs met. No wonder this period is often called the "terrible twos."

As children gain control over their impulses, they move into the **imperial stage** in which needs, interests, and wishes become primary and impulses can begin to be controlled. For instance, children begin to recognize what they want, can begin to reflect on their needs, and can control impulses to meet these needs (see Box 5.6). The child who wants a new toy, perceives the toy, and recognizes the desire for it now has some control over how to obtain the toy.

The last three stages occur primarily in adulthood and were noted in Chapter 1. Briefly, during the **interpersonal stage,** the individual is embedded in relationships. Here, one's relationships with other people become primary, and needs and wishes are met through the relationship. In this stage, there is a beginning awareness of other people's feelings. This is manifested by the ability of individuals to show

BOX 5.6 | Garrett: Responding from the Imperial Stage

Garrett is a 12-year-old son of a friend. Recently, when he wanted to spend time with a friend of his, he was told that this friend had already made plans to spend time with another boy. Garrett felt rejected and left out. If Garrett had still been in the impulsive stage, he might have thrown a temper tantrum. Instead, having passed into the imperial stage, he had control over his impulses and devised a way to have his needs met. He manipulated a way to spend time with both of them, disregarding their need to be with each other. In the imperial stage, one can control impulses and develop plans to have one's needs met. However, in this stage, there

is little empathy for other people's desires. Therefore, Garrett did not yet have the ability to talk over his feelings with his friends. I suspect that when he is a little older, he will be able to share his feelings of being left out and understand his friends' desire to be with each other. When his father was explaining this situation to me, he said that at first he was going to try to talk to his son about the other boys' feelings, but then he realized that Garrett just could not hear that yet. If someone is in the imperial stage and not yet ready to give it up, there is little anyone can do to make that person move to the interpersonal stage.

empathy because it helps them understand the other with whom they are embedded. The Stage 3 need for relationships is highlighted by many of the songs of this and past generations, songs that say, "Without you, I can't go on living."

As the individual moves out of embeddedness in another, he or she moves into the **institutional stage** where a sense of autonomy and self-authorship of life is acquired. Relationships in this stage are still important but no longer seem to be the essential ingredient for living. In this stage, the individual's understanding of his or her values and interests becomes important. Here the individual may choose a partner because this person shares similar values; however, the person in this stage does not need the partner as he or she does in the interpersonal stage.

Kegan's final stage, the **interindividual stage,** highlights mutuality in relationships; that is, the individual can share with others and learn from others in a nonembedded, nondependent way. Here there is a sharing of selves without a giving up of self. In this stage, differentness is tolerated and even encouraged at times.

Kegan's model offers an important departure from the other life span developmental models in that it stresses the interpersonal nature of development. Growth is based on our ability to interact with others and to let go of past, less effective types of relating. Although Kegan gives some general timelines for when movement into higher levels could occur, it is not unusual to find older adults who have not moved out of the interpersonal and sometimes even the imperial stages. Knowing the developmental stage of a person can help human service professionals provide an environment conducive to the personal growth of the client.

Knowledge of Life Span Development: Applications for the Human Service Professional

Whereas knowledge of child development and personality development can be crucial to understanding the person, these views tend to stress early development instead of changes in the individual throughout the life span. On the other hand, the life span approaches acknowledge that growth and struggles continue after puberty and on through older age in a predictable manner. Knowledge of some of the life span stages can help the human service professional facilitate the expected transitions through which the individual will pass. Therefore, the human service professional is better able to make appropriate referrals, counsel adequately, and provide educational materials to help the client.

OTHER MODELS OF DEVELOPMENT

There are many models of development that try to explain the gradual progression of the manner in which individuals understand the world. For instance, **Jane Loevinger's** theory of ego development examined how individuals develop interpersonally, cognitively, and morally over the life span. **Arthur Chickering** developed a theory to help us understand the major changes students go through while in college. Like Erik Erikson and Robert Kegan, **Roger Gould, George E. Vaillant,** and **Daniel and Judy Levinson** all examined adult development. **Mary Field Belenky** came up with a developmental model that described "women's ways of knowing," and **Carl Stoltenberg's** supervision model gave us a perspective on changes that helpers go through as they are supervised. **Donald Super's** model of career development helped us understand that career counseling is a lifelong process, beginning at the moment we are born and lasting to the day we die, and **Michael D'Andrea's** stages of racism helped us understand that racism is learned and that attitudes can change over time. Finally, **James Fowler's** theory of faith development helped us see that faith is much more than just being religious and can mature over time. Although not examined in this chapter, some of these theories will be explored elsewhere in this book. But, keep in mind that what you have in this chapter is simply a sampling of some of the more popular theories that impacted our understanding of the development of the person.

COMPARISON OF DEVELOPMENTAL MODELS

The varying models of development discussed in this chapter offer differing dimensions to our understanding of the person. Figure 5.2 outlines the varying stages of the theories we examined. Keep in mind that many individuals become fixated in stages. This will hinder their passage through the later stages.

NORMAL AND ABNORMAL DEVELOPMENT

While I was employed as an outpatient therapist at a mental health center, I was working with a 35-year-old married woman who had a history of several acute psychotic episodes. This meant that for short periods she lost touch with reality, had auditory hallucinations, and her thinking process became disorganized or unclear. I saw her for a few months and she seemed rather coherent, warm, and relatively normal. One day I received a call from her panicked husband who stated his wife was "out of control." He brought her to the mental health center, and I was startled to see a woman I hardly recognized. She thought she was possessed by the devil, was in a panicked state, and was screaming about some unusual sexual acts in which she stated she had participated. It was difficult to follow her line of

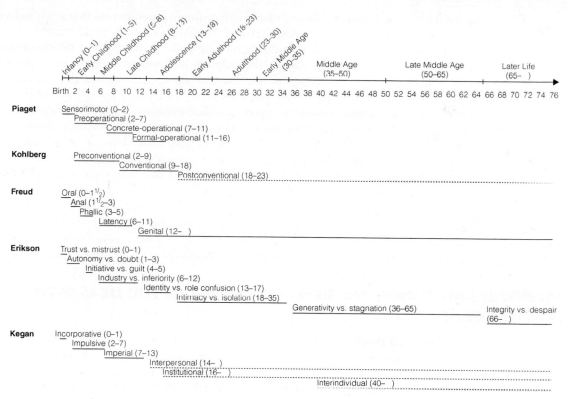

Figure 5.2 | Varying Models of Human Development Offer Different Ways of Understanding the Person Through the Life Span

Note: The onset of certain stages can vary by several months in childhood and several years in adulthood. In fact, Kegan and Kohlberg state that individuals may never reach the later stages of possible development. A dashed line represents the age range in which an individual could *potentially* attain a particular stage. A solid line represents the age range in which an individual is more *likely* to attain a particular stage. *Remember:* Attainment of a particular age may *not* mean attainment of a particular stage.

reasoning. In fact, little of what she said seemed to make sense. This once warm, coherent, lucid woman seemed like a different person. She was placed on medication to calm her and to help her regain stability and lucidity.

As a young counselor, I wondered how much of what she stated was real, how much was fantasy, how a seemingly "together" person suddenly lost it, and what I could do to help her get back in touch with reality. This woman was very scared and desperately wanted help. To this day, this woman represents to me the difference between what we call "normal" and "abnormal," as well as how fragile that line can sometimes be.

The various models we examined in this chapter each offer us a unique perspective on the development of the person and how that development could potentially affect an individual's understanding of reality. Each approach has its place. In addition, today, there is growing evidence that genetics and the individual's unique experiences both assert an essential role in the expression of personality: "it is largely through gene-environment interactions that each individual's unique personality develops" (Clark & Watson, 2008, p. 277).

The linking of biology, including genetics, with environmental factors in the development of personality moves the helping professions toward an approach that is truly holistic. Understanding the intricate interaction among these variables can be very powerful in effectively helping clients. Helpers in today's world should no longer be shy about consulting experts familiar with genetics and biology as these efforts can help them provide the most broadly based treatment for their clients.

It is my hope that you will leave this chapter with some deeper understanding of how a person becomes who he or she is. So, when you are working with a client who seems a bit "off," or, if you work with a client like I did, who suddenly walks into your office one day and is clearly out of touch, you will consider these models and be able to make some sense out of the individual's behavior. And, perhaps, you can offer your sense of the client's behavior to the client. This is a gift to the client in that it can help the client understand himself or herself in a little different way and perhaps offer a bit of peace of mind as the client begins to understand who he or she is.

DIAGNOSIS AND ABNORMAL BEHAVIOR: WHAT IS THE *DSM-IV-TR* AND THE *DSM-5*?

The **American Psychiatric Association** (APA), in consultation with the other mental health associations, has developed the *Diagnostic and Statistical Manual (DSM)* to help in the diagnosis of mental disorders. The current manual, the *Diagnostic and Statistical Manual of Mental Disorders-IV-TR (DSM-IV-TR)* (APA, 2000), is a complex manual that describes a full range of behaviors that epitomize different types of mental disorders. It can be of great assistance in our understanding, diagnosis, and treatment of individuals. This manual has also become extremely important for the payment of mental health benefits because most health insurance companies will not pay for mental health counseling unless there is an appropriate diagnosis from a duly licensed clinician. If you remember from Chapter 4, *DSM-IV-TR* has five axes: Axis I describes "Clinical Disorders and Other Conditions That May Be a Focus of Clinical Attention." Axis II delineates "Personality Disorders and Mental Retardation." Axis III explains "General Medical Conditions." Axis IV describes "Psychosocial and Environmental Problems," and Axis V offers a "Global Assessment of Functioning Scale" (see Box 4.4).

As of the writing of this text, *DSM-5* is scheduled to be published in 2013. This revised classification system will have many changes from its *DSM-IV-TR* cousin, with the most dramatic being the likelihood that Axis I and Axis II (the mental disorders) and Axis III (medical conditions) will be combined (APA, 2010). Such a collapsing of the axes would remove the stigma that has sometimes been associated with the personality disorders located on Axis II and would imply a closer link between mental disorders and medical problems. Many other changes are also likely; however, the APA is currently seeking feedback about potential changes and we probably won't know the outcome until the book is actually published.

The *DSM* has its critics. Some say that it is too reductionistic—that is, it tries to reduce mental illness and emotional problems into very neat categories, categories that some believe do not really exist. Others say a diagnosis tends to be a

Table 5.3 | Advantages and Disadvantages of *DSM*

Disadvantages	Advantages
1. Does not predict outcomes of counseling	1. Can help with case conceptualization
2. Does not examine etiology	2. Proper diagnosis can lead to good treatment planning including proper use of medication
3. Use can reinforce the helper's tendency to use a medical model of treatment	3. Allows mental health professionals to communicate more effectively to one another
4. Does not fully account for contextual and social factors	4. Fosters research on diagnostic categories
5. Can lead to labeling and stigmatization of client	5. Helps clients understand their emotional problems
6. Can be dehumanizing to client	6. Offers a model to test hypotheses concerning treatment outcomes
7. Fosters an objective view of client and minimizes the helping relationship	7. Provides a sense of what is "normal" for most people
8. Problems with the "scientific" evidence supporting diagnostic categories	8. Provides a forum for professionals to discuss nomenclature and treatment

self-fulfilling prophecy in that once a client is given a diagnosis, others tend to see the client in that light and will tend to reinforce those behaviors in the person (see Table 5.3). Despite its critics, the *DSM-IV-TR*, and the soon-to-be-published *DSM-5*, offer us one additional means of understanding emotional problems and is an important step toward our treatment of various mental health concerns.

ETHICAL, PROFESSIONAL, AND LEGAL ISSUE: MISDIAGNOSIS AND CULTURAL COMPETENCE

Unfortunately, it has become clear that clients from nondominant groups are misdiagnosed at higher rates than Whites (Mwaba & Pedersen, 1990; Yeh & Hwang, 2000). Why is this so? Perhaps it is partly because people from different cultures may express feelings in different ways, and symptomatology may differ as a function of culture (Kress, Eriksen, Rayle, & Ford, 2005). Thus, some have argued that although the use of diagnosis and the *DSM* can be helpful in treatment planning, it can lead to the misdiagnosis of clients from nondominant groups because it does not fully take into account these differences. Others have noted that the *DSM* tends to view mental disorders as residing in the individual and largely ignores external forces that can produce and exacerbate psychological problems (e.g., racism, poverty) (Atkinson, 2004a). An even more radical view held by some is that a diagnosis is a way of giving those in positions of power the ability to legally oppress the culturally different by "officially" defining some of their behaviors as being socially unacceptable (Eriksen & Kress, 2005, 2006, 2008; Halstead, 2007; Horwitz, 2002; Kress et al., 2005; Madsen & Leech, 2007).

Diagnosis is complicated, and as a human service professional it is critical that you take into account all of the previous factors when diagnosing a client or being given a diagnosis of a client by another professional. In other words, you must become culturally competent (Maramba & Nagayama Hall, 2002); that is, acquire the attitudes, skills, and knowledge to be able to work with a wide variety of ethnically and culturally diverse clients. It is only through your competence that our brothers and sisters from nondominant groups will be understood and afforded appropriate treatment goals.

THE EFFECTIVE HUMAN SERVICE PROFESSIONAL: CONSTANTLY CHANGING, CONSTANTLY EXAMINING

> What is it about my development that I have lived 42 years, never married, yet now so want a family? Why did I end up in the field of human services and teaching? Why do I sometimes feel an emptiness inside that seems insatiable and at other times feel so totally filled with joy and excitement that I wonder how I could ever feel empty?

This is what I wrote for the first edition of this book. My own personal development has changed dramatically since that time. Where I was single, I now am married. Where I was not a parent, I now am a father, twice. Where I was not a son-in-law, I now am one. Then I was in what Donald Super calls the establishment stage of career development; now I have moved into my maintenance stage (see Chapter 9). I have developed—moved on. We all are constantly changing. If we do it with relative ease and a little support, we can cherish each moment and enjoy our aging process. In a sense, each new developmental milestone brings with it a new birth and new growth ahead.

We all have unique developmental stories related to how we go through developmental stages. By reflecting on our developmental history, we can better understand ourselves and the underlying reasons why we have developed in our unique ways. As there are reasons why I waited until my 40s to get married, there are explanations for all aspects of your personality development. In fact, not attempting to understand our own developmental histories can negatively affect our work with our clients through **countertransference**. It is our responsibility to put ourselves in situations that help expand awareness of self. Vehicles such as counseling, self-help groups, meditation, and reading literature on personal development are just a few of the many ways in which we can better understand self.

SUMMARY

This chapter presented an overview of human growth and development from birth through old age. The chapter started by defining some themes common to most developmental schemes. Thus, we noted that developmental models are continual; orderly, sequential, and build upon themselves; are a natural change process; are painful yet growth producing; tend to be hopeful; and are preventive and wellness oriented.

After offering some basic definitions of development, we briefly reviewed the importance of knowing about the physical development of a child, especially as compared with the child's peer group. We noted that although the rate of children's physical development is fairly consistent, the scope of a specific child's development is based on the genetic predisposition of the child in interaction with the environment. We gave some examples of how a nurturing environment will result in a very different child than a problematic environment.

We next presented some models that spoke to the development of knowing in children. Starting with cognitive development presented by Piaget, we pointed out that he found that children pass through specific, identifiable stages of cognitive growth that he identified as sensorimotor, preoperational, concrete-operational, and formal-operational. We also noted that Piaget stated that children either assimilate new information or accommodate to it. We next examined the moral development models of Kohlberg and Gilligan. Kohlberg identified three levels of moral development with six stages. These include the preconventional, conventional, and postconventional levels. Gilligan, who also studied moral development, challenged some of Kohlberg's ideas and noted that she believed women's moral development was different from boys and men's, which Kohlberg's theory was mostly based upon. Gilligan stated that in making moral decisions women use a "standard of care" and care more about interconnectedness with others. We pointed out the relationship between Piaget and Kohlberg and Gilligan.

This chapter then moved on to discuss a number of personality models of development. Although many exist, we highlighted the theories of Freud, the learning theorists, the humanists, and the postmodernists. We noted that Freud identified five stages of psychosexual development: oral, anal, phallic, latency, and genital and that early child-rearing affects personality development. He noted that the development of defense mechanisms is important through these stages and affects the formation of the id, ego, and superego (the psychosexual stages of development). The learning theorists, on the other hand, stress the role of operant conditioning, classical conditioning, and modeling in the development of the person. Some of the more important learning concepts that we reviewed included positive reinforcement, negative reinforcement, schedules of reinforcement, discrimination, generalization, extinction, and spontaneous recovery. More recently, cognitive theorists such as Ellis and Beck, have added a cognitive perspective to how personality is formed through conditioning of our thinking. Learning theory today incorporates both cognitive and behavioral views. From the humanistic perspective, we noted that Rogers believed that the development of the person has to do with the kinds of nurturing received from significant others in the form of empathy, congruence, and unconditional positive regard, and that conditions of worth can dramatically affect the development, or lack thereof, of the "real self." We noted that the humanistic approach is a departure from the deterministic views of Freud and the reductionistic ideas of the learning theorists in that the humanists stress the importance of significant relationships to our understanding of personality development. The newest perspective, offered by such individuals as Michael White and David Epston, is called postmodernism. This approach is more radical than the others and suggests that realities are socially constructed, realities are constituted through language, realities are organized and maintained through narrative, and there are no essential truths.

Finally, viewing development as a life span model, we presented the stage models of Erikson and Kegan. Erikson offered eight developmental tasks that individuals must deal with as they go through life: (1) trust versus mistrust, (2) autonomy versus shame and doubt, (3) initiative versus guilt, (4) industry versus inferiority, (5) identity versus role confusion, (6) intimacy versus isolation, (7) generativity versus stagnation, and (8) integrity versus despair. Erikson's model highlights certain virtues or strengths that are associated with each stage. Kegan, on the other hand, believes that life span development is a function of how we construct reality as a result of our interactions with others as we pass through life. Kegan's theory includes six stages and is similar to Erikson's in its belief that almost all people have the capability to pass through all stages.

However, contrary to Erikson, he notes that passage through the adult stages may occur at different rates, or not at all, as a function of environmental factors such as education and the kinds of nurturing received. His stages are called incorporative, impulsive, imperial, interpersonal, institutional, and interindividual.

We pointed out that a number of other developmental models exist, some of which will be highlighted within the text and all of which offer the human service professional a better understanding of the developing person. We then presented a comparison of some of the major models of development we examined in this chapter. This chapter then pointed out the fine line between what is sometimes considered normal and abnormal and that developmental theories can be a way for us to understand our clients and for our clients to understand themselves.

This chapter moved on to discuss the *Diagnostic and Statistical Manual*. We noted that in 2013 the *DSM-IV-TR* is supposed to be replaced by the *DSM-5* and that these diagnostic manuals give us one additional mechanism to understand a person who is struggling with an emotional disorder. We offered some advantages and disadvantages to the *DSM*. This chapter then moved on to point out some possible reasons that clients from nondominant groups tend to be misdiagnosed more frequently than others and the importance of human service professionals to acquire the attitudes, skills, and knowledge to be able to work with a wide variety of ethnically and culturally diverse clients. This chapter concluded with the importance of understanding our own unique development so that we have better clarity when working with our clients.

Experiential Exercises

I. Reflecting on Your Personality Development

Refer to the personality theories of Freud, Rogers, the learning theorists, and the postmodernists and social constructionists, and reflect on your personality development as it might be described from each of those perspectives.

1. How does each perspective explain characteristics of your personality?
2. In explaining your personality development from the differing perspectives, what commonalities do you see between the varying theories?
3. In explaining your personality development from the differing perspectives, what differences do you see between the varying theories?

II. Examining the Development of an Adult with a Developmental Disability

The following is the story of Gloria. From a developmental perspective, describe Gloria from the following viewpoints:

1. Child development
2. Personality development
3. Life span development

Gloria's life story: Gloria, a 53-year-old developmentally disabled adult, was born with a moderate intellectual disability and with cerebral palsy. Soon after her birth, her parents hospitalized her in an institution for the developmentally disabled. She lived in this institution until she was 31, at which time she was placed in a group home for individuals with intellectual disabilities. During childhood, Gloria's language development was delayed. She could not speak in sentences until she was 4 years old. She was not toilet trained until age 7. Although her parents would visit her periodically, her main caretakers were the social service workers at the institution. Gloria was schooled at the institution, where she acquired the equivalent of a second-grade education. Gloria had few friends in the institution and was considered a loner. Despite working on socialization skills while in the institution, Gloria still prefers to be alone and spends much of her time painting. She has become a rather good artist, and many of her paintings are found in the institution and in the group home. Visitors often comment on the paintings and are usually surprised that a person with an intellectual disability can paint so well. Gloria has a part-time job at a local art supply company where she generally does menial work.

Although Gloria does have some friends at the group home and at the art supply store, when she spends much time with someone, she often ends up having a temper tantrum. When this happens she will usually withdraw—often to her painting. Gloria generally blames other people for her anger. Gloria is a rules follower. She feels very strongly about the list of rules on the bulletin board at her group home. She methodically reports people who break the rules. She always feels extremely guilty after having a temper tantrum because she sees herself as breaking the rule stating that one should "talk things out rather than get into a fight." In a similar vein, Gloria feels that laws "are there for a purpose." For instance, at street crossings she always stops at red lights and waits for the light to change.

Gloria has no sense of her future. She lives from day to day, and, despite periods of depression, generally functions fairly adequately. She states that she wants to get married, but her lack of social skills prevents her from having any meaningful relationships with men. Overall, the human service professionals who have contact with Gloria describe her as a rigid, conscientious, talented person who has trouble maintaining relationships. They note that, despite being in individual counseling and in a socialization support group, she has made little progress in maintaining satisfying relationships. Their feeling is that she probably will maintain her current level of functioning, and they see little hope for change.

III. Examining the Development of a Gifted Child

The following is the story of Joe. From a developmental perspective, explain Joe's development from the following viewpoints:

1. Child development
2. Personality development
3. Life span development

Joe's life story: Joe is 13 years old and is the only child, grandchild, and niece or nephew on his mother's side of the family. Joe's parents separated when his mother was five months pregnant with him. His parents, both of whom are highly educated, went through a tumultuous separation and divorce but now have a cordial relationship. Following his birth, his mother was distraught over the breakup of her marriage but subsequently has maintained a strong sense of self and high self-esteem. Following Joe's birth, his mother, who works fulltime, was fortunately able to afford a live-in nanny. This woman still lives with them and has been a significant help for the family and an additional source of comfort for Joe.

Joe's mother remarried when Joe was 10 years old, and his father has been involved in a long-term relationship. Joe lives with his mother but spends every other weekend, some weekdays, and extended periods during the summer and holidays with his father. Joe seems to have a good relationship with both parents, his stepfather, and his father's girlfriend.

Joe, who has always done well in school, currently attends a private school. He maintains very high grades and has a high IQ. Joe is at ease in relationships, as evidenced by his many friends and his ability to relate to people of all ages. He has many skills and is just beginning to examine those things that he is best at. He is just entering puberty, and girls are becoming more important to him. Overall, most people would describe Joe as a bright, personable, and thoughtful young man who is at ease with himself.

Although sometimes Joe may appear a little "spoiled," he generally is thoughtful and can recognize other people's feelings. He can think abstractly, and it would not be difficult to have a conversation with him concerning such philosophical matters as death and the existence of God.

IV. Counseling Gloria

If you were to counsel Gloria, how would your knowledge of her development help you in the strategies you used?

V. Counseling Joe

If you were to counsel Joe, how would your knowledge of his development help you in the strategies you used?

VI. Understanding Defense Mechanisms

Provide an example of each of the following defense mechanisms:

1. Repression
2. Denial
3. Projection
4. Rationalization
5. Regression

VII. Examining Defenses People Use

Can you think of other kinds of defenses people use to protect themselves from past pains and current hurts?

VIII. Developmental Differences Between Men and Women

Using the concepts presented by Kohlberg and Gilligan, discuss your views on how men and women approach moral reasoning. What differences and similarities do you see in how men and women approach morality?

IX. Examining Differing Perspectives on Abnormal Behavior

Respond to the following statements concerning abnormal behavior:

1. Using a situational point of view, make an argument for abnormal behavior being a function of one's surroundings.
2. Using a personality development perspective, make an argument for abnormal behavior being a function of early child rearing.
3. Using the perspective of postmodern perspective, make an argument that there is no such thing as abnormal behavior.
4. Using a genetic and biological orientation, make an argument for abnormal behavior being determined.

X. Using the *DSM*

Obtain a copy of the most recent *DSM* (e.g., purchase one, go to reference desk at library). Pick one diagnostic category and review the behavioral characteristics of that disorder along with a possible etiology of that disorder. In class, discuss the varying diagnostic categories you found.

XI. Ethical and Professional Vignettes

Reflect on the following ethical vignettes and discuss them in class:

1. A colleague with whom you work continually uses pathological language in describing her clients. You believe that this behavior is demeaning to her clients and wonder about her ability to work with them. Is the colleague acting ethically? Professionally? What, if anything, should you do?

2. A human service professional who does not believe in mental illness insists on treating clients with severe pathology in a proactive, humanistic manner and refuses to explore the possibility of medication as an adjunct to counseling. Is this ethical? Professional? Legal?

3. A human service professional who is working with a severely depressed client tells the client that she needs to seriously consider taking some anti-depressant medication. She then refers the client to a psychiatrist. Is this ethical? Professional? Legal?

4. A human service professional offers, for a fee, educational workshops to help individuals understand developmental tasks and unique developmental issues. Can the helper ethically and legally do this without being licensed?

5. A psychologist places an ad in the local newspaper that states, "Holistic, nonintrusive, nonpsychopathologically oriented counseling. See a helper who cares and can offer hope to all individuals." Is this type of ad ethical? Professional? Legal?

6. A human service professional who is a colleague and a friend has had little training in developmental stages and normal transitions in life. You notice that often the treatment planning for his clients is based on a medical model, and you believe that some of his clients are being served poorly because normal developmental struggles are being viewed as pathology. What is your responsibility to this professional? To his clients? What should you do if you explain your concerns and he does not do anything differently?

7. You realize when working with a colleague that she often views clients from nondominant groups in a negative light and pathologizes them more than she does White clients. You believe that her misdiagnosis leads to poor treatment, and you are concerned about her lack of cultural competence. What actions should you take?

Human Systems:
• Couples and Families
• Groups
• Organizational and Community
• Administrative and Counseling Supervision

CHAPTER **6**

CHAPTER CONTENTS

The concept of system thus treats people and events in terms of their interactions rather than their intrinsic characteristics. The most basic principle underlying the systems viewpoint has been understood for some time. An ancient astronomer once said, "Heaven is more than the stars alone. It is the stars and their movements." (Baruth & Huber, 1984, p. 19)

My sister is five years older than I, my brother five years younger. My father, who died when I was 26 years old, was a hard-working, kind, thoughtful man, somewhat on the quiet side and not particularly expressive of his feelings. My mom was a strong, nurturing, sometimes opinionated, yet mostly supportive woman on whom we could always rely in time of need. Both my parents were college-educated and first generation in this country. Dinner was a very special time for my family. My mother (and sometimes my sister) would prepare dinner while the rest of us would watch television in the den. During dinner, we would often have lively discussions about politics or other contemporary issues. As much as I loved these family interactions, I clearly remember being both overwhelmed by, and particularly in awe of, my sister's ability to argue her point of view. Because I had struggled with a childhood illness and was overweight, my self-esteem was not very high. Although I loved the family interactions, I had a sense that I could not hold my own in the nightly discussions; I would often find myself going inward to my feelings rather than relying on my intellectual ability. I remember arguing over issues such as capital punishment and the war in Vietnam. My arguments often became very passionate because I had become comfortable in the feeling world and less comfortable presenting a factual argument. It seems as if we began to take on particular roles in the family—my father being the strong yet quiet debater; my sister, the verbally fluid family member; my mom, the mediator; me, the passionate member; and my brother, being the youngest and perhaps because the feeling and verbal roles were already taken, seemed on the quiet side. There was a kind of balance in the family. Things seemed a little off if we suddenly were out of our family roles. Perhaps it's not surprising that my sister became a lawyer; I, a mental health professional; and my brother, an engineer—professions that match the personality characteristics of the roles we lived in our family.

My first therapeutic experience was in a counseling group in college. It is not accidental that I was the advocate for "expression of feelings," for invariably the roles we took on as children in our families are repeated in these groups. A woman of that same group, who had always taken on what might be considered male qualities, wanted to experiment with her feminine side. Therefore, she decided to try to act more feminine in the group. A third member of the group was always considered the outcast in school. He quickly took on this role in the group, and the group leader helped him examine why this continually happened to him.

My first job as a mental health professional was at a storefront crisis and drop-in center. There, we would often have homeless people seeking shelter. These people, many of whom had abusive or deprived childhoods, were often unkempt and uneducated, and many had emotional problems. Unfortunately, because of their inability to communicate effectively, which many times was a function of early roles played out in their families of origin, they would sabotage their attempts to receive aid from local social agencies. I remember how effective Vanessa, a woman who had been on welfare herself, was in helping these individuals work with the local social service systems.

When I accepted my current job at Old Dominion University, I discovered that a colleague of mine, Garrett, had grown up in an Irish-American neighborhood a few miles from my predominantly Jewish neighborhood in Queens. I had not even known that his neighborhood existed. Despite the fact that we grew up close to each other, our neighborhoods were so insulated that there was little shared between these cultures. These closely knit neighborhoods had somewhat rigid boundaries that prevented a sharing of cultural wealth.

What do all these vignettes have in common? They all are expressions of the complex interactions in systems. From the family systems in which we grew up, to the groups in which we now interact, to the organizational and community systems in which we live and work, to the kinds of supervision we receive at our work, systems play an important role in our lives. Thus, it is not surprising that "human systems" is one of the mandated curriculum areas listed in the accreditation standards of the **Council for Standards of Human Service Education** (CSHSE, 2010).

In this chapter, we will examine how human service professionals can use knowledge of systems to enhance their work with clients. We will begin by reviewing general systems theory and examining how this theory can help us understand all kinds of systems. Then, we will take a look at a number of systems in which we have or will participate—families, groups, communities, and work. We will examine how the human service professional can affect change in each of these systems. In addition, we will discuss ethical and professional issues related to working in systems. Finally, we will examine the importance of understanding the complex interactions of systems for the effective human service professional.

GENERAL SYSTEMS THEORY

> Living systems are processes that maintain a persistent structure over relatively long periods despite rapid exchange of their component parts with the surrounding world. (Skynner, 1976, pp. 4–5)

Although knowledge of the amoeba may seem like a far cry from our understanding of systems, in actuality there is much we can learn from this one-celled animal. The amoeba has **semipermeable boundaries** that allow it to take in nutrition from the environment. This delicate animal can not survive if its boundaries are very **rigid** or extremely **permeable**. Boundaries that are too rigid would prevent it from ingesting food, and boundaries that are too permeable would not allow the amoeba to maintain and digest the food it has found.

General systems theory was developed to explain the complex interactions of all types of systems, including living systems (e.g., the amoeba in its environment), family systems, and community systems (von Bertalanffy, 1934, 1968). Each system has **boundaries** that define its information flow and allow it to maintain its structure while the system interacts with other systems around it. Thus, the action of the amoeba, a small living system, affects the surrounding environment. Similarly, the action of a family unit will affect other families with which it interacts, and the action of a community group will affect other aspects of the community.

Components in a system tend to maintain their typical ways of functioning, whether those actions are functional or dysfunctional. A much-used analogy is that of the thermostat in the house (Nichols & Schwartz, 2009; Turner & West,

2006). When the temperature drops in the house, the thermostat, based on the temperature setting, switches on. If the thermostat is set for 70 degrees and the temperature drops below that, the heater turns on. However, if the thermostat is set for 40 degrees, the heater will not turn on until the temperature drops below 40 degrees. This tendency is called **homeostasis**.

In families, groups, and even social systems, members take on typical ways of behaving, regardless of whether these typical patterns are dysfunctional. Because these systems become comfortable with their typical ways of behaving, members of these systems will exert covert or overt pressure to have atypical behaviors suppressed. For instance, it was unusual for any member of my family to express anger. When I was a teenager, the few times I got very angry I distinctly remember my mother saying, "I don't understand why you're so angry; maybe we should take you to see a psychologist." My anger was atypical (rather than wrong), and the family system was attempting to deal with my "unusual" behavior. You may have experienced something similar to what I experienced at school or in a work setting. For instance, in either of these settings have you ever noticed someone who seemed "odd" or out of place? Did that person get labeled as different in some fashion and eventually become an outsider to the system? In actuality, the reaction to the "odd" or atypical behavior is an important statement about what the system can tolerate. In fact, people's response to the individual probably says more about the system than about the behavior. From a systems perspective, sometimes individuals who exhibit atypical behaviors are said to be the **scapegoat** of the system.

General systems theory views a healthy system as one that has semipermeable boundaries that allows new information to enter the system and be processed and incorporated. When a system has rigid boundaries, information cannot flow easily into or out of the system, and the system has difficulty with the change process. Alternatively, a system that has extremely permeable boundaries allows information to flow too easily into and out of the system, resulting in the individual components of the system having difficulty maintaining a sense of identity. Although American society allows for much variation in the permeability systems, systems that have particularly rigid or very loose boundaries have a tendency toward dysfunction. Sometimes these systems undergo disastrous results when breakdown occurs (see Box 6.1).

COUPLES AND FAMILIES

Today, about half as many people get divorced as get married (Centers for Disease Control and Prevention, 2011). So great is the impact of divorce on the family that Wallerstein and Blakeslee (2004) found that following a divorce, a great majority of the children were negatively affected by it years later and many struggled with issues from the divorce well into adulthood. Divorce affects everyone in the family and many outside of it. Couples and families are living systems, and each unique system affects other systems around it. In this section, we will explore couples and families, how they function, how they become dysfunctional, and the role of human service professionals in their encounters with couples and families.

BOX 6.1 | Jim Jones and the Death of a Rigid System

In the 1950s and early 1960s, Jim Jones was a respected minister in Indiana. However, Jones became increasingly paranoid and grandiose, believing he was Jesus. He moved his family to Brazil and later relocated to California where approximately 100 of his church followers from Indiana joined him. In California, he headed the People's Church, and he began to set more rigid rules for church membership. Slowly, he became more dictatorial and continued to show evidence of paranoid delusions. He insisted that church members prove their love for him, by demanding sexual intercourse with female church members, having members sign over their possessions, sometimes having them give their children to him, and having members inform on those who broke his rules. In 1975, a reporter uncovered some of the tactics Jones was using and was about to write a revealing article about the church. Jones learned about this and, just before publication of the article, moved to Guyana, taking a few hundred of his followers with him. As concerns about some of the church practices reached the

United States, California Congressman Leo Ryan and some of his aides went to Guyana to investigate the situation. Jones and his supporters killed the congressman and some of the aides. Jones then ordered his followers to commit suicide. Hundreds killed themselves. Those who did not do so were murdered.

Jones had developed a church with a rigid set of rules. The publication of a revealing article and the congressman flying into Guyana were threats to the system. As in many rigid systems, attempts at change from the outside were seen as potentially lethal blows to the system. Jones dealt with the reporter's threat to the system by moving his congregation to Guyana. Then, rather than allowing new information into the system, Jones killed off the system, first killing the congressman and then ordering church members to commit suicide. The members had become so mired in the rules of the system that nearly 900 of them committed suicide or were murdered. This is a tragic example of how dysfunctional a rigid system can become.

Key Rules That Govern the Functioning of Couples and Families

Communication and general systems theorists have developed a number of rules or common elements that can help professionals understand the basic functioning of couples and families. These include the following (Barker, 2007; Turner & West, 2006):

1. The interactional forces between couples and in families are complex and cannot be explained in a simple, causal fashion.
2. Couples and families have **overt and covert rules** that govern their functioning.
3. Understanding the hierarchy in a family (e.g., who's "in charge"; who makes the rules) can help one understand how couples and families communicate.
4. Understanding the unique subsystems of couples or families (e.g., spousal, sibling) can help one understand how couples and families communicate.
5. Understanding the effects on couples and families when boundaries are rigid, semipermeable, or extremely permeable.
6. Understanding the language used by couples and family members can give insight into how couples and families maintain their way of functioning.
7. Each couple and family has its own unique homeostasis that describes how its members typically interact. This homeostasis is not "bad" or "good." It simply is.
8. Change occurs by changing the homeostasis, or the usual patterns in the couple and in the family.

Through the lens of the common elements just noted, we can begin to understand the development of healthy and dysfunctional families.

Healthy Couples and Families

Healthy couples and families have semipermeable boundaries that allow information to flow in and be evaluated, and through healthy communication channels, make change as needed. Such couples and families have open and honest communication patterns. They are aware of their feelings and go to lengths to take ownership of their feelings. They are aware of how negative feelings can reverberate through a system, and they try not to let their negative feelings deeply affect others in the couple and in the family. Healthy couples and families are largely successful at not blaming others for their problems and tend to not scapegoat other members.

A healthy family has parents or guardians who are the main **rule makers** (a healthy family system can also have a single parent or guardian). Although rules will differ from family to family, healthy families have a clear sense of **hierarchy**, with the parents being in charge and the children, although possibly consulted, being the recipients of those rules.

Dysfunctional Couples and Families

Dysfunctional couples and families do not take ownership for their feelings or actions and do not take responsibility for problems in their relationship. They will easily scapegoat others. Some dysfunctional couples and families will have a tendency to see problems as residing in other people, not in themselves, and thus play the "blame game." Others will only see the problem as residing within themselves and reject the notion that the couple or the system shares the problem. Dysfunctional couples and families have a tendency toward very rigid boundaries that

Virginia Satir (1967), a well-known family therapist, noted that when one member of the family feels pain, the whole family is affected in some manner.

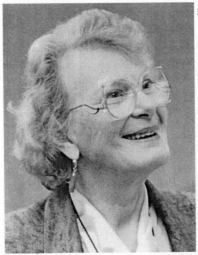

hold in secrets about the couple or family, or extremely permeable boundaries that do not allow for adequate development of separate identities.

Since all husbands and wives bring **unfinished business** to their marriage, the more serious the unfinished business, the greater the likelihood it will negatively impact the couple or family. For instance, a wife who was sexually molested as a child and has not worked through her pain will undoubtedly bring this unfinished business into the relationship. She might have developed mistrust of men and therefore unconsciously have chosen a man who is distant (and safe). Perhaps he is a workaholic. Alternatively, a man who has difficulty with intimacy might unconsciously pick a wife who allows him to be distant (and safe). As the relationship unravels, each spouse's issues are played out on one another or on one or more children. The husband may become stressed at work and take this out on his wife, children, or both. The wife may crave more intimacy, become discontent with the marriage, and take this out on her husband or children. Is it surprising that there are so many affairs and divorces?

When spouses are discontented with each other, they will sometimes unconsciously take out their anger on a child. In such a case, the child is said to be the **scapegoat** (Nichols & Schwartz, 2008, 2009). Often, when an individual is scapegoated, he or she becomes the **identified patient** (IP), or the member that is identified as the "one with the problem." In actuality, it is the couple or the family that has the problem. When a scapegoated child acts out in the family, in school, or in the community, the child is often said to be the member carrying the pain for the family (see Box 6.2).

BOX 6.2 | An Example of a Dysfunctional Family

A school counselor referred a 12-year-old boy to me because the boy's grades had dropped considerably and he was acting out in school. I asked him and his parents to come in for family counseling. For the first two months, the parents insisted that everything was fine in their marriage. As I continued to explore the situation, I could not understand why this boy was doing so poorly in school and was demonstrating such a dramatic personality shift. Then, during one session, the father revealed to me that he was extremely depressed—in fact, suicidally depressed. His depression stemmed from events that had occurred during his childhood. Soon, the mother revealed that she was bulimic, and later I discovered she was having an affair. The secrecy of the father's depression and the mother's bulimia and affair were symptoms of deep discontent in the marriage, and all stemmed back to issues in the parents' childhoods.

Rather than dealing with these very painful issues with each other, the couple had taken out their discontent on their oldest child. They did this through the mother becoming overly protective, the father becoming overly distant, and, whenever they would get angry at each other, both focusing on their son's problems. When the school tried to involve them in assisting the boy, they sabotaged whatever they were asked to do, as if they had something at stake in keeping him the identified patient. In essence, as long as he was seen as the one with the problem, they did not have to deal with their own problems. As soon as they became aware of what they were doing, the mother became less protective, the father became closer to his son, and the couple stopped scapegoating their son and began to deal with their own issues. The son's acting-out behaviors immediately stopped, and his grades improved dramatically.

Situational and Developmental Stress in Couples and Families

Salvador Minuchin (1974) believes that all couples and families are stressed by **situational** (unexpected) problems and by problems that are predictable **developmental** struggles as the couple or family passes through its life stages. For example, when a couple has their first child, the spousal dyad faces its first predictable developmental crisis. The couple will face a disruption in their relationship because rules in their family change to deal with the new family member. As children age, families will continually face other developmental crises (see Chapter 5) that necessitate changes in family rules. In other cases, families will be faced with stress from a number of unexpected events, such as an unforeseen illness, natural disaster, accident, or job loss. Healthy couples and families have the mechanisms to successfully deal with such stressors (see Box 6.3).

Family Guidance, Family Counseling, and the Role of the Human Service Professional

Over the years, a number of approaches to **family counseling** (often called "**couple and family counseling**") have been developed (see Nichols & Schwartz, 2006). Some of these include strategic family therapy (Haley, 1973, 1976, 2009), family therapy from a communication perspective (Satir, 1972a, 1972b), structural family therapy (Minuchin, 1974, 1981), multigenerational family therapy (Bowen, 1976, 1978), experiential family therapy (Napier & Whitaker, 1978; Whitaker, 1976), psychodynamic family therapy (Skynner, 1981), cognitive–behavioral family therapy (see Foster & Gurman, 1985), and more recently, narrative family therapy

---

BOX 6.3 | A Situational Family Crisis

With the recession, James lost his job of 16 years at the auto plant. He is mildly depressed but is mostly concerned about his three children, Lillian, Akira, and James, Jr., who are 15, 13, and 10, respectively. His wife, Patrice, is a part-time nursing assistant at a nursing home. The loss of income and benefits (e.g., health insurance) weighs heavily on James and Patrice; however, they have always been able to communicate to one another their worries. And, communication has led to a plan. Patrice will look for full-time work, and James will look for another job and go to the community college to be trained in a new field—being a chef, which he has always secretly wanted to do.

James is not a big talker, but he does say what he needs to say, and although Patrice has not had courses in communication theory, she knows how to care for someone when he is down. They are able to share their worries with one another, care for one another, and although the children know about their dad's job loss, James and Patrice have successfully kept the additional stress they are feeling out of their children's lives. As far as the children are concerned, things are pretty much as they have always been, except for a few "cutbacks" here and there.

This scenario could have ended very differently. In some families, James's loss of a job would have yielded stress that resulted in yelling and screaming and/or chaos. Other families may have seen a father or mother retreat into deep depression. However, James and Patrice have something special—in moments of stress they can rely on one another and talk enough to one another about how to handle their current situation.

(White, 1995; White & Epston, 1990). Although each of these approaches has its unique take on the family counseling process, they all follow, to some degree, the common elements noted earlier in this chapter.

Training in family counseling and family therapy is rigorous and requires at least a master's degree. Although human service professionals do not have the background to do family counseling, they can do **family guidance** in the sense that their knowledge of family systems allows them to recognize when to refer clients to family counselors, suggest workshops to attend, offer reading materials regarding how families interact, and give basic advice on family matters. It is important that the human service professional make an assessment about the seriousness of the family dysfunction and act accordingly.

Individual Counseling Versus Family Counseling

When should a family member be referred for individual counseling rather than the whole family being referred for family counseling? Although some would suggest it is always appropriate to refer the whole family for counseling rather than just one member (Napier & Whitaker, 1978; Satir, 1967), most helpers today agree that it is often a matter of making a decision based on an assessment of the situation. For instance, a child from an extremely dysfunctional family may be better off seeing a counselor individually because working with the family may be an extremely long process, whereas individual counseling may give the child some immediate relief. Or, it may be prudent to refer a spouse for individual counseling to work on his or her unfinished business because this could quicken the pace of change in the individual and facilitate change in the whole family. Also, individual members in a family will often seek out individual counseling while the family undergoes family treatment. If you are unsure what might be the best referral for a client, seek advice from a more experienced human service professional.

GROUPS

Groups, like families, can be viewed from a systemic perspective in which individuals in the group can be understood by examining the dynamic interaction of its members and how that interaction results in specific communication patterns, power dynamics, hierarchies, and the system's unique homeostasis (Agazarian, 2008; Connors & Caple, 2005; Napier & Gershenfeld, 2004). Like members of families, group members will bring in their unfinished business, which may cause problems in the healthy functioning of the group. Groups tend to create their own homeostasis, and members may be scapegoated in this process. Therefore, when a group member is scapegoated, he or she is reflecting problems within the whole system. When a group has a trained leader, it is up to him or her to create an atmosphere that will prevent scapegoating and allow group members to interact in healthy, functional ways—ways in which they may have never interacted before. Although community and social groups have always existed, groups whose intent is to explore human interactions are relatively new.

A Brief History

Gladding (2008) notes that prior to 1900, the purpose of group treatment was to assist individuals in ways that were functional and pragmatic. This often revolved around helping people with daily living skills and arose out of the social group work movement in which individuals, such as **Jane Addams**, organized group discussions that centered on such things as personal hygiene, nutrition, and self-determination (Andrews, 2001; Pottick, 1988). Using groups as their vehicle, social reformers like Addams were also concerned with community organizing as an effort to assist the poor.

At the turn of the century, some high schools began to offer "Vocational and Moral Guidance" in group settings. These efforts were often preachy in their nature, and group members had little opportunity to discuss personal matters in reflective ways. Soon after, with the spread of psychotherapeutic theory and with the beginnings of sociological concepts concerning group interactions, the first use of counseling and therapy groups that had more of an introspective nature arose in the 1920s and 1930s (Gladding, 2008).

In the 1940s, the modern group movement emerged. During this decade, **Carl Rogers** was asked by the Veterans Administration to run training sessions for counselors who might be working with returning GIs from World War II. Running the group training using his person-centered style, he found that there was increased self-disclosure, deepening of expression of feeling, and increased awareness of self. Thus began the **encounter group** movement (Rogers, 1970). At about the same time, **Kurt Lewin** and other nationally known theorists developed the **National Training Laboratory** (NTL) to examine **group dynamics**, or the ways in which groups tend to interact (NTL, 2008). NTL still exists and continues to train individuals in understanding the special dynamics of groups.

Groups became more popular during the 1960s and 1970s, and there were even places, like **Esalen** in California, where one could specifically go to experience an in-depth group experience (see www.esalen.org). Today, accrediting bodies and ethical codes acknowledge and attest to the importance of group work. The use of groups at social service agencies, or the referral of individuals to groups as an adjunct of counseling, is now an important, and sometimes essential treatment mode. Three of the more popular types of groups that human service professionals run or refer to include: **self-help, psychoeducational,** and **counseling and therapy groups.**

Defining Self-Help, Psychoeducational, and Counseling and Therapy Groups

Although systems dynamics occur in all groups, there are some differences in the functioning of **self-help groups, psychoeducational groups,** and **counseling and therapy groups** (Capuzzi & Gross, 2010; Gladding, 2008). Regardless of the type of group, however, all groups have rules regarding membership behavior, leadership style, technical issues (e.g., when and where to meet, number of group members, length of meeting times), and ground rules (e.g., limits of confidentiality, limits on socializing outside of the group, nature and purpose of the group).

Self-Help Groups   Although self-help groups have been around for more than 50 years, their growth has been phenomenal over the past 30 years (Southern, Erford, Vernon, & Davis-Gage, 2011). From Alcoholics Anonymous (AA), to codependency groups, to eating disorder and diet groups, to men's and women's groups, to groups for the chronically mentally ill, the kinds of self-help groups that have emerged seem endless. Self-help groups tend to espouse a particular philosophy or way of being in the world and generally attract individuals who share a particular diagnosis, symptom, experience, or condition (Lieberman & Keith, 2002). Their purpose is the education, affirmation, and enhancement of existing strengths of the group members. Generally there is a nonpaid volunteer leader who focuses the discussion and assists in defining the rules of the group (Humphreys, 2004). However, sometimes there may be no leader at all. Self-help groups are generally free or have a nominal fee and can be facilitated by a trained layperson or mental health professional (see Box 6.4).

Self-help groups are not in-depth psychotherapy groups and generally do not require a vast amount of member self-disclosure. In fact, because self-help groups tend to be open groups, which means members may come and go as they please, it is sometimes difficult to build group cohesion, a critical element for in-depth work. Usually, individuals in self-help groups are encouraged to share only the amount that feels comfortable. Some self-help groups even discourage intense self-disclosure, as that would be seen as more appropriate for individual or group counseling.

BOX 6.4 | **Bill Comes to His First AA Group**

Bill is at his first AA meeting. The meeting begins with an introduction by the secretary of the local AA group who makes an announcement that the meeting is "open" and that all new members are welcome. Open meetings are such that anyone can come, as long as he or she follows the rules. The secretary notes that the only requirement for being in AA is the desire to stop drinking. The secretary then opens the meeting with a moment of silence followed by the Serenity Prayer.

> "God, grant me the serenity to accept the things
> I cannot change, courage to change the things
> I can, and the wisdom to know the difference."

After the Serenity Prayer a definition of AA is read. An announcement is then made that invites any members who have had 30 days of sobriety, or are at their first meeting to introduce themselves by their first name. No one is pressured to talk.

Bill stands up and says, "My name is Bill—this is my first meeting." Although nervous, he is glad he is there. Other people introduce themselves and then a member volunteers to read a chapter from the Big Book of AA. This book suggests ways of staying sober and of living in the world as opposed to being preachy. Afterward, the 12 traditions of AA are read. These traditions explain the general rules of AA.

A discussion is then led by the chairperson on ways that people have been successful in staying sober. As the meeting continues, Bill realizes he has found others in a similar situation to his and that he is feeling increasingly comfortable and willing to share more about himself with others. Before he knows it, the group is ending, and a basket is being sent around for donations to continue to support the group. Bill leaves having gained some insight into his disease, some support from others, and with the names of people he can call if he feels like drinking. He has a sense that he will come back to the group.

With self-help groups, the number of group members, length of meeting times, and atmosphere of the group setting can vary considerably. Some groups might have 200 members, while others might be limited to just a few people. Some groups might meet in the basement of a church, while others might meet in the comfort of the office of a counselor who has loaned the group space. Some self-help groups may be ongoing, while others may be time limited; some might demand confidentiality, while others might not.

Self-help groups have become an increasingly important referral source and are often used as an adjunct to the helping process (Klaw & Humphreys, 2004). For these reasons, it has become increasingly important for human service professionals to be aware of the types of self-help groups available in their communities.

Psychoeducational Groups   Psychoeducational groups attempt to increase self-understanding, promote personal and interpersonal growth, and prevent future problems through the dissemination of mental health education in a group setting (Aasheim, 2010; Association for Specialists in Group Work, 2000). In the past, these groups were called **guidance groups,** but in recent years the term psychoeducational groups has become more popular because the word *guidance* has been misconstrued as being too highly advice-oriented, has held negative connotations for people, and has been particularly associated with the schools (Brown, 1998; Gladding, 2008). A few examples of the many topics that psychoeducational groups have focused on include sex education, conflict resolution, AIDS awareness, career awareness, communication skills, diversity issues, chemical dependence, stress management, and lifestyle adjustment.

Compared with self-help groups, psychoeducational groups always have a designated, well-trained group leader, and generally, their purpose is the education and support of the group members. Leaders will usually offer a didactic presentation, and although there is not much in-depth self-disclosure, there may be an opportunity for some sharing of personal information. With their purpose being more educational than psychotherapeutic, the result of this group is to increase members' knowledge. Such groups may be ongoing or can meet for just one session. Psychoeducational groups can vary in their length, and other technical issues can also vary, depending on the focus of the group. Like self-help groups, psychoeducational groups may be free of charge; however, some psychoeducational groups involve a fee (see Box 6.5).

BOX 6.5 | **An AIDS Psychoeducational Group**

Jonathan is a human service professional who works for the local AIDS awareness center. His main job is to visit local schools, businesses, and community centers, and present workshops on how one contracts HIV, current diagnostic procedures for HIV, and treatment of AIDS. His two-hour workshop is information based, and he allows time for questions and self-disclosure when appropriate. When requested, he will extend his presentation for one to four additional meetings. He also provides referrals to AIDS self-help groups and to therapists who work with HIV-positive individuals, their families, and their friends.

Counseling and Therapy Groups As with individual counseling and therapy, many people differentiate a counseling group from a therapy group by the depth of self-disclosure and the amount of personality reconstruction expected during the therapeutic process (Capuzzi & Gross, 2010; Gazda, 1989; Gladding, 2008). However, counseling groups and therapy groups probably have more similarities than differences. For instance, both counseling and therapy groups have a designated, highly trained leader. Generally, there are between 4 and 12 group members. Such groups usually meet for a minimum of eight sessions, and some continue on an ongoing basis.

Most counseling and therapy groups meet at least once a week for 1–3 hours. Confidentiality of the group is critical, and individual members are asked not to reveal information about other members outside the group. Although leadership styles may vary, members usually will have the opportunity to freely express their feelings and to eventually work on behavioral change. Leaders must therefore be equipped to handle clients who might have extreme emotional responses to a group meeting (Jacobs, Masson, & Harvill, 2009). Many of the counseling and therapy approaches noted in Chapter 3 have been adapted for these types of groups (see Box 6.6).

Group Membership Behavior

We all have typical ways of behaving in life. These typical patterns are repeated in groups as they are in our daily interactions with friends and acquaintances. Therefore, groups are often called minilabs of our world, and they give us the opportunity to look at how we present ourselves to others. In addition, they allow us to obtain feedback about our typical ways of interacting. In counseling, therapy, and self-help groups, we will often be given the opportunity to examine these behaviors and work on changing those that we might identify as maladaptive. As members pass through the stages of group development, their typical patterns of behavior will emerge. Some group specialists have identified certain characteristics or roles taken on by members (Gladding, 2003; Vander Kolk, 1990). For instance, some

---

| BOX 6.6 | **William's Therapy Group** |

William has been struggling his whole life with mild depression. When he married 2 years ago, he thought he would feel better. However, after an initial period of being pretty mellow, his depressive feelings again began to emerge. He entered individual counseling and began to work on some of his issues, discovering that he often had expectations that women in his life would bring him happiness. He found that he often relies on them for comfort and nurturing and becomes upset when they do not meet his needs. After some initial gain in self-awareness during individual counseling, his therapist suggested that he might want to enter a mixed (male and female) counseling group to experiment with new ways of relating to women. Although he has found this to be difficult, as he continues to build trust in the group, he is beginning to examine his behaviors more closely and explore new ways of relating.

members may be dominators, mediators, manipulators, caretakers, nurturers, or facilitators, whereas other members may be withdrawn, hostile, blockers, or opinionated. These are just a few of the types of roles members assume. Can you think of others?

As the group process continues, **group membership behaviors** (the roles that members take on) may vary. For example, whereas some members might be withdrawn near the beginning stages of the group, others might become withdrawn at later stages. Whether a member is withdrawn, manipulating, or nurturing, I prefer to not place a value judgment on the behavior. Instead, I view group membership roles as a statement about the individual, a statement about the needs of the group, and a role that can be beneficial or harmful to the group process. For instance, consider the individual who is a great nurturer near the beginning of the group. Such a role may come easily to a particular member of the group and thus be a statement about the member's way of being in the world. Also, the group may need a member to be the nurturer, so the group allows this behavior to emerge so all the members can build a sense of trust. Finally, although such a role can be beneficial as it helps to build group cohesion, it can also be harmful if it is used by group members to avoid focusing on other issues or if the nurturer uses this behavior as a means of avoiding other behaviors (e.g., expressing anger, deep hurts).

Group Leadership Styles

Group leadership styles will vary based on the leader's personality and theoretical orientation, and prior to running the group, a good leader should consider the impact of his or her leadership style on the group (Corey, 2008; Gladding, 2008). For instance, a leader who is more comfortable with a person-centered approach that includes expression of feelings might want to consider whether he or she would be the best person to run a weight loss or bridge phobia group, both of which generally do better with a cognitive–behavioral focus. In addition, good leaders consider the composition of their group and have adjusted their style to the needs of the group members. Finally, research suggests that an effective group leader "will want to be positive, supportive, provide sufficient structure, attend to the development of group cohesion, allow group members to take ownership of their group, and provide a meaningful context for what occurs in the group" (Riva, Wacthel, & Lasky, 2004, p. 45). Others (Corey, 2008) have suggested that good leadership also entails being emotionally present, having personal power and self-confidence, being courageous and willing to take risks, being willing to confront oneself, being sincere and authentic, having an identity or strong sense of self, being enthusiastic and believing in the group process, and being inventive and creative.

Stages of Group Development

The development of a group has been shown to occur in predictable stages (Brabender & Fallon, 2009; Yalom, 2005). Although group experts differ on the terms they use to identify these stages, they tend to describe the characteristics of the stages in fairly consistent ways. One popular series of words, still very much in use today, that describes these stages was developed by Tuckman (1965; Tuckman & Jensen, 1977). Tuckman suggested that the beginning stages have to do with **forming** the group, as members move from a number of separate individuals to the realization that they are together in a group. The group then moves into the **storming** stage as defensiveness and intragroup struggles heighten as members test the waters to see if they can trust one another. Slowly as trust is built, the group moves into the **norming** stage, where the group becomes a cohesive unit. Soon after, the group members are in the **performing** stage, and the members begin to work on their issues. Finally, as members wind down and begin to deal with their feelings about leaving the close-knit relationships they have built in the group, they move into the last stage, **adjourning**. As you read through the following stages I have identified, take particular note of how Tuckman's stages might apply.

The Pregroup Stage (Forming)   Before forming a group, the leader has to decide on a method to prescreen potential group members (ACA, 2005). This pregroup stage can be accomplished in many ways. Some group leaders will have a pregroup meeting attended by all potential members. Other leaders will provide potential members with thorough written or even videotaped descriptions of the expectations of the group in an effort to have potential members screen themselves (see Box 6.7). Members can then give their **informed consent** to these rules or decide that they do not want to participate under such conditions.

Probably the most effective and common screening method is the individual interview. Couch (1995) notes that the interview can accomplish many things, including (1) identifying needs, expectations, and commitment of the potential group member; (2) challenging myths and misconceptions of the potential member; (3) conveying information to and procuring information from the potential member; and (4) screening out (or in) potential members.

The Initial Stage (Forming)   The beginning of a group is often highlighted by anxiety and apprehension by group members (and to a lesser degree, by the group leader). Members are learning about the rules and goals of their group and are wondering whether they can trust the other members.

BOX 6.7 | **Important Rules That Potential Members Should Know Prior to Joining a Group**

1. The limits of confidentiality
2. The limits to socializing and dating outside the group
3. Attendance expectations, including showing up on time and staying the whole time
4. Expectations about self-disclosure
5. Repercussions and limits of physical acting out during group sessions
6. Expectations about topics to discuss
7. Expectations about the responsibility of members to others if a member suspects another member is at danger of harming self or others
8. Any agency rules that might determine specific conduct within the group

During this initial stage, group members are often self-conscious and worried about how others might view them. Because of this initial apprehension and lack of trust, group members will often avoid talking about feelings in depth, and discussions will stick to topics that are relatively "safe." Therefore, it is common for conversations to be superficial, for members to talk about things not related to their lives, and for discussions to revolve around past feelings rather than current feelings. Corey, Corey, and Corey (2010) call this a "self-focus" as compared with an "other focus."

The major task for the group leader in this stage is to define the ground rules and to build trust. In building trust, it is crucial for the leader to have the ability to set limits, to use empathy, and to show unconditional positive regard. As members become comfortable with the ground rules and as they begin to feel at ease with one another, they move on to the next stage of group development.

The Transition Stage (Storming–Norming)   During the early transition stage, group members understand the goals and rules of the group but continue to remain anxious concerning the group process. Issues of control, power, and authority become increasingly important in this stage as members position themselves within the system (Corey et al., 2010; Yalom, 2005). Hostility during this stage can be viewed as a type of resistance that gives members a way to avoid dealing with their issues. The leader needs to be aware of any scapegoating that could occur as one manifestation of this hostility. Although empathy is still crucial, the leader must actively prevent a member from being scapegoated or attacked. Therefore, the leader will often take an active role in preventing coalitions from forming and in preventing verbal attacks on members.

Groups can offer a safe environment in which one can share feelings and gain feedback about self.

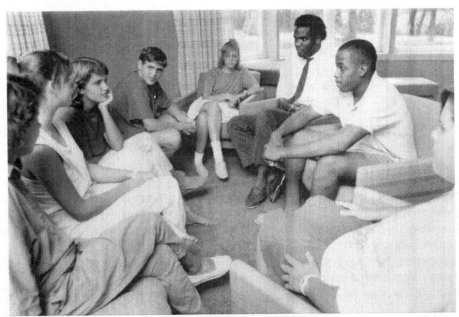

Joel Becker

As this stage continues, group members begin to settle in and can focus more on themselves (Higgs, 1992). This is highlighted by a sense of self-acceptance of the member's life predicaments. Members now demonstrate the ability to take ownership of their feelings, to talk in the here and now, and to not blame others for their problems. This is an important step toward the next stage, which involves actually making change. As members move into this part of the transition stage and begin to take more responsibility for their feelings and actions, the leader's role becomes much easier. No longer is it necessary for the leader to "protect" members, and during this part of the transition stage, the leader can usually relax and let the group develop on its own.

The Work Stage (Performing) As group members gain the capacity to take ownership of their feelings and life predicaments, a deepening of trust and a sense of cohesion emerge within the group (Corey, 2008). Now, group members experience a sense of readiness to work on their identified problems. During this work stage, the group has developed its own homeostasis. Now it is important that the group leader prohibit members from becoming too comfortable in their styles of relating because this can prevent change and growth. Members readily give feedback to other members, and as they identify problem areas, they begin to take an active role in the change process. At this point, members might attempt new ways of communicating, acting, or expressing feelings. The leader can best facilitate movement by asking questions, using problem-solving skills, giving advice, offering alternatives, encouraging feedback by members, and affirming members' attempts at change.

As members accomplish their goals, they begin to gain a sense of heightened self-esteem. This is a product of receiving positive feedback from other members as well as a personal sense of accomplishment for the work that they have done. As members meet their goals, they are near the completion of the group process.

The Closure Stage (Adjourning) As group members reach their identified goals, there is an increased sense of accomplishment and the beginning awareness that the group process is near completion (Corey, 2008; Gladding, 2008). During this closure stage, the leader will often summarize the learning that has taken place and begin to focus on the separation process. Because members typically have shared deep aspects of themselves, a sense of togetherness, cohesion, and warmth has developed. Therefore, saying good-bye can be a difficult process for many, and it is important that the leader facilitate this process in a direct yet gentle fashion. Often this is done by members sharing what they have learned about themselves and one another, expressing feelings toward one another, and defining future goals for themselves. This important final stage in the group process allows members to feel a sense of completion and wholeness about what they have experienced.

In this stage, the leader might actively encourage members to express their feelings concerning the group process as well as their feelings about ending the group. Asking questions and encouraging members to express their feelings might accomplish this. Of course, using empathy to listen to members' feelings regarding the closure of the group is extremely important.

Conclusion Whereas psychoeducational and self-help groups may not pass through all of the stages, or may pass through them with less intensity, there is an expectation that counseling and therapy groups should pass through all these stages to be successful. Since the goals and process are different as a function of the type of group, when conducting groups, expectations of group behavior should be partially based on the type of group being offered.

Individual Counseling Versus Group Counseling

When does one refer a client to group counseling as an alternative or adjunct to individual counseling? With the most current research indicating that group counseling is as effective as individual counseling, some suggest that group work should always be considered as an alternative to individual treatment (Burlingame & Krogel, 2005; Burlingame, MacKenzie, & Strauss, 2004). Although there is no easy method of determining when to use group or individual counseling, a few guidelines might help. For instance, it might be smart to refer to group counseling when:

- A client cannot afford the cost of individual counseling.
- The benefits for a client of individual counseling have gotten so meager that an alternative treatment might offer a new perspective.
- A client's issues are related to interpersonal functioning, and a group might facilitate working through these issues in a real-life manner.
- A client needs the extra social support that a group might offer.
- A client wants to test new behaviors in a system that will support him or her while simultaneously receiving realistic feedback about the new behavior.
- The experiences of others who are working through similar issues can dramatically improve the client's functioning (e.g., alcoholism or depression).

ORGANIZATIONAL AND COMMUNITY SYSTEMS

One way that American culture has tried to equalize the inequities found throughout various communities in our society is to provide social service agencies that offer services to the poor, disabled, and disenfranchised. Many of these agencies offer free or low-cost aid to individuals in need. In almost any community today, we find local, state, and federally supported programs such as mental health centers, shelters for the homeless, vocational rehabilitation, child protective services, Medicare and Medicaid programs, food stamp programs, and Aid to Families with Dependent Children (AFDC). To offer these services effectively, human service professional must understand the intricacies of **organizational systems** and **community systems**. They must know how to work within an organization *and* also be able to effect change from outside of the agency—in the community (Foster-Fishman & Behrens, 2007).

Working Within Agencies

I've worked in enough human service agencies to know they are not always the comfortable, nurturing places we idealize them to be. Sometimes they run well, but sometimes, as in a dysfunctional family, there are problems. A systems perspective offers insight into understanding an agency where you might work. In particular, assessing an agency's boundaries, rules, and hierarchy can go far in deciding whether or not you want to work at an agency and also help you understand the complex dynamics that occur at an agency.

We hope that, like a family, an agency in which a human service professional works is healthy in that it has semipermeable boundaries that allow for open communication, flexibility, and change. Boundaries that are too rigid are indicative of an agency struggling with issues of power and control. Boundaries that are too loose are often a sign that the agency has not yet gotten its act together and needs to formulate rules to help govern itself effectively.

Human service professionals need to understand the unique overt and covert rules of the agency in which they work and, at times, make difficult ethical and moral decisions about whether or not they will follow the rules. In fact, sometimes, the system's rules may be contrary to the ethical guidelines of the human service profession. For instance, a system may have an overt rule stating that any use of illegal substances by a client should be reported to the police. Because this overt rule is contrary to the ethical guidelines of confidentiality, the human service professional may struggle with ways of dealing with this conflict. An example of a covert rule might be an agency that verbally states that it has no dress code, yet looks askance at those professionals who come to work dressed in blue jeans.

Knowing who's in charge is critical if one is to be a "team player" at an agency. For instance, in every agency there is a pecking order, which generally needs to be respected if a person is to survive at the agency. In healthy agencies, this pecking order is of a collaborative nature, where those in charge are willing to listen to others, particularly when "underlings" have opposing points of views. However, hierarchies can also be abusive, such as the supervisor who harasses his or her supervisee.

Sometimes, the human service professional has to decide whether to listen to his or her supervisor or "buck the system." Although rebuking a person in authority can result in the loss of one's job, it is a decision that some professionals will periodically make if they believe there is a moral reason for doing so. Whatever decision is made, you can see how the "wrong" decision can lead to improper treatment of clients, lowering one's liability risk, and relationships issues at work. Of course, it is always important to try and work toward bridging differences:

> When a conflict arises between fulfilling the responsibility to the employer and the responsibility to the client, human service professionals advise both the employer and client of the conflict, and work conjointly with all involved to manage the conflict. (See Ethical Standards of Human Service Professionals, Appendix A, Statement 34)

In short, in healthy agencies there is a clear understanding of the rules, semipermeable boundaries that allow open communication, and respect for the hierarchy because the hierarchy deserves that respect (e.g., an administrator or supervisor who is a strong, knowledgeable, ethical, collaborative, and flexible). If there are, however, problems in the agency, the human service professional has an ethical obligation to work on improving conditions (see Box 6.8):

> Human service professionals participate in efforts to establish and maintain employment conditions which are conducive to higher quality client services. (See Ethical Standards of Human Service Professionals, Appendix A, Statement 33)

| BOX 6.8 | Some True Stories in Agencies and Organizations |

The following are four of a number of true stories I have witnessed over the years. What would you do if you were in any of these situations?

1. A female human service professional is sexually harassed at her internship, and the harasser ends up "stalking her"—following her to her car, and sometimes even following her home. She says little and waits for her placement to end.

2. A human service professional is told by his supervisor that he is doing inferior work. He believes his supervisor is doing inferior supervision. He continues doing what he has been doing with clients. He is fired.

3. A psychiatric aide sexually harasses clients, and the administration covers it up for years. When one of the clients sees a counselor at the agency years later and tells him that she was molested by this aide, the counselor reports it to the new administration. This new administration refuses to act on it, saying she's "making it up."

4. A male faculty member is harassed by a drunk male colleague, with the colleague yelling and screaming and saying: "You'll never make it here, I'll make sure of that." When the faculty member complains to the Dean, it is discovered that the same colleague had "informal" sexual harassment complaints made against him but the women were "too scared" to move forward on them.

Working with the Community to Effect Client Change

> We also know that the social environment has a significant impact on individual behavior and development. Therefore, we must create programs that attend to the development and enhancement of the community and its climate. This will require that substantial attention be given to addressing systemic and environmental issues. (McMillen, 2001, p. 234)

Change tends to spread from the larger system to the smaller system, and often in very complex ways. Thus, if we are to positively impact our clients, we must consider making inroads in the community. A number of strategies for changing the community have been suggested over the years; however, today, it is clear that whatever intervention one makes, it should be undertaken with an attitude of respect and collaboration with community members (Chang, Hays, & Milliken, 2009; Close, 2001; McMillen, 2001). Six steps for implementing community change are as follows:

1. **Accurately Define Your Problem.** A clear understanding of the problem is necessary before one attempts to make change. If a community has a widespread drug problem, one needs to make sure the problem is indeed drugs and not a high unemployment rate.

2. **Collaborate with Community Members.** Before developing strategies for change, it is critical that the agency staff not be seen as a group of "outsiders" pushing their ideas for change on the community. Individuals in the community will have vital ideas about how to develop change strategies that can be incorporated into a broader plan. Human service professionals should keep

informed about current social issues as they affect the client and the community. They need to share that information with clients, groups, and the community as part of their work. (See Ethical Standards of Human Service Professionals, Appendix A, Statement 11)

3. **Respect Community Members**. Human service professionals must not have a "better than" attitude if change is to occur. Only when the professional is seen as respectful of the community, and even a part of the community, can effective change take place:

> Human service professionals need to be knowledgeable about the cultures and communities within which they practice. They should be aware of multiculturalism in society and its impact on the community as well as individuals within the community. They should respect individuals and groups, their cultures and beliefs. (See Ethical Standards of Human Service Professionals, Appendix A, Statement 18)

4. **Collaboratively Develop Strategies for Change**. In consultation with the community, the human service professional should develop strategies for change, make sure these strategies are attainable, and publicize them.

5. **Implement Change Strategies**. The next step is for the human service professional to develop a timeline for implementing the change strategies, and with the help of community members, apply the strategies.

6. **Assess Effectiveness**. In consultation with community members, the human service professional needs to evaluate whether or not the change strategies have had a positive impact on the community. If not, why? And if not, the process should start over.

Unfortunately, human service professionals have been reticent to advocate for changes in systems. If we are to be effective at what we do, assist clients to the best of our ability, and ensure quality services, we must learn how to both work within the system and affect change to broader systems. Regardless of whether you're working with an individual client at an agency or with the community at large, understanding the complexity of systems will help you work effectively toward creating positive change.

ADMINISTRATIVE AND COUNSELING SUPERVISION

Agencies are dramatically impacted by two kinds of supervisors—administrative and counseling. How these individuals carry out their duties reverberates throughout the agency. When supervisors are collaborative, flexible, fair, willing to listen to others, and willing to be leaders and take a stand, then the agency will flourish. On the other hand, when supervisors are dogmatic, mean-spirited, and noncollaborative, there will be discontent at the agency and an increased likelihood of rapid turnover of employers. At times, the roles and functions of the administrative supervisors can be at odds with counseling supervisors, such as the administrator who wants employees to spend less time with clients in an effort to cut costs, and the counseling supervisor who views this as a disservice to clients. However, good supervisors can and do discuss these issues, and they work out their differences in a collaborative fashion. Sometimes, the administrative and counseling supervision are the same person! This can be a difficult position for a supervisor who has to straddle two different roles.

Administrative Supervision

Those who are involved with the administration of an agency are focused on how their leadership will promote the smooth running of the agency. These individuals are often concerned with a number of mundane tasks, such as strategic planning, human resource management (hiring, firing, benefits, etc.), planning and operating programs, developing and maintaining budgets, obtaining grants, ensuring professional development, managing volunteers, lobbying for programs, and addressing legal concerns related to risk management (CSHSE, 2010). Although such administrators may be concerned about the well-being of their employees and the employees' clients, there is another concern which at times takes precedence: the "bottom line" (Kadushin & Harkness, 2002). In other words, will the agency be able to survive, and hopefully thrive, given its budgetary constraints and operating expenses? Thus, those who conduct **administrative supervision** are sometimes found in the position of encouraging tasks that some employees may not like, such as:

- Requesting that employees see more clients to better manage cost
- Developing evaluation techniques that some employees may feel are a "waste of their time," yet provide administrators with needed evidence for funding sources that the agency is meeting its goals
- Suggesting that some employees change their roles and functions
- Encouraging the development of new client services and/or the elimination of older ones
- Suggesting new and "better" ways of case management
- Insisting on some forms of professional development (e.g., substance abuse training, mandated reporting of abuse, affirmative action)

Counseling Supervision

Counseling supervision has been defined as an intensive, extended, and evaluative interpersonal relationship in which a senior member of a profession (1) enhances the professional skills of a junior person, (2) assures quality services to clients, and (3) provides a gatekeeping function for the profession (Bernard & Goodyear, 2009). Whoever the supervisor is, he or she should have obtained knowledge and competency in a number of areas, including the following (ACES, 1990):

1. Counseling skills
2. Ethical and legal issues
3. Nature of the supervisory relationship
4. Knowledge of the developmental nature of helping
5. Case conceptualization
6. Assessment and evaluation of clients
7. Oral and written report writing

8. Current research in counseling
9. Cross-cultural and social justice issues
10. Evaluation of helpers

The supervisor has a number of roles and responsibilities, including assuring the welfare of the client; meeting regularly with their supervisee; assuring that that ethical, legal, and professional standards are being upheld; overseeing the clinical and professional development of the supervisee; and evaluating the supervisee (ACA, 2005, Section F; NOHS, 1996, Appendix A, Statements 4, 5, 21, and 27). Like the effective helper, the good supervisor is empathic, flexible, genuine, open, concerned, supportive, and able to build a strong supervisory alliance; is willing to evaluate the supervisee; and knows appropriate boundaries for supervision (Borders & Brown, 2005; Corey, Haynes, Moulton, & Muratori, 2010).

Counseling supervision is a skill unto itself, and often individuals who are supervisors have taken courses and/or workshops on how to be effective in this role. It is a critical role in an agency as it is the final step to ensuring that clients are treated well and can be the reason why a helper is terminated. Supervisors are also often called on to write recommendations for credentialing boards to attest to a helper's ability. Clearly, counseling supervision is an important aspect of working in an agency.

ETHICAL, PROFESSIONAL, AND LEGAL ISSUES

The System and Confidentiality

Human service professionals have a responsibility to protect the confidentiality of the client, whether information is shared in individual, group, or family counseling.

> Human service professionals protect the client's right to privacy and confidentiality except when such confidentiality would cause harm to the client or others, when agency guidelines state otherwise, or under other stated conditions. (See Ethical Standards of Human Service Professionals, Appendix A, Statement 3)

At the same time, human service professionals have a responsibility to the broader system, as noted in the Ethical Standards of Human Service Professionals:

> Human service professionals understand the complex interaction between individuals, their families, the communities in which they live, and society. (See Ethical Standards of Human Service Professionals, Appendix A, Statement 12)

Therefore, the ethical guidelines recognize the complexity of the system and acknowledge that a person is not an island unto himself or herself. Human service professionals are responsible for being aware of any agency regulations and of laws that could affect their work with clients relative to confidentiality and for making wise decisions when dealing with complex issues related to confidentiality.

Although human service professionals can assure clients that *they* will not break confidentiality except in the situations noted in Chapter 3, they cannot ensure that group or family members will uphold such standards. Therefore, when working with groups or families, stressing that confidentiality be maintained is important. When the human service professional becomes aware that a group or family member has broken confidentiality, appropriate action must be taken. Such action may be simply to discuss the breaking of confidentiality; however, with more extreme cases in a group, a specific action might be taken (e.g., a member may be asked to leave the group). Any such action should be taken after careful reflection and with sensitivity to the client and the group.

In social service systems, client confidentiality also must be maintained. This means that your work with clients should not be discussed with your colleagues unless it is for consultative or supervisory reasons, and in those cases, your consultation must be kept in confidence:

> All consultations between human service professionals are kept confidential unless to do so would result in harm to clients or communities. (See Ethical Standards of Human Service Professionals, Appendix A, Statement 25)

and

> Human service professionals protect the integrity, safety, and security of client records. All written client information that is shared with other professionals, except in the course of professional supervision, must have the client's prior written consent. (See Ethical Standards of Human Service Professionals, Appendix A, Statement 5)

Finally, if human service professionals are sharing information concerning their clients with other mental health professionals, a signed release-of-information form should be obtained from the client before the information is shared. In addition, all client records should be secured so that only employers and supervisors have access to such records.

> Human service professionals protect the integrity, safety, and security of client records. All written client information that is shared with other professionals, except in the course of professional supervision, must have the client's prior written consent. (See Ethical Standards of Human Service Professionals, Appendix A, Statement 5)

Training and Competence

The Ethical Standards of Human Service Professionals states,

> Human service professionals know the limit and scope of their professional knowledge and offer services only within their knowledge and skill base. (See Appendix A, Statement 26)

When working with families or conducting groups, or when working with community members, human service professionals need to know the limits of their professional competence. For instance, although many human service professionals have the training to lead psychoeducational and self-help groups, generally, counseling and therapy groups should be left to more highly trained professionals. Similarly, human service professionals are not trained to do family counseling and family therapy but may offer family guidance as an aspect of the human service professional's job function. In either case, when human service professionals believe that their training is not at the level to work effectively with specific clients, they need to either refer those clients to other mental health professionals, seek out supervision and consultation, or gain additional training (Cogan, 1989; Corey et al., 2010).

Finally, it should be remembered that training can take place outside the classroom setting. Depending on the circumstances, additional training can be gained through workshops or other continuing education activities. Ultimately, human service professionals need to carefully review the helping relationships in which they are working and decide whether their training is adequate for each specific situation.

THE EFFECTIVE HUMAN SERVICE PROFESSIONAL: USING A SYSTEMS APPROACH TO UNDERSTAND THE COMPLEXITY OF INTERRELATIONSHIPS

Effective human service professionals do not view clients in isolation, unaffected by the systems in which they interact but, instead, understand the complexity of the interactions in the clients' world. Effective human service professionals understand that families, groups, and social systems have a large impact on the client. Therefore, they view depression, anxiety, economic deprivation, acting-out behavior, and so forth as symptoms of client problems and as issues related to the systems in which clients interact. Many times, I have seen human service professionals make statements such as, "That client just has no motivation to change; he will do nothing for himself." If one were to take an individualistic view of this client, then such statements may seem to be true. However, human service professionals who view clients as being affected by their systems understand the power such systems have on their clients.

SUMMARY

In this chapter, we examined the complex interactions of systems. We noted that general systems theory states that all systems have regulatory mechanisms that maintain their unique homeostasis. In addition, we learned that all systems have boundaries that can range from being rigid to semipermeable to extremely permeable. In an effort to maintain a system's unique homeostasis, members will act covertly or overtly to maintain the homeostasis of the system. We highlighted the fact that healthy systems change by permitting information to flow into the system and allowing this information to be evaluated by the system.

Relative to couples and families, we listed some key rules related to systems theory that most couples and family counselors adhere to. We then went on to distinguish dysfunctional couples and families from healthy couples and families, highlighting elements related to boundaries, rule making, hierarchies, unfinished business, and scapegoating. We also showed how situational and developmental stress can impact couples and families. We noted that most human service professionals practice couples and family guidance, not couples and family counseling; listed a number of well-known family counseling theories and theorists; and suggested the importance of referring to couples and family counseling when needed.

In addition to the family system, in this chapter we examined groups and noted that as in all systems, groups develop a homeostasis with rules that govern their behavior. We then presented a brief history of the development of group treatment and suggested that crude types of groups started during the 1800s with the purpose of dispensing "moral guidance" but have evolved over the years. We mentioned the role of Jane Addams, Carl Rogers, and Kurt Lewin in the history of groups, and noted that today, the three major categories of groups include self-help groups, psychoeducational groups, and counseling and therapy groups and gave basic descriptions of each.

We next pointed out that each of us has typical ways of behaving in life and that these patterns are repeated in groups as they are in our daily interactions with friends and acquaintances. Therefore, we noted that groups are often called minilabs of our world, and they give us the opportunity to look at how we present ourselves to others. We talked about the importance of good leadership style if a group is to be successful and identified a number of qualities of the good group leader.

We next identified five typical stages of group development including the pregroup stage (forming), the initial stage (forming), the transition stage (storming–norming), the work stage (performing), and the closure stage (adjourning). We noted typical behaviors that occur within each stage and pointed out that leadership styles will vary as a function of the stage of the group. We identified typical patterns of group membership behavior in each stage and some skills that may be helpful for the leader to use in each stage.

The chapter then moved on to a discussion of organizational and community systems. We noted that like families, agencies can be healthy or unhealthy and noted that within a social service agency, the human service professional must have a clear understanding of the boundaries, rules, hierarchy, and information flow within the system. We then suggested six steps for effecting change in the community: accurately defining the problem, collaborating with community members to acquire information, respecting community members, collaboratively developing strategies for change, implementing change strategies, and assessing effectiveness.

The last part of the chapter examined administrative and counseling supervision. We noted that both kinds of supervision have a dramatic affect on the system in which we work and our clients visit and pointed out some of the similarities and differences between the two types of supervision.

As we neared the end of the chapter, we examined ethical and professional issues involving the system and confidentiality and the training and competence of group leaders. We highlighted the importance of protecting confidentiality in systems, exceptions to confidentiality, and the difficulty of ensuring confidentiality when working with systems. Finally, we noted that the effective human service professional can use a systems approach in understanding the complexity of the interrelationships within clients' lives.

Experiential Exercises

I. Reflecting on Your Family of Origin
After reflecting on your family of origin, write responses to the following questions:

1. What roles did your family members take as you were growing up?
2. Do you think your family had rigid boundaries, loose boundaries, or boundaries that allowed for healthy communication?
3. Were there predictable patterns of behavior that you could identify in the various members of your family?
4. What would happen if the behavior of a member in your family deviated from expected patterns?
5. Was there a family member who was scapegoated or an identified patient?

6. How did your family handle conflict?

7. When your family experienced periods of stress, how were they handled?

8. What situational crises did you or members of your family experience? How were they handled?

9. Reflect on the developmental cycles of your family. How were they handled?

II. Developing a Psychoeducational Group Program

Develop an outline of a psychoeducational program on a topic of your choice. Discuss the following issues in the development of your program:

1. The title of the program
2. A brief outline of your program
3. Technical issues related to your program
   a. Number of sessions
   b. Number of clients
   c. Ground rules
   d. Type of meeting place
4. Expected responses of clients as they pass through the group stages of development
5. How you would handle closure of the program
6. Any follow-up you might do

III. Developing a Self-Help Group Program

Using the outline in Exercise II, develop a self-help group program on a topic of your choice.

IV. Working with a Family in Need

Read the following description of a family that sought aid from your agency. Then respond to the questions that follow.

The Family: David, Jan, and their three children have just moved to the area. They made the move because David thought he would have an easier time finding a job. Having left family and friends, they no longer have the support that they had at their prior residence. They noted that, when they first moved, they were living out of their car and then at the "hotel from hell," but they recently moved into a low-income subsidized housing project. David is an unemployed construction worker, and Jan works part time at a local convenience store. David is 28, and Jan is 29. They have been married for 10 years. Jan states that David "sometimes drinks too much"; David denies this.

David states that Jan has "gotten too fat"; Jan admits having gained some weight but states, "David should love me anyway." During your meeting with them, you find that they often argue with each other about work, the children, and Jan's weight. Mark, the oldest child, is 11 and has been autistic and unable to form relationships since birth. Jan and David have received disability payments for him in the past and previously placed him in a residential treatment center. They are unsure about how to care for him now that they have moved. Jordan, who is 9 years old, has had behavioral problems in school and has been involved in some vandalism in his neighborhood. Jan thinks he may be "drug running" for some of the older kids in the neighborhood. Jordan is entering the third grade (he was held back one year at his previous school). David and Jan are do not know how to register Jordan in his new school. In fact, they're not sure where his new school is located. They describe their youngest child, Jessica, as "their gem." She is 6 years old and entering the first grade. They state that she is the only one who has not caused them problems.

As you work with this family, respond to the following questions:

1. Do you think this family's boundaries are healthy (not too rigid or too loose)?
2. Do you think any member(s) of this family is (are) being scapegoated?
3. Is there an identified patient in this family?
4. What helping skills would you need to have in order to work effectively with this family?
5. How would you diagnose the problem areas in this family?
6. What needs does this family have?
7. What goals would you help the family set for itself?
8. What referrals would be appropriate for this family?
9. What type of follow-up would you want to do?

V. Working with an Individual in Need

Read the following description of an individual who sought aid from your agency. Then respond to the questions that follow.

Alice: Alice is a 16-year-old single female who is three months pregnant. She seeks your advice concerning her pregnancy. She lives with her parents and her 15-year-old sister. She has not told her parents about the pregnancy and is concerned that they will find out before long. Her family has little money, and she is concerned about paying for the pregnancy and birth. Her parents do not have medical insurance.

Alice has come to your agency because she is depressed and feels at the "end of her rope." She is looking for help. When you meet with her, she sobs throughout the interview and at times seems to whine. Alice's father, Arnold, who is 34 years old, is a part-time truck driver. Alice states that he has rigid views and tends to be rather "authoritarian." She also thinks that he will "lose it" if he learns she is pregnant and will want to "take care of the situation" to make it go away. Although he has not abused her in the past 2 years, Alice says that when she was younger, he would often "take a belt to me." At times, he drinks too much, and there seem to be conflicts between him and his wife. He was married at age 18.

Alice states that her mother "cares a lot about me"; however, Alice also notes that her mother would never go against her father's wishes. Alice's mother, Linda, is 35 years old, works part time at a fast-food restaurant, and is very concerned about her daughter's well-being. Because her parents were married when her mother was pregnant with Alice, Alice thinks that her mother will probably understand her situation.

Joan is Alice's 15-year-old sister. Alice states that Joan is a good student but at times acts like a "wise-ass." She feels as if Joan has always received all the attention in the family; now that Alice is pregnant, she is concerned that she will be even more of an outcast. Alice notes that Joan has many friends and is often out of the house, doing things rather than staying home with her "drunk dad" and her mom.

As you work with Alice, respond to the following questions:

1. What helping skills would you need to use in order to work effectively with Alice?
2. How would you diagnose Alice's problems?
3. What needs does Alice have?
4. What goals would you help Alice set for herself?
5. What referrals would be appropriate for Alice?
6. Would you consider a referral for family counseling or family guidance for Alice and her family?
7. Do you think this family's boundaries are healthy (not too rigid or too loose)?
8. Do you think any member(s) of this family is (are) being scapegoated?
9. Is there an identified patient in this family?
10. Would you consider a referral to a group for Alice?
11. If you were to consider a referral to a group for Alice, what type of group might you consider? Why?
12. What type of follow-up would you want to do?

VI. Wearing Labels

Using the following phrases or other terms your instructor lists, do the following exercise in class. Have the instructor cut out the phrases and tape one on each student's forehead (students should not know which phrase they have on their foreheads). Then find an open space and "mill around," responding to one another based on the phrase an individual has on his or her forehead. After a few minutes, sit in a large circle and, without removing the phrase, discuss your response to how people interacted with you.

Look at me intensely.	Walk away from me.
Tell me you like what I'm wearing.	Look at my shoes.
Frown at me.	Act as if I don't exist.
Be loving toward me.	Yell at me when I speak.
Speak softly to me.	Be angry at me.
Look at my stomach.	Treat me humanely.
Touch me when you talk to me.	Act disgusted toward me.
Be nice to me.	Disagree with anything I say.
Be rude to me.	Reflect back anything I say.
Talk to me but don't listen to me. Treat me like an object when talking.	Act as if you like me even though you don't.

After you have finished the exercise, discuss the following questions:

1. What's it like being labeled?
2. Do we all wear labels as we go through life? (Are there certain personality characteristics that we tend to exhibit?)

3. If we do exhibit certain personality characteristics, is it possible that we create other people's responses to us by the personality characteristics that we exhibit?

4. How can the group process help us understand the labels (personality characteristics) that we tend to exhibit?

VII. A Detailed Examination of an Agency

To fully understand the nature of an agency system, a thorough review of its policies and practices is needed. Using the following guidelines, you and a partner pick a social service agency and interview someone who can respond to the items. Write down the individual's responses and compare agencies in class.

1. What is the name of the agency?
2. What is the agency's address?
3. How many total staff members does the agency have?
4. How many administrative staff are there, and what are their roles?
5. What are the approximate salaries of administrative staff?
6. How many direct-service personnel (mental health professionals who work with clients) are there?
7. What are the types of direct-service personnel (e.g., mental health aides, therapists, supervisors, program coordinators, group leaders, family counselors)?
8. What degrees are held by direct-service personnel?
9. What are the approximate salaries of direct-service personnel?
10. What are the number and type of support staff (e.g., secretaries, clerical staff)?
11. Is this a private or a public agency?
12. Where does the agency get its funding?
13. Does the agency have a policy and practices statement (a written statement that explains the functions of the agency and the roles of the staff)?
14. Who are the clients of this agency?
15. How does the agency obtain its clients?
16. What happens when a client initially contacts this agency?
17. Is there a process in which client problems are diagnosed, client needs are assessed, goals are established, referrals are made, and follow-up is accomplished?
18. How do clients pay for services?
19. What types of counseling or assistance take place at this agency (e.g., individual, group, family)?
20. How long are typical counseling/interviewing sessions?
21. What kind of paperwork do the direct-service personnel have to fill out?
22. How many hours, days, weeks, months, or years would a typical client spend at this agency?
23. How are services for the typical client terminated?
24. How does the agency evaluate itself?
25. Does a staff development effort take place at the agency (e.g., in-house workshops, guest speakers, monetary support for conferences)?

26. How does the agency deal with ethical concerns related to confidentiality, counselor training, and competence?

27. Does the policy and practices statement of the agency match what is actually going on within the agency?

VIII. Ethical and Professional Vignettes

Reflect on the following vignettes and then share your thoughts in class. You may want to refer to the NOHS Ethical Standards in Appendix A.

1. Before meeting with a family for a family guidance session, a human service professional gives the parents a written document explaining the limitations of confidentiality and the general direction the session will take. After reading this informed consent document, the parents sign it and bring the family in. The informed consent document is not given to or described to the children. Has the helper acted ethically? Professionally?

2. You are seeing a family in family guidance when you realize the father is extremely depressed, perhaps suicidally so. You decide to refer him for individual counseling. Is this ethical? Is this the professional thing to do? Is this a wise thing to do?

3. In deciding on how to act on an ethical concern with a family, a human service professional notices that the code of ethics of the American Association for Marriage and Family Therapy (AAMFT) handles the situation differently from the Ethical Standards of Human Service Professionals. The human service professional decides to go with the code of ethics that best matches her view of the situation. Is this ethical? Is this the professional thing to do?

4. You are aware of a human service professional who is practicing family counseling even though she doesn't have advanced training in this area. Is this ethical? Professional? Legal? What, if anything, should you do?

5. A few months after working with a family on some parenting issues, you are subpoenaed to testify against one of the spouses. You believe she has major unresolved issues from her family of origin. Is it ethical to testify? Is this professional? Legal?

6. While running a psychoeducational group for substance abusers, you realize that a couple of the members of the group are using illegal substances. What should you do?

7. After setting a ground rule that group members cannot date, a group leader finds that two members of a group are seeing each other. He immediately throws them out of the group. Is this ethical? Is this professional?

8. Despite the fact that a group leader stresses the importance of confidentiality, the leader discovers that some intimate information about a group member has been "leaked" by another member. The group member asks who in the group broke confidentiality, and no one answers. Therefore, the leader decides to meet individually with each member in an attempt to find out who broke confidentiality. Is this ethical? Professional? Do you have other ideas about what the leader should do?

9. A group member shares that he has committed a robbery. Subsequently, the police arrest him, and the group leader is subpoenaed to court to testify to what she heard in the group. Can she be forced to testify?

10. When you are running a psychoeducational group on safe sex, a 16-year-old member of the group reveals that he committed a date rape when out with a "friend." The human service professional does not act on this knowledge because he wants to protect the confidentiality of the student. Is this ethical? Professional? Legal?

11. A human service professional decides to run a short-term group for at-risk students. While running the group, some of the girls ask him where they can get information on birth control. He gives them the phone number and address of the local Planned Parenthood agency. Is this ethical? Legal?

12. After learning that a girl in a teen responsibility group is pregnant and wants to have an abortion, a group leader encourages the girl to consider keeping the child or adopting it out. Most of the group members concur, and the group leader gets them to promise that they will support her. Is this ethical? Professional? Legal?

13. The director of the agency in which you work tells all employees to report any client who is using illegal substances to the police. Can the director do this? Is this ethical? Professional? What, if anything, should you do?

14. After working at an agency for a few months, you realize that there are many breaches of confidentiality. What, if anything, should you do?

15. After working at an agency for a few months, you realize that many of your co-workers tend to make fun of their clients during break. What, if anything, should you do?

16. Your agency is meeting with individuals from the community to discuss a proposal to offer an HIV prevention program at a number of after-school programs. An irate member of the community accuses you of promoting sexual promiscuity and endorsing the use of condoms even though you didn't mention any specifics of the program. You then ask the rest of the individuals at the meeting to raise their hands if they had heard you promoting these values. Is this ethical? Is this professional? Was this the best way to respond? What are some other ways you could have responded?

Diversity, Cultural Competence, and Social Justice

CHAPTER CONTENTS

You scorn us, you imitate us, you blame us, you indulge us, you throw up your hands, you tell us you have all the answers—now shut up and listen. (Lamar, 1992, p. 90)

Growing up in New York was a world unto itself—the ethnic foods, the multicultured music, the people; oh, how I loved to watch the people. Walk down a Manhattan street and you could watch a sea of endless people, a sea that seemed to change color as it flowed by you. A sea whose shape transformed constantly, and if you flowed with it long enough, you could visit every part of the world. Unquestionably, New York gave me a multicultural perspective that many people don't have an opportunity to obtain. However, despite this exposure to a variety of cultures and ethnic groups, I really never got "below the surface." I could taste the foods, I could see the people, and I could listen to the music, but that experience alone was still from a detached perspective. Even though I might see the brightly colored clothes of a Nigerian, I still didn't know that person. Even though I could taste the sushi, I didn't understand the world of the Japanese. And even though I could listen to the Latino music, I didn't really understand the people.

When I lived in New Hampshire, I learned to adapt. No longer would I be this brash New Yorker. I mellowed. New Hampshire's population has a very large percentage of Catholics. My friend John, a priest at the Catholic college at which I worked, would often tell me that some of the nuns thought I was on the verge of a conversion. They saw me as searching. Maybe I was... a little, but not enough to convert to another religion. These nuns could not understand how a person with my values could not be more religious. They didn't really know me. Perhaps, if they had taken the time to find out who I was, they could have understood me better.

From New Hampshire, I moved to Norfolk, Virginia, from an area that was mostly Catholic to a part of the country that had many fundamentalist Christians. I found that a small minority of these fundamentalist Christians would confront me on my religious orientation. For instance, one day I was eating lunch with a friend and a friend of hers. As my friend momentarily got up from the table, her friend slowly reached into her purse, pulled out some flyers, and placed them in front of me without saying a word. I looked down and was aghast to see that they were "Jews for Jesus" flyers. I said to her, "Are you trying to tell me something?" She responded that perhaps I would be interested in this. I felt intruded upon. I felt disrespected. Not unlike the nuns in New Hampshire, here was another person trying to place her values on me. If she had tried to talk with me, tried to understand me, tried to have a conversation regarding different approaches to religion, I would have talked with her.

At my current university, a friend of mine had a colleague who was increasingly losing weight and growing his hair longer. I asked him if he was "okay," and he always came up with some minor medical reason why he was losing weight. One day, out of the blue, it came to me—he was preparing his body for sex change therapy. He was becoming a woman. I must admit that I was very surprised, and it took me a while to understand that he, in many ways, was always a she, and was becoming congruent with how she saw herself. She is now content working at another university.

As you can see, diversity issues have permeated my life, as it does in all of our lives. And, for the human service professional, issues related to diversity and being a culturally competent helper are critical. Thus, in this chapter, we will first describe some of the diversity in the United States and in the world. Then, we will offer eight reasons why human services professionals need to become culturally competent helpers. Next, we will provide you with some definitions of culturally competent helping which will be followed by a model of social justice work, an important aspect of culturally competent helping. Definitions of a variety of words and terms related to culturally competent helping will follow, and this chapter will highlight varying aspects of the human services professional's ethical code that focus on culturally competent helping. This chapter will conclude by suggesting that becoming an effective culturally competent helper is a developmental process that occurs throughout one's career.

CULTURAL DIVERSITY IN THE UNITED STATES AND THE WORLD

America is the most diverse country in the world—a country that is truly a conglomerate of ethnic groups, races, cultures, and religions (see Table 7.1). In addition to the data in Table 7.1, some additional select groups include nearly 58 million people (26.2%) who have a diagnosable mental disorder (National Institute of Mental Health, 2008), 54 million Americans (19%) age 5 or older who have a disability (U.S. Census Bureau Commerce, 2008a), about 40 million people (13%) who are over 65 (U.S. Department of Health and Human Services, 2011), about 700,000 people who are homeless (National Coalition for the Homeless, 2009), 44 million people (14.3%) who are poor (U.S. Census Bureau, 2010a), and over 1 million people who are HIV-positive (Centers for Disease Control and prevention, 2010). We are truly a diverse nation, and thus human service professionals are called to offer services to individuals from many diverse backgrounds.

As can be seen in Figures 7.1 and 7.2, the world, too, is a diverse place. Sometimes, when we become sheltered within our communities or become focused on our own country, we lose sight of the great diversity that exists on this planet. As we become increasingly more worldly, not only will we have to acknowledge diversity within our country, but we will also have to understand the diversity that exists on this place we call earth.

THE NEED FOR CULTURAL COMPETENCE

Diversity challenges human service professionals to do good work with *all* clients by embracing **cultural competence** and **cross-cultural sensitivity**. Unfortunately, this is often not the case as clients from diverse cultures are frequently misunderstood, often misdiagnosed, sometimes spoken down to and other times patronized, have the impact of negative social forces minimized by the helper, find the helping relationship less helpful, seek mental health services at lower rates, and terminate helping relationships earlier (Buckley & Franklin-Jackson, 2005; Constantine & Sue, 2005; Evans, Delphin, Simmons, Omar, & Tebes, 2005; Neukrug & Milliken, 2008; Sewell, 2009; U.S. Department of Health and Human Services, 2001). It should not be surprising that many clients from nondominant groups are distrustful of helpers, are confused about the helping process, or feel worlds apart from their helper. Why is the helping relationship unappealing to so many clients from nondominant groups? Oftentimes it is helper incompetence because the helper holds one or more of the following viewpoints (Buckley & Franklin-Jackson, 2005; Constantine & Sue, 2005; McAuliffe, Gómez, & Grothaus, 2008; Sue & Sue, 2008; Suzuki, Kugler, & Aguiar, 2005):

1. *The melting pot myth.* Some helpers view the United States as a **melting pot** when in actuality American society is more of a **cultural mosaic**. These human service professionals are less likely to honor their clients' unique cultural heritage.
   Example: The helper who challenges a client to move to a "better" ("Whiter") community because she believes the client's children will gain a better education. This "advice" ignores the client's comfort level in his own community.

Table 7.1 | Number and Percentage of Individuals from Select Racial, Ethnic, Religious, and Sexual Identity Backgrounds in the United States

Ethnicity/Race*	Number (in Millions)	Percentage	Religion**	Number (in Millions)	Percentage
White	199.8	65.1	Christian	173	76.0
Hispanic	48.4	15.8	Christian (non-Catholic)	116	50.9
Black or African-American	41.8	13.6	Catholic	57	25.1
Asian	16.0	4.3	Select religions (Christian and non-Christian)		
American Indian and Alaska Native (AIAN)	5.0	1.6	Baptist	36	15.8
			Christian Generic	32	14.2
Native Hawaiian and other Pacific Islander (NHPI)	1.1	<1	Mainline Christians (Methodist, Lutheran, Episcopalian, United Church of Christ)	29	12.9
Two or more races	5.4	1.7	Pentecostal	7.9	3.5
			Mormon	3.2	1.4
			Jewish	2.7	1.2
			Eastern religions (e.g., Buddhist)	2.0	.9
SEXUAL ORIENTATION[†]			Muslim	1.3	.6
Gay		2.8	Other		
Lesbian		4.8	Atheist/Agnostic	3.5	1.6
Gay, lesbian, or bisexual		4.9	None	34	15.0

*Figures from U.S. Census Bureau (2009a). Hispanics are treated as one group, and they identify as 92% White, 4% African-American, 1.6% AIAN, 1.5% two races, 0.6% Asian, and 0.3% NHPI. Group members may identify with more than one race. Thus, the groups add up to more than the total population of the United States. Whites listed are non-Hispanic. White, including White Hispanic, equals 84% of the population.

**From Kosmin, B. A., & Keysar, A. (2008). Number of Jews is based on religious identification and is a smaller number than those who identify as Jewish. The number of Muslims is probably much higher, as many mosques do not officially affiliate as a religious demonization.

[†]Gay and lesbian figures are based on the percentage of individuals, between the ages of 18 and 44, who reported being "only" or "mostly" attracted to the same sex. Gay, lesbian, or bisexual figure includes those who had same sex activity within 1 year (Centers for Disease Control and Prevention, 2011b).

2. *Incongruent expectations about the helping relationship.* The helping relationship tends to be based on Western values and consequently stresses the importance of expression of feelings, self-disclosure, cause-and-effect thinking, "open-mindedness," and internal locus of control. A helpee who does not

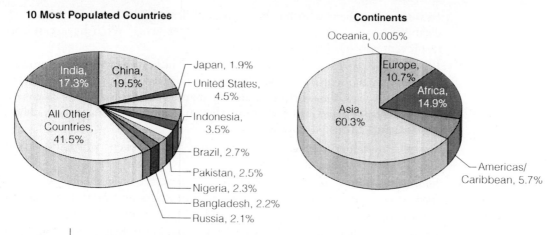

Figure 7.1 | Ten Most Populated Countries of the World and Population of the Continents

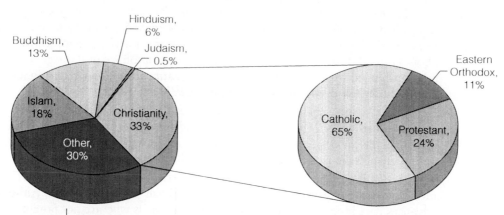

Figure 7.2 | Percentage of Select Religions from Around the World

embrace these characteristics might be viewed as resistant or pathological and feel disappointed, angry, or guilty when he or she does not live up to the helper's expectations.

Example: The helper who does not realize that many Asian clients pride themselves in their ability to restrict their emotions, pushes an Asian client to express her feelings. The Asian client ends up leaving the helping relationship and feels like she has disappointed her helper.

3. *De-emphasizing social forces.* Some helpers attribute most problems to internal conflicts and de-emphasize environmental issues. By de-emphasizing social forces, human service professionals are likely to have a difficult time building a relationship with a client who has been considerably harmed by external factors.

Example: The client who has been illegally denied jobs because of his disability becomes discouraged when the helper says, "What have you done to prevent yourself from obtaining a job?"

4. *Ethnocentric worldview.* Culturally incompetent helpers who are **ethnocentric** tend to view the world through the lens of their own culture. They falsely assume clients view the world in a similar manner to themselves or believe that when clients present a differing view, they are emotionally disturbed, culturally brainwashed, or just simply wrong.

Example: A helper inadvertently turns off a Muslim client when she says to her: "Have a wonderful Christmas."

5. *Ignorance of one's own racist attitudes and prejudices.* The helper who has not spent time examining his or her own racist attitudes and prejudices will unconsciously project negative and harmful attitudes onto clients.

Example: The heterosexual helper who unconsciously believes that being gay is a disease but consciously states he is accepting of all sexual orientations tells an antigay joke to a colleague. The colleague, who is heterosexual but "gay friendly," walks out of his office angry and upset.

6. *Inability to understand cultural differences in the expression of symptomatology.* What may be seen as "abnormal" in the United States may be considered usual in another culture. The human service professional's lack of knowledge about cultural differences in the expression of symptoms can damage a helping relationship and result in misdiagnosis, mistreatment, and early termination of culturally diverse clients from the helping relationship.

Example: A Latina client describes a series of bodily complaints (somatic problems) to her helper. The helper assumes that the client is a hypochondriac. In actuality, the client's mother had recently passed away, and like many Latino/Latina clients, she is dealing with her grief through somatizations.

7. *The unreliability of assessment and research procedures.* Over the years, assessment and research instruments have been notoriously culturally biased. Although advances have been made, human service professionals who are not familiar with these biases may utilize instruments that may be inappropriate for certain clients or make assumptions about test results and research results that may be incorrect.

Example: A helper encourages a child to take a self-esteem inventory, not realizing that the instrument was normed on a sample of White children and that children of color often score lower on it. In actuality, they don't have lower self-esteem; they simply interpret the questions differently.

8. *Institutional racism.* Because **institutional racism** is embedded in society, and some would argue, even within the professional organizations, materials used by human service professionals may be biased, and helpers will unknowingly have a skewed understanding of culturally different clients.

Example: A human service program has a very large percentage of White students in it. Students of color are wary of applying to it because all of their recruiting materials show White students in the pictures.

In summary, the eight reasons that the helping relationship does not always work for clients from diverse cultures are (1) the melting pot myth, (2) incongruent expectations about the helping relationship, (3) de-emphasizing social forces, (4) ethnocentric worldview, (5) ignorance of one's own racist attitudes and prejudices, (6) inability to understand cultural differences in the expression of symptomatology, (7) unreliability of assessment and research instruments, and (8) institutional racism.

DEFINING CULTURALLY COMPETENT HELPING

Having looked at common reasons why some helpers are *not* culturally competent, let's now define **culturally competent helping.** One definition by McAuliffe (2008) suggests that the culturally competent helper has "a consistent readiness to identify the cultural dimensions of clients' lives and a subsequent integration of culture into counseling work" (p. 5). Such helpers are willing and ready to examine the lives of their clients, learn about the uniqueness of their clients' cultures, and make the effort to find the necessary skills that would most effectively work with clients from different cultures. Another definition by Sue and Torino (2005) suggests that culturally competent helping

> can be defined as both a helping role and process that uses modalities and defines goals consistent with the life experiences and cultural values of clients, utilizes universal and culture-specific helping strategies and roles, recognizes client identities to include individual, group, and universal dimensions, and balances the importance of individualism and collectivism in the assessment diagnosis and treatment of client and client systems. (p. 6)

Sue and Torino's definition, shown in Figure 7.3, suggests that helpers should understand both culture-specific skills and universal skills when working with clients from nondominant groups. This means that some skills will be effective with all clients, while some skills will be effective only with certain clients, as a function of their culture. Knowing the difference and when and how to use these skills is essential. They go on to suggest that the helper should consider three aspects of the client's

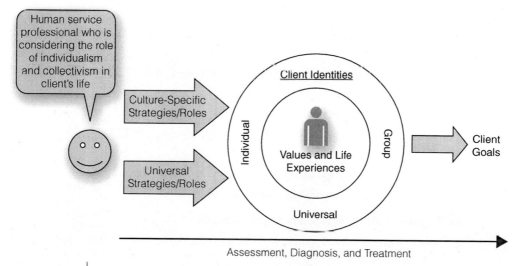

Figure 7.3 | Sue and Torino's Definition of Multicultural Counseling and Helping

life; they call the client's identities. First, the helper should understand that he or she has unique issues and concerns (individual identity). Second, they propose that all clients have a cultural background that impacts them and partially defines their problems and concerns (the group identity). Third, the helper should recognize that as humans, we all share common experiences (the universal identity). In assessing and helping the client, Sue and Torino suggest that the culturally competent helper determines if the client relies more on an **individualistic perspective** (focus more on self) or a **collective perspective** (focuses more on community) and then works to understand the client's identities in order to set goals for the helping relationship.

SOCIAL JUSTICE WORK

> Working towards the liberation of society's most vulnerable, marginalized, and discarded people—not on a one person crusade of charity, but *with* the people, seeking justice together—is ... the historical vocation of human beings. For the human service professional, it is a privilege and a gift. (Marchand, 2010, pp. 43–53)

In recent years, it has become clear that working for **social justice** is a critical part of the cross-cultural helping relationship and of the human service professional's work in general (Marchand, 2010; Pieterse, Evans, Butner, Colins, & Mason, 2009). Whereas culturally competent helping has traditionally been seen as a face-to-face meeting with a client, social justice work broadens culturally competent helping by including a wide range of activities that affect the client's broader system in some profound manner and ultimately creates a better life for the client. One framework to view social justice work is **advocacy** (Wark, 2008). Recent **advocacy competencies** provide a mechanism for human service professionals to understand their work on social justice issues.

The advocacy competencies encompass three domains: the client, community, and public. Each of these domains is divided into two levels that include a focus on whether the helper is "acting on behalf" of the domain or is "acting with" the domain (see Figure 7.4). For instance, within the client domain, a helper might

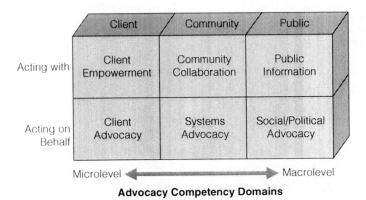

Advocacy Competency Domains

Figure 7.4 | Advocacy Competencies

Source: Adapted from: Toporek, R. L., & Lewis, J. A., & Crethar, H. C. (2009). Promoting systemic change through the ACA advocacy competencies. *Journal of Counseling and Development, 87,* p. 267.

"act with" a client to help him or her identify strengths and resources, so that he or she can feel empowered and advocate for himself or herself; *or*, the helper might "act on behalf" of the client by finding and contacting needed services. The competencies run from the *microlevel* (focus on client) to the *macrolevel* (focus on system). The following offers examples of each of the competencies and how you, as a human service professional, might implement them.

Acting with the Client, Community, and Public

Client Empowerment: Through the helping relationship, the helper assists the client in identifying external barriers that are impeding growth and offers skills to the client, so the client is empowered to make specific changes in his or her life.

Example: A client who is being sexually harassed at work is taught assertiveness skills and shown how to file a complaint at the Equal Employment Office where she works.

Community Collaboration: Helpers are often aware of issues within the community and can identify concerns that specific agencies and organizations might be interested in working on collaboratively. As a result of their knowledge and efforts, helpers can bring together agencies and organizations to work toward common goals.

Example: A human service professional at a homeless shelter collaborates with local churches, mosques, and synagogues to develop a "shelter system" during the winter months where homeless individuals can stay. The churches, synagogues, and mosques each take a week offering shelter and food for the homeless. They also jointly seek funding from local governments for their work.

Public Information: Due to the human service professionals' knowledge of how environmental factors can deleteriously affect people, they have a unique ability to inform the public about issues that have far reaching affects. In some cases, they may reach out to the public, communicate their concerns, and work with the public toward making change.

Example: Recognizing that many individuals returning from war, as well as their family members, have unique mental health concerns, a human service program places an ad in the local newspaper, inviting the public who have been affected by this issue to work on the passage of a statewide bill that will provide free mental health for war veterans and their families.

Acting on Behalf of the Client, Community, and Public

Client Advocacy: Because human service professionals work with clients who are frequently faced with external barriers to growth, they are in a unique position to advocate for client services that will reduce these barriers.

Example: In working with a mother and her daughter at the city social services office, the human service professional learns that the ten-year-old girl is suspected of having a learning disability. The mother and daughter had been homeless, but they have recently found housing, and the girl is attending the local public school. The school has procrastinated on having the girl testing for a learning disability. Realizing that the law states that the school must test the girl within 60 days, the human service professional calls the principal and advocates for the testing, citing the law.

Systems Advocacy: Human services professionals have an understanding of system wide barriers that negatively impact clients and can develop a plan for eliminating such barriers through social action and political power.

Example: A human service educator realizes that the university in which she works has not replaced curbs with ramps for individuals with disabilities. Realizing the illegality of the nonaction, the human service professional contacts the vice-president for building and physical management who was unaware of the law. He immediately suggests a committee look into it further and devises an action plan for change.

Social/Political Advocacy: Human service professionals are sensitive to the concerns of nondominant groups and, when they recognize that a particular group is being discriminated against, will take action to eliminate such discrimination.

Example: Concerned that gay, lesbian, bisexual, and transgendered (GLBT) individuals are being discriminated at the workplace, a human service professional joins the local GLBT action committee to work toward passing a federal law against such discrimination (see Box 7.1).

BOX 7.1 | **Scott King**

Forty-five-year-old Scott was born the eldest of four children in a small town in Maine. He remembers his early years as being almost a stereotype of the early 1960s American family: His father worked, and his mother stayed at home and raised the children. Scott remembers being raised with the expectation that he would grow up, get married, and have children. He was not aware of any individuals who were gay or lesbian when he grew up.

After graduating from high school, Scott attended Bates College, a liberal arts school where the world outside Maine made its first impact. Although for years he had realized that he found men much more attractive than women, he dated the opposite gender mainly because that was the only option that he felt was possible. Soon after college, he began graduate school and for the first time started to realize there was a gay community out there. During a summer job in Texas, he began to come to terms with his own homosexuality and in the process left graduate school and decided to start living what he saw as a more truthful life. Shortly after his coming out, Scott met and moved in with the man who would become his partner for 15 years, Lee. Scott subsequently began working in international student services and has remained in this profession for almost 20 years.

Being in an openly gay relationship caused difficulties and was a significant factor in Scott's departure from jobs at three universities. Although no supervisor ever directly raised the issue of sexual orientation, some supervisors created an uncomfortable atmosphere that made work unpleasant. In 1991, Scott accepted a university job in Virginia, a decision that was to some extent made because of the school's inclusion of sexual orientation in its antidiscrimination statement. During the first year at the university, he was, for the first time, fully open about his sexual orientation and took leadership positions in gay/lesbian/bisexual issues on campus. In 1992, Lee died of AIDS, and the support provided by the campus community cemented Scott's desire to work toward equality for gay, lesbian, and bisexual people.

Recognized as a leader within the Association of International Educators, Scott founded a gay/lesbian/bisexual caucus and led that for the first two years of its existence. In addition, Scott advises the campus gay/lesbian/bisexual student organization, has taken leadership within the local gay/lesbian/bisexual community through such activities as cochairing the annual Pride festival and chairing the area chapter of the gay/lesbian/bisexual ministry of the Episcopal Church. Scott King is a true leader who happens to be gay.

IMPORTANT DEFINITIONS

The culturally competent helper is familiar with a wide range of diversity issues and understands basic definitions of words and terms that give them a common framework within which to communicate. Thus, the following offers basic definitions of culture; prejudice, stereotypes, and racism; discrimination and microaggressions; ethnicity; minority and nondominant group; power differentials; race; religion and spirituality; sexism, heterosexism, and sexual prejudice; and social class ("class"). We'll conclude this section with a short piece about political correctness relative to when one should use which words and terms.

Culture

Shared values, symbols, language, and *ways of being in the world* are some of the words and phrases I think of when reflecting on the word **culture**. Culture is expressed through common values, habits, norms of behavior, symbols, artifacts, language, and customs (McAuliffe, 2008; Sewell, 2009; Spillman, 2007). For instance, despite great diversity in the United States, most Americans share a similar cultural heritage because there is a shared language, symbols that most of us recognize, and patterns of behavior with which most are familiar. Traveling throughout this country we find many symbols of a common culture (e.g., fast-food restaurants, music, laws, basic values, shared language). Yet, even as I acknowledge this common culture, I am acutely aware of the bicultural, or even tricultural nature of many individuals in the United States. For instance, there are those who share the culture of urban gays and lesbians; of their racial, ethnic, and religious groups; of their gender; and of their region (e.g., "the South"). Whitfield, McGrath, and Coleman (1992) suggest considering 11 elements that can be used in helping to understand specific cultural patterns. For instance, they suggest that helpers should understand how each cultural group:

- Defines its sense of self
- Dresses and values appearances
- Embraces specific beliefs and attitudes
- Relates to family and significant others
- Plays and makes use of leisure time
- Learns and uses knowledge
- Communicates and uses language
- Embraces certain values and mores
- Uses time and space
- Eats and uses food in its customs
- Works and applies itself

Prejudice, Stereotypes, and Racism

Generalizing, falsehoods, irrational fears, and *anger* are what I think of when I consider the terms **prejudice**, **stereotypes**, and **racism**. Generally, all three of these words are related to preconceived ideas or attitudes people have toward others. Whereas prejudice has to do with judging a person or a group based on preconceived notions about the group (e.g., gays are no good; therefore, I hate John because he's gay), stereotypes are rigidly held beliefs that most or all members of a group share certain characteristics, behaviors, or beliefs (e.g., Asians are intelligent people, American Indians are alcoholics) (Jennings, 2007; Lum, 2004). Racism is a specific belief that one race is superior to another (e.g., Whites are better than Blacks) and is considered a social construction that leads to prejudice, stereotyping, discrimination, and microaggressions (McAuliffe et al., 2008).

Discrimination and Microaggression

Active, harmful, conscious and *unconscious acting out* are what I think of when I reflect on **discrimination** and **microaggressions**. Whereas the words *stereotypes, prejudice,* and *racism* refer, in some capacity, to attitudes held by people, discrimination is an active behavior, such as gay bashing or unfair hiring practices, that results in differential treatment of individuals within specific ethnic or cultural groups (Law, 2007; Lum, 2004).

Although we have undoubtedly made progress, there is still quite a bit of discrimination in our country. For instance, the most recent hate crime statistics from the FBI (United States Department of Justice, 2008) indicate that 51% of the 9,168 hate crime offenses were for racial bias, while religious and sexual orientation each represented about 18% of the crimes, ethnicity/national origin about 13%, and disability approximately 1% (United States Department of Justice, 2008). Perceptions by Americans seem to verify the notion that, as a country, we still discriminate, with fairly high percentages of Americans believing that the following groups face "a lot" of discrimination: gays and lesbians (64%), Muslims (58%), Hispanics (52%), Blacks (49%), women (37%), Jews (35%), Evangelical Christians (27%), atheists (26%), and Mormons (24%) (The Pew Forum on Religion and Public Life, 2009).

Although discrimination is generally thought of as obvious transgressions against a group, in recent years, a more subtle form of discrimination, called microaggression, has been identified. This type of discrimination is conscious or unconscious and includes brief, subtle, and common put-downs or indignities directed toward individuals from diverse cultures (Constantine, Smith, Redington, & Owens, 2008; Sue, 2010). Some examples include statements like "You don't seem 'gay' (or Black, or...)," "My ancestors made it in this country without anything, I don't see why your family can't." Other types of microaggressions include poor or slow service at a restaurant or store and differential treatment by individuals, such as police or others in positions of power. Such discrimination is probably more commonplace by those who "know" that outward discrimination is wrong, yet carry with them subtle, embedded feelings of prejudice toward others.

Ethnicity

Heritage, ancestry, and *tradition* are some of the words that come to mind when I reflect on the word **ethnicity**. More specifically, when a group of people share a common ancestry, which may include specific cultural and social patterns such as a similar language, values, religion, foods, and artistic expressions, they are said to be of the same ethnic group (Jenkins, 2007). Ethnicity, as opposed to race, is not based on genetic heritage but on long-term patterns of behavior that have some historical significance and may include similar religious, ancestral, language, and/or cultural characteristics. Therefore, many (but not all) Jews share a common ancestry, religion, and cultural practices, and are often considered an ethnic group, while people of Asian heritage, given the diverse religious, political, historical, and cultural experiences of this region of the world, may not share the same culture or ethnic background (see Box 7.2).

BOX 7.2 | Dr. Sylvia Nassar-McMillan

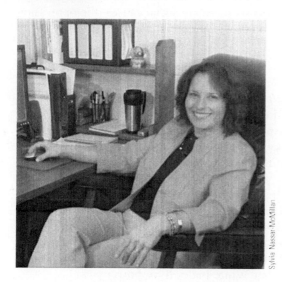

Sylvia Nassar-McMillan

Dr. Sylvia Nassar-McMillan was born in Detroit, Michigan. Her mother and father were both foreign-born immigrants. Her father immigrated into the United States from Palestine, via Lebanon, in the early 1950s. Her mother came from Germany in the late 1950s, and her maternal grandmother followed several years later. Her parents both immigrated as refugees—they came to the United States to seek relief from political situations that had resulted in loss of their respective homelands.

Sylvia's paternal family changed its name to a more anglicized version shortly after resettlement in the United States and quickly became immersed in the American way of life. For a variety of reasons, she did not have much contact with her paternal relatives during her childhood years. Had she not been referred to as Sand Nigger and Camel Jockey by elementary school classmates, she might not

have realized the extent to which her ethnicity contributed to her inability to "fit in." At the same time, she was strongly rooted in German traditions, events, and also the German language, which was the predominant one spoken at home.

Sylvia has distinct memories of being in public with her father when people approached him, speaking in Arabic. Her father would pretend not to understand them, and sometimes even tell them he was Italian. He believed that his family's ethnicity was no one's business. In later years she came to understand the wide range of stigmas associated with being of Arab descent. For example, she had several romantic relationships with men whose families did not accept her because of her Arabic heritage. In the early 1990s, during the U.S. offensive stances toward Iraq (Operations Desert Storm and Desert Shield), she lived for 2 years near a large military base. During that time, she never talked about Arab American issues, and in fact, it was the only time in her adult life that she did not have a support network of Arab American family and friends. In hindsight, she realized how much she emphasized her Germanic heritage and connected with the German community during that time, as if in denial of her other "half."

Today, Sylvia is highly aware of the complexity of her ethnic identity. Personally, she is involved with Arab American and German American communities, practices traditions from both cultures, and has a support network of friends from each. Professionally, she is a faculty member teaching in the helping professions and specializing in ethnic, gender, and career identity development issues. In addition, she is a passionate advocate for the Arab American community nationally.

Minority and Nondominant Group

Oppression of one group over another is my immediate reaction to the word **minority**. A minority is any person or group of people who are being singled out due to their cultural or physical characteristics and are being systematically oppressed by those individuals who are in a position of power. Using this definition, a minority could conceivably be the numerical majority of a population, as was the case for many years for Blacks in South Africa and as is the situation with women in the United States (Atkinson, 2004b; Macionis, 2009). In recent years, we have seen the helping professions increasingly use the term **nondominant group** rather than the word minority because of the negative connotations the word holds and because the term nondominant group suggests there are social causes (the oppression by dominant groups) that causes distress on other (nondominant) groups.

Power Differentials

Potential abuse, force, control, and *superior/underling* are some of the words and phrases that come to my mind when I think of the term **power differential**. Power differentials may represent greater disparities between people than culture, ethnic group, race, or social class (Kuriansky, 2008). Power can be a function of race, class, gender, occupation, socioeconomic status, and a host of other factors and can easily be misunderstood. Whether perceived or real, power can be abused. For instance, a professor may abuse his or her power by sexually harassing a student. An upper-management Mexican-American female who does not abuse her power may still be disliked because the workers believe that Hispanic females should not hold positions of power. And a White male may be given a leadership position in a management group, not because of his expertise, but because it is unconsciously believed by the other group members that White males have power.

Race

Genetic heritage, skin color, and ambiguity are some of the words and phrases I think of when reflecting on the word **race**. Whereas the concept of culture has been based on such characteristics as shared, learned characteristics generally agreed upon by those in the culture, race has traditionally been defined as permanent physical differences as perceived by an external authority (Arthur, 2007). Although traditionally this notion was based on genetics, in recent years this concept has been challenged. For instance, research on the human genome shows that genetic differences between any two people are only 0.1% (1/1000!) (National Human Genome Research Project, 2010). In fact, gene pools throughout the world, and especially in the United States, have become increasingly mixed due to migration, exploration, invasions, systematic rape as a result of wars and oppression of minorities, and intermarriage. Also, behaviorally, there seem to be more differences within racial groups than among them (Atkinson, 2004c). With some sociologists saying there are no races, others saying there are three, and still others concluding that there are as many as 200, the issue of race is cloudy and perhaps doesn't matter. However, it is undeniable that race and the perception of race have effected

BOX 7.3 | What Race Are You Anyway?

Although most people tend to think of themselves as one race or another, take a look at what happened in this one study that examined the genetic makeup of a group of students at Pennsylvania State University:

About 90 students took complex genetic screening tests that compared their samples with those of four regional groups. Many of these students thought of themselves as "100 percent" White or Black or something else, but only a tiny fraction of them, as it turned out, actually fell into that category. Most learned instead that they shared genetic markers with people of different skin colors. ("Debunking the Concept of Race," 2005)

every level of society. At its best, race represents perceived differences; at its worse, those perceived differences become translated into real differences that result in oppression of "racial" groups. This is why I have tried to avoid the use of the word *race* (see Box 7.3).

Religion and Spirituality

Religion is seen as an organized or unified set of practices and beliefs that have moral underpinnings and define a group's way of understanding the world (Cipriani, 2007; McAuliffe, 2008). In contrast, **spirituality** is seen as residing in a person, not in a group, and defines the person's understanding of self, self in relationship to others, and self in relationship to a self-defined higher power or lack thereof. Because religion is concerned to some degree with values from an external referent group and spirituality has to do with internal processes, there are important differences with how one would assist a person who is struggling with religious concerns (e.g., value differences between self and a self-chosen religious group) versus how one would work with a person who is struggling with spiritual concerns (e.g., finding meaning in life).

Sexism, Heterosexism, and Sexual Prejudice

Denigrating and *consciously putting another person down* due to his or her gender and/or sexual orientation are some of the terms and phrases I think of when I hear **sexism, heterosexism,** and **sexual prejudice.** Whenever a person discriminates, denigrates, or stigmatizes another due to his or her gender, that person is said to be sexist. In a similar fashion, when a person discriminates, denigrates, or stigmatizes a person for nonheterosexual behaviors, that person is said to be heterosexist. The word heterosexism has become preferred over **homophobia** as homophobia implies there is a "phobia" or "disorder" within a person that makes the person act in a stigmatizing or denigrating fashion, while heterosexism suggests that such behaviors are more of a conscious choice about the kinds of language and behaviors we exhibit (Adam, 2007). Finally, sexual prejudice is a more inclusive term that refers to negative attitudes targeted toward homosexual, bisexual, heterosexual, or transgendered individuals (Herek, 2000).

Sexual Orientation

Sexual orientation refers to the predominant gender "for which a person has consistent attachments, longings, and sexual fantasies" (McAuliffe, 2008, p. 14). One's sexual orientation, therefore, can be toward the same sex, the opposite sex, or both sexes. Common terms associated with sexual orientation include being **gay, lesbian, bisexual, or transgendered (GLBT)**. In recent years some have even questioned the use of the words *gay* and *lesbian*, suggesting that they reinforce existing power structures in society. Some now advocate for the use of the word **queer** instead of lesbian or gay as a means of regaining power and not buying into existing ways of seeing the world. Meanwhile, it should be noted that in 1975 the American Psychological Association did away with the notion that homosexuality was a disorder and just about all professional associations in the social services have supported this notion. Today, the words gay, lesbian, bisexual, or heterosexual simply define a person's sexual orientation and do not connote a disorder.

Social Class ("Class")

Money, power, status, and *hierarchy*—these are the words that come to mind when I think of the term **social class**. If *class* represents "a person's position in a society's hierarchy based on education, income, and wealth" (Mcauliffe, 2008, p. 13), *social class* represents the perceived ranking of an individual within a society and the amount of power an individual wields (Macionis, 2009). An individual's social class may cut across a person's ethnicity, cultural identification, or race. Therefore, even though individuals may share a similar culture, ethnicity, or race, they may have little in common with one another due to differences in social class. For instance, it is not unusual to find a poor, undereducated African-American who may have little in common with a well-to-do, highly educated African-American.

Political Correctness, or, Oh My God, What Do I Call Him or Her?

Hispanic, Latino, Latina, Chicano, Chicana, Black, Negro, African-American, Afro-American, Oriental, Asian American, Chinese American, Japanese American, Native American, Indian, Eskimo, Inuit, Aleut, native, American Indian, Asian Indian, Jew, Hebrew, Jewish American, Protestant, WASP, Muslim, Moslem, Islamic, Born Again, Fundamentalist Christian, Christian, Catholic, White, Caucasian, European American, American, gay, homosexual, heterosexist, straight, heterosexual, bisexual, lesbian, queer, transgendered, transsexual, cross-dresser, transvestite, disabled person, individual with disability, mentally retarded, intellectual disability, handicapped person, physically challenged, and on and on. Did I offend anybody? I hope not, but in these days of political correctness, finding the correct term is often difficult. And, even once you find the correct term, you will offend somebody.*

Although there is great variety in how individuals prefer to be addressed, nomenclature is an important statement of who we are and what we stand for. For example, words like *Negro* and, to a lesser degree, *Hispanic* are reflective of a long history of oppression for African-Americans and Latinas/Latinos and are not commonly used by many people these days. And we all know words that we dare not even print because of the prejudicial and racist overtones they represent. More than simple "political correctness," naming conventions can represent a way for people to assert their identity. For instance the reclaiming of the words *Black* and *Indian* was a mechanism that some used to assert their identity, and the recent embracing of the word *queer* by gays and lesbians has helped to defuse the negative connotations that it has held. That said, the next paragraph describes some terms that have been used recently.

For Americans with African heritage, the term *African-American* is generally used, although Black is still acceptable and even preferred in some circles. *Asian American* refers to any of a number of individuals with heritage from Asia and the Pacific Islands, including approximately 40 distinct subgroups that differ in language and cultural identity (Sandhu, 1997). The word *Hispanic* is sometimes used to refer to Mexican Americans, Puerto Ricans, Cuban Americans, individuals with Central and South American heritage, and individuals with roots from Spanish-speaking countries in the Caribbean. However, not all individuals from these countries are comfortable with these terms, especially many Cuban Americans, as it refers to anyone with Spanish roots and connotes a history of colonialism. Latino or Latina is sometimes a preferred nomenclature. Islam is a religion whose followers are called Muslims (less commonly called Moslems). Homosexuals today generally use the terms *gay* for men and *lesbian* for women, although, as noted earlier, some have now moved to the word *queer* to define their sexual orientation. The term *straight* is becoming less acceptable to describe heterosexuals because of the implication that it is better than another type of orientation (e.g., "on the straight and narrow"), and *heterosexist* is now the preferred term over *homophobic*. Individuals who have been born in this country and identify with their cultural or ethnic background often place the word *American* following their heritage. Therefore, it is not unusual for us to find individuals referring to themselves as Irish American, Italian American, Arab American, and so forth. Individuals who are naturalized citizens generally do not use the term *American* following their country of origin. For instance, a colleague of mine who was raised in Mexico and became a U.S. citizen refers to herself as "Mexican" (see Box 7.4). Rather than saying handicapped or disabled person, generally people now say *individual with a disability* although some prefer the term *physically challenged*. (Notice the importance of placing the word *individual* prior to the word *disability*.) Finally, although the term *mentally retarded* has been used in recent years, the new *Diagnostic and Statistical Manual* (5th ed.) is replacing that term with *individual with an intellectual disability*, and we are likely to see the term *mentally retarded* used less frequently.

Although it is not within the scope of this text to exhaust in detail the accepted nomenclature for all cultural groups, I have attempted to use commonly accepted terms throughout this text, but particularly highlight these terms in Chapters 7 and 8. Of course, people vary in how they wish to be addressed. However, I believe that making an effort to use terms correctly shows our sensitivity to individuals from diverse cultures.

Dr. Martha Muguira: A Woman of Mexican Heritage

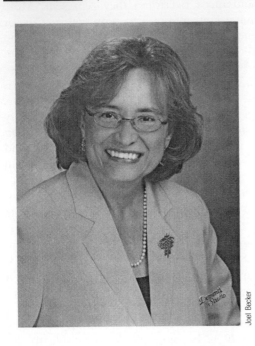

Joel Becker

Dr. Martha Muguira was raised in Mexico City in a family that included her parents and three younger siblings. Marty, who is a naturalized citizen, considers herself Mexican, rather than Mexican American, because she was raised in Mexico.

Marty's paternal and maternal great grandparents were of Spanish and Mexican-Indian descent. Marty notes that the population of Mexico is mostly Catholic, and the rituals include many Indian customs that are not ordinarily found in the United States. She comments that, until recently, light-skinned Mexicans (usually Mexicans of Spanish heritage) were treated preferentially in the country. She mentions that Mexico has tended to be a male-oriented society with preferential treatment toward men, particularly concerning careers.

As a female, Marty remembers that she received mixed messages from her parents. On the one hand, they valued education, particularly bilingual education, and sent her to an American school in Mexico City. In fact, when Marty was 17 years old, she received a scholarship to live in North Carolina with a banker's family and go to a private school. On the other hand, even though Marty received this scholarship, her father encouraged her to stay in Mexico, pursue a more traditional education, and have a family. Despite these mixed messages, Marty went on to finish her doctorate, raise a family, and now works at a counseling center at a university in Virginia.

Although Marty states that she has not experienced overt discrimination, she notes that throughout her life people would have expectations of her because of her Mexican heritage. For instance, while living in North Carolina, she was asked to fit in better by wearing American rather than Mexican-style clothes. Also, when she worked at a Veterans Administration hospital, she was chosen to run a special program for Spanish-speaking employees mostly because she was Mexican. Dr. Muguira is proud of her Mexican heritage, values her bilingual education, and is another prime example of the diversity in the United States.

ETHICAL, PROFESSIONAL, AND LEGAL ISSUES: THE CLIENT'S RIGHT TO DIGNITY, RESPECT, AND UNDERSTANDING

The client from a nondominant culture deserves a culturally competent human service professional who is knowledgeable about cultural differences and is sensitive to the needs of the clients from nondominant groups. The importance of these attributes should not be underestimated. Examples of how knowledge deficits, biases, and prejudices have negatively affected clients from nondominant cultures were highlighted throughout this chapter and abound in the literature. All clients deserve the respect and understanding of the professionals with whom they are working.

Our prejudices are often beyond our awareness; even though a human service professional may think he or she is unbiased, unconscious prejudicial attitudes may seep out during interviews with clients. This is why ethical guidelines stress the importance of having the knowledge and skills to work effectively with a wide range of clients *and* of knowing one's own beliefs and possible prejudices (National Organization for Human Services, 1996; also see Appendix A):

> *Statement 16:* Human service professionals advocate for the rights of all members of society, particularly those who are members of minorities and groups at which discriminatory practices have historically been directed.

> *Statement 17:* Human service professionals provide services without discrimination or preference based on age, ethnicity, culture, race, disability, gender, religion, sexual orientation or socioeconomic status.

> *Statement 18:* Human service professionals are knowledgeable about the cultures and communities within which they practice. They are aware of multiculturalism in society and its impact on the community as well as individuals within the community. They respect individuals and groups, their cultures and beliefs.

> *Statement 19:* Human service professionals are aware of their own cultural backgrounds, beliefs, and values, recognizing the potential for impact on their relationships with others.

> *Statement 20:* Human service professionals are aware of sociopolitical issues that differentially affect clients from diverse backgrounds.

> *Statement 21:* Human service professionals seek the training, experience, education and supervision necessary to ensure their effectiveness in working with culturally diverse client.

THE EFFECTIVE HUMAN SERVICE PROFESSIONAL: BEING OPEN TO THE CONTINUAL DEVELOPMENT OF A MULTICULTURAL PERSPECTIVE

Effective human service professionals are culturally competent in that they are able to work with clients of diverse backgrounds, attempt not to be prejudiced or to hold stereotypic views, approach each client as unique, understand their limitations, strive to learn about the culture or ethnic background of clients with whom they are working, and work toward making changes in society to help those who are disenfranchised. However, for most professionals, getting to this point is a process.

Today, many believe that becoming a culturally competent helper is a developmental process. For instance, D'Andrea (1996) and D'Andrea and Daniels (1991, 1992) suggest that there are a number of stages that most professionals will pass through. These stages range from an **affective/impulsive stage** of racism, where a professional may respond impulsively and in a hostile fashion when discussing issues of diversity; to a **dualistic rational stage,** where professionals learn to monitor their prejudices but still feel them; to the **liberal stage,** where professionals can begin to see different viewpoints when understanding clients from nondominant cultures; to the **principled activist stage,** where one can understand and accept that all people hold varying values and beliefs and may behave in ways different from the helper. In this stage, the helper is willing and ready to embrace social justice actions in order to work toward systemic change, so that all individuals can gain true equality. Moving along these stages is a process and occurs throughout one's career. Where are you in these stages?

SUMMARY

This chapter examined diversity, cultural, competence, and social justice. We started by showing the wide range of diversity that exists in the United States and the world. Then, we pointed out the need for cultural competence in human service work and listed eight viewpoints that some human service professionals hold that prevent them from working effectively with clients from nondominant groups. These are the melting pot myth, incongruent expectations about the helping relationship, de-emphasizing social forces, ethnocentric worldview, ignorance of one's own racist attitudes and prejudices, inability to understand cultural differences in the expression of symptomatology, unreliability of assessment and research instruments, and institutional racism.

The next section of this chapter offered two definitions of culturally competent helping, including one that suggested it is "a consistent readiness to identify the cultural dimensions of clients' lives and a subsequent integration of culture into counseling work" and a second that stated it was important for the human service professional to look at three client identities (individual, group, and universal) and to develop culture-specific and universal strategies and roles as he or she works toward treatment goals.

The next part of this chapter examined the importance that social justice work plays in becoming culturally competent. It was suggested that whereas culturally competent helping has traditionally been seen as a face-to-face meeting with a client, social justice work broadens culturally competent helping by including a wide range of activities that affect the client's broader system in some profound manner and ultimately creates a better life for the client. One model of social justice work, the advocacy competencies, was presented. The advocacy competencies encompass three domains: the client, community, and public. It was noted that each of these domains is divided into two levels that include a focus on whether the helper is "acting on behalf" of the domain or is "acting with" the domain.

As this chapter continued, we noted that the culturally competent helper is familiar with a wide range of diversity issues and understands basic definitions of words and terms which give them a common framework within which to communicate. Thus, basic definitions of the following were offered: culture; prejudice, stereotypes, and racism; discrimination and microaggressions; ethnicity; minority and nondominant group; power differentials; race; religion and spirituality; sexism, heterosexism, and sexual prejudice; sexual orientation; and social class ("class"). This section concluded with a short piece about political correctness relative to when one should use which words and terms.

As this chapter neared its conclusion, we discussed various aspects of the human service professional's ethical code that highlight culturally competent helping and then noted that becoming a culturally competent helper is a process that encompasses four stages: the affective/impulsive stage, the dualistic rational stage, the liberal stage, and the principled stage.

Experiential Exercises

I.   **The Culturally Competent Helper**
     Your instructor will divide you into small groups where you will be asked to discuss your view of the culturally competent helper. What is different about this helper as compared to the helper who cannot work effectively with culturally

different clients? Share your answers with the class, and have your instructor make a list, on the board, of the qualities of the culturally competent helper.

II. The Alligator River*

Read "A Loving Story," and then fill in the grid as instructed.

A Loving Story: Lovey is in a committed relationship with Fine who lives on the other side of the Alligator River. Lovey wants to see Fine, but the bridge is out due to a recent flood. Lovey could swim across the river but would get eaten by the alligators. Therefore, Lovey goes to Popeye, who is the only person with a boat on the river, and asks Popeye for a ride to the other side of the river. Popeye has always been infatuated with Lovey from a distance. Popeye has a severe speech impediment, low self-esteem, and has rarely dated. Popeye earns a meager living taking people across the river. When Lovey asks Popeye for a ride across the river, Popeye states, "Lovey, I've always been infatuated with you, and I'll take you across the river if you'll make love with me." Lovey is initially disgusted and goes to a close confidant named Friend for advice. Friend states, "This is your problem, and you're going to need to work it out on your own." Lovey ponders the situation and thinks, "What the hell, I've slept with lots of people; one more won't make a difference." After they have sex, Popeye, as promised, takes Lovey across the river. When Lovey gets to the other side of the river, out of a sense of honesty, Lovey tells Fine the whole story. Becoming enraged, Fine states, "Get out of my life. I never want to see you again." Lovey becomes distraught and seeks advice from a friend named Slug. Slug becomes infuriated and punches out Fine.

1. **Examining Values as a Function of Gender and Ethnicity Scoring your results:** Using the grid at the end of this exercise, rate each of the five characters in the story. Place an X under number 1 and across from the name of the person you like most; then place an X under number 2 and across from the name you like second most; and so forth. Your instructor will then collect all the grids and count all the 1s, 2s, 3s, 4s, 5s, and place them on a master grid on the board.

	1	2	3	4	5
Lovey					
Fine					
Slug					
Friend					
Popeye					

---

*This exercise is adapted from the book by Simon, Howe, & Kirschenbaum (2006). *Values clarification: A handbook of practical strategies for teachers and students.* Ellington, CT: Values Realization (see www.valuesrealization.org).

Then, as a class, respond to the following questions:

    a. What does the distribution tell you about how students in your class view individuals with differing values?

    b. Based on the characters' roles, did you assume that certain characters in the story were male and others were female?

    c. Consider how you might rate the characters if you changed their genders.

    d. If the characters in the story were of differing ethnic, cultural, or religious backgrounds, would you have responded differently to them?

    e. If you were in a helping relationship with any of the characters in the story, how would your positive and negative stereotypes affect your work with them?

2. **Alternative to the Previous Exercise**

Instead of having the class complete Exercise II.1, the instructor will divide the class into six groups and have each group make assumptions about the characters as noted in a through f that follows. Then, using the scoring instructions in Exercise II.1, collect the aggregate data in each of the six groups and compare the responses of the six different groups. (Feel free to create other groups of different gender and ethnic mixes.)

    a. Group 1 (all characters are White): Lovey is female, Fine is male, Popeye is male, Friend is female, Slug is male.

    b. Group 2 (all characters are African-American): Lovey is female, Fine is male, Popeye is male, Friend is female, Slug is male.

    c. Group 3 (female characters are White, male characters are African-American): Lovey is female, Fine is male, Popeye is male, Friend is female, Slug is male.

    d. Group 4 (male characters are White, female characters are African-American): Lovey is female, Fine is male, Popeye is male, Friend is female, Slug is male.

    e. Group 5 (all characters are female).

    f. Group 6 (all characters are male).

III. Examining Our Heritage

In class, form groups of four or five persons. Within your group, state your full name (if you're married and use your husband's last name, include your maiden name). Then discuss the origins of your name. Note such things as the origins of your last name, why you were given your first name, and any other information about how your full name relates to your family history. If you are not familiar with the history of your family name, ask a parent, guardian, or relative and see what he or she knows.

IV. Acknowledging Our Cultural/Ethnic/Religious Affiliations

In class, the instructor will ask each student to anonymously write on a piece of paper all ethnic, cultural, and religious groups to which each student belongs (e.g., Irish-American, Catholic, gay, lesbian, individual with a disability). Then, have the instructor gather all papers and write on the board all the diverse groups found in your class. (Note to instructor: It is important to maintain anonymity.)

V. Finding Out About Other Cultural Groups (Follow-Up to Exercise III)

After the various cultural, ethnic, and religious groups are written on the board, have each student anonymously write any question he or she would like to ask about any of the diverse groups on the board. Have the instructor collect the questions, and, as a class, all help answer the questions as best you can. It is important that any person in class can respond to the question posed and that no one person has to take ownership of the question.

VI. Interviewing a Person from Another Cultural Group

Using the following questions, interview a person from a different cultural, ethnic, or religious group. In class, share what you learned about that person.
1. What benefits does he or she attribute to being a member of that group?
2. What drawbacks does he or she attribute to being a member of that group?
3. What history does he or she know about his or her group?
4. What are the individual's feelings concerning stereotypes of the group?
5. What prejudice has he or she experienced?
6. How would he or she feel about seeing a helper of a differing ethnic, cultural, or religious background? Of the same background?

VII. Experiencing Prejudice

Have the class divide into groups based on some physical attribute (e.g., hair color, eye color, height). In addition, have the instructor randomly pick some of the groups to be of below-average, average, and above-average intelligence. Within your group, come up with stereotypes of the other groups. During class, respond to one another based on your stereotypes and on the chosen intelligence level. At the end of class, process how the experience felt to members of the groups.

VIII. Counseling Myths Questionnaire*

Using the following scale, write the number to the left of each statement that best represents your view. When finished, the class can discuss their varying responses. Allow different points of view to be expressed and heard. Your instructor might want to obtain a mean from the class for each item so you can compare your answers to others.

1	2	3	4	5
strongly agree	agree	no opinion	disagree	strongly disagree

1. _____Certain clients should be avoided because of their past experiences.
2. _____Cultural myths and stereotypes cannot be avoided when working with culturally different clients.
3. _____Cultural myths and cultural stereotypes are often a reality.
4. _____Large behavioral differences exist between clients as a function of their culture.
5. _____Helpers have fewer problems when they understand their clients' backgrounds.

---

*Adapted with permission from Dr. Richmond Calvin, **Indiana University—South Bend.**

6. _____Helpers work best within their own cultural group.

7. _____Clients from the same ethnic background, religion, or culture have similar issues to work on.

8. _____Culturally different clients should usually be referred to helpers from the same cultural group.

9. _____Cultural differentness of client and the helper is a significant factor in the helping relationship.

10. _____Cultural variations exist regarding verbal and nonverbal communication.

11. _____Everyone is culturally different; therefore, helpers need a model that will serve all clients.

12. _____All types of social services are available for all persons who desire them.

13. _____All cultures receive fair treatment in the helping relationship.

14. _____Clients from nondominant groups use profanity more often than White clients.

15. _____White clients are more likely to respond to helping interventions than non-White clients.

16. _____Generally, clients from low-income backgrounds are very difficult to help.

17. _____Many culturally different persons have shown they do not trust helping professionals.

18. _____Family ties are extremely weak for many culturally different clients.

19. _____Value systems for many culturally different clients are inferior.

20. _____Clients from a low socioeconomic status do not trust middle-class helpers.

21. _____Sociocultural history represents the most important ingredient in the helping relationship.

22. _____Culturally different clients do not possess qualities such as boldness, initiative, and assertiveness.

23. _____Clients from nondominant groups tend not to be logical thinkers, problem solvers, or good decision makers.

24. _____All helping relationships have a cross-cultural component.

25. _____Religious differences are not as important as racial differences in the helping relationship.

26. _____Age differences are not as important as racial differences in the helping relationship.

27. _____Gender differences are not as important as racial differences in the helping relationship.

28. _____Sexual-orientation differences are not as important as racial differences in the helping relationship.

IX. Ethical and Professional Vignettes

After reflecting on the following vignettes, discuss your thoughts with other students in your class.

1. Because of cross-cultural differences, you believe that your work with an Asian client has not been successful. Rather than referring the client to

another human service professional, you decide to read more about your client's culture in order to gain a better understanding of him. Is this ethical? Is this professional?

2. You discover some fellow students making sexist jokes. What should you do? Have you encountered such behavior? What was your response?

3. You find some family members making ethnic/cultural slurs. What should you do? Have you encountered such behavior? Have you acted?

4. You discover that a colleague of yours is telling a gay client that he is acting immorally. Is this ethical? Professional? Legal? What should you do?

5. A friend of yours advertises that she is a Christian counselor. You discover that when clients come to see her, she encourages reading parts of the Bible during sessions and tells clients they need to repent and ask God to forgive them for their sins. Is this ethical? Is this professional? Is this legal?

6. An African-American human service professional who has expertise in running parenting workshops decides he should work only with African-American clients. A White client has heard about his workshops and calls to sign up for one. The human service professional refers him to someone else and tells the client he works only with African-Americans. Does this human service professional have a responsibility to see this client? Is he acting ethically? Professionally? Legally?

7. Your client wants to obtain her GED diploma but felt demeaned when she went to the local high school to ask about the process of obtaining her GED. You decide to go with her to help empower her and advocate for her in obtaining the information. Is this ethical? Professional?

8. You have a client with a panic disorder, and as a result, he is fearful of looking for a job. You have decided to help him identify potential jobs and go to possible job interviews with him and wait outside of the office as he interviews. Is this ethical? Professional?

9. A female client of yours has been sexually harassed by her supervisor. She is fearful of reporting him. You encourage her to report him and tell her that if she allows him to continue with this behavior, he will likely harass others. Is this ethical? Professional?

10. Using the same scenario as in number 9, this time you decide, after talking with your client, to report the client's superior yourself. Is this ethical? Professional?

11. An African-American client tells you that the realtor he has been working with has refused to show him certain properties in mostly White neighborhoods. Your client says, "that's the way it is, and that's the way it always will be." You encourage your client to report the realtor, but he refuses. You therefore report the realtor anonymously. Is this ethical? Professional?

12. A gay high school student you have been working with is bullied by others in his school because of his sexual orientation. Without asking for permission from your client, you decide to contact the school counselor and ask her to provide a series of workshops on understanding gay and lesbian youths and on bullying. Is this ethical? Professional?

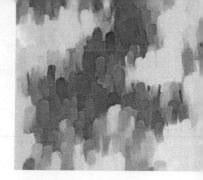

Working with Diverse Clients

To say I was a novice helper when I first started in this profession is probably an understatement. Sure, I wanted to help people, but my way of helping undoubtedly was ethnocentric, and was at times problematic with clients who were from non-dominant groups as compared to the White clients with whom I worked. Being White meant that I could probably relate better to those who were like me than my other clients. This does not mean that I was necessarily incompetent or unhelp-ful, but it did mean that I had a lot to learn. And, when I entered this field, there was not a lot written to help me learn. With the vast majority of helpers having been White, I think a lot of helpers were in the same boat that I was in. As a result, a lot of clients from nondominant cultures were probably getting inferior services. Again, this is not to blame all of those White helpers who so wanted to adequately serve all clients; however, it does describe the state of affairs—in the past.

Today, things have changed. First, there are significantly more helpers of color entering the human service field. Second, becoming a culturally competent helper has become a critical piece of becoming a well-rounded human service professional. That is why I have spent two chapters on this important aspect of the human service professional. Today, we all must learn how to become culturally competent—the

White human service professional and the human service professional who is from a nondominant culture.

Whereas Chapter 7 offered reasons why it is important to be culturally competent and provided definitions that could help us understand culturally competent helping, this chapter will provide us with some models to help us work effectively with clients from diverse backgrounds and will also offer a number of practical guidelines when working with a variety of clients. But let's first start by looking at how much the United States has changed over the years as well as some predictions as to how our country will look in years to come.

THE CHANGING FACE OF AMERICA

America is the most diverse country in the world and is becoming increasingly more so. In fact, today, well over one-third of Americans are racial and ethnic minorities, and nondominant groups are expected to become the majority by the year 2042 (U.S. Census Bureau, 2008b). By the year 2050, the makeup of America will be quite different than it is today (see Figure 8.1).

Changing demographics are a function of a number of factors, including higher birth rates of culturally diverse populations, the fact that most immigrants no longer come from Western countries, and immigration rates that are the largest in American history. Today, the great majority of immigrants are Latin American (53.6%) and Asian (26.8%) (U.S. Census Bureau, 2010b) as compared to past immigrants who were mostly White European, and today's immigrants have a tendency to want to assert their cultural heritage rather than be swallowed up by the Western-based American culture. In actuality, this has always been the case, as Italian Americans, Irish Americans, Jewish Americans, German Americans, and others all developed their own communities and maintained their unique heritages when they first came to this country. After all, there is some sense of safety when you live with those who are familiar in a new, yet strange land.

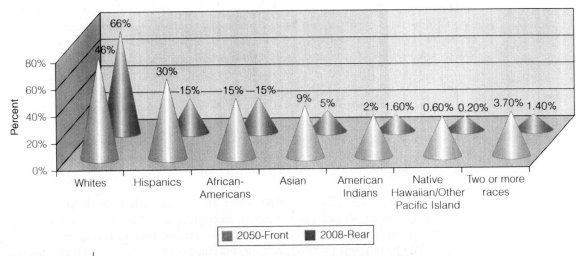

Figure 8.1 | Changes in Population by Race/Cultural Background

Changes in the racial, ethnic, and cultural makeup of Americans bring with it changes in the religious composition of the country. As increasing numbers of Asians, Latinos/Latinas, and people from the Middle East arrive at our shores, we will more frequently encounter religions that were previously rare in America. But diversity in religion is not just brought to us by our immigrants. Although America is a country that is largely Christian, diversity in Christianity is now greater than ever. From a multitude of generic and mainline Christian faiths, to Roman Catholics who are increasingly varied in their beliefs, to Eastern Orthodox, Mormons, Christian Scientists, Seventh-day Adventists, Amish, Mennonites, and on and on, Christian religion in America is a religious mosaic in and of itself.

In addition to the changing ethnic, cultural, and religious diversity in America, today there are changes in sex-role identity. The macho male is no longer considered the model for maleness, while expectations concerning the role of women in the workplace and as childcare providers have changed dramatically. Also, in America today, we see increased awareness and increased acceptance of sexual minorities, such as those who are gay, lesbian, bisexual, and transgendered (Gallup, 2010). Whereas in the past many individuals felt a need to hide their sexual preference for fear of discrimination, today we find an increasing number of gays, lesbians, and bisexuals coming out. In addition, changes in federal, state, and local laws as well as a gradual move toward more tolerance of differences have given us an increased sensitivity to and awareness of a number of special groups, including the physically challenged, older persons, the homeless and the poor, individuals who are HIV positive, the mentally ill, and others. Let's spend a little time examining each of these groups.

DEVELOPING CULTURAL COMPETENCE

If human service professionals are to work effectively with *all* clients, then they must graduate from training programs with more than a desire to help all people (Neukrug & Milliken, 2008). Human service professionals will have achieved competence in working with clients from nondominant groups when each training program graduates students who have worked with clients from diverse backgrounds; who have an identity as a human service professional that includes a multicultural perspective; and who have the attitudes and beliefs, knowledge, and skills to be effective with a variety of clients. The following section provides the Multicultural Counseling Competencies model that suggests competencies that all human service professionals should develop if they are to become culturally competent. This is followed by the RESPECTFUL model and the Tripartite model, two models that can help us better understand clients from non-dominant groups.

Multicultural Counseling Competencies Model

The **Multicultural Counseling Competencies** offer us a framework to develop our skills at becoming culturally competent (Arredondo, 1999; Sue & Sue, 2008). These competences focus on the importance of helpers having: (1) the appropriate **attitudes and beliefs** in the sense that they are aware of their assumptions, values, and biases; (2) the **knowledge** needed about their clients' culture so that they can better understand their clients; and (3) a repertoire of **skills** or tools that can be effectively applied to clients

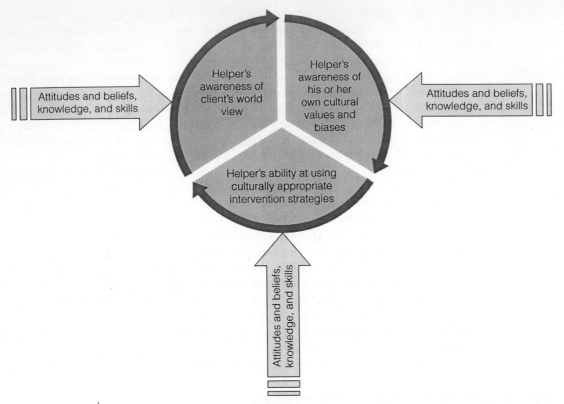

Figure 8.2 | Focus of Multicultural Competencies

from diverse backgrounds. These attitudes and beliefs, knowledge, and skills should be applied in three areas: the helper's awareness of the client's world view, the helper's awareness of his or her own cultural values, and the helper's ability to use culturally appropriate intervention strategies (see Figure 8.2).

Let's examine how the attitudes and beliefs, knowledge, and skills can impact each of these three domains in a little more detail.

Attitudes and Beliefs The culturally competent helper has an awareness of his or her own cultural background and has actively pursued gaining awareness of his or her own biases, stereotypes, and values. Although this helper may not hold the same belief system as his or her client, he or she can accept differing world-views as presented by the helpee. In other words, "Differences are not seen as being deviant" (Sue & Sue, 2008, p. 48). Being sensitive to differences and tuned into his or her own cultural biases allows the culturally competent helper to refer a client to a helper of the client's own culture when the helper realizes that his or her beliefs are such that they do not respect the client's beliefs. Nonreferral in this case would result in the misuse of skills and intervention strategies. Unfortunately, as shown in Chapter 7, examples of how mental health professionals have failed clients who are culturally different from themselves have been common (see Chapter 7, "The Need for Cultural Competence").

Knowledge   Culturally competent helpers have knowledge of their cultural heritage and how that might impact their relationship with clients. Culturally competent helpers also have knowledge of the group from which the client comes and do not jump to conclusions about the client's ways of being. In addition, he or she shows a willingness to gain a greater depth of knowledge of various cultural groups. This helper is also aware of how sociopolitical issues such as racism, sexism, and heterosexism can negatively affect clients. In addition, this helper knows how different theories of counseling carry values that may be detrimental for some clients in the helping relationship. This culturally competent helper understands how institutional barriers can affect the willingness of clients from nondominant cultures to use mental health services. Unfortunately, lack of knowledge of a cultural group can cause the human service professional and others to jump to incorrect conclusions (see Box 8.1).

Skills   The culturally competent helper is able to apply, when appropriate, generic interviewing and helping skills and also has knowledge of and is able to employ specialized skills and interventions that might be effective with clients from specific nondominant groups. This helper also understands the verbal and nonverbal language of the client and can communicate effectively with the client. In addition, the culturally skilled helper understands the importance of having a systemic perspective, such as an understanding of the impact of family and society on clients. Thus, this helper can collaborate with extended family members, individuals in the community, folk healers, and other professionals, and knows when to advocate for his or her clients. Finally, culturally competent helpers know the limit of their skills and what steps they have to take to pick up new skills vital in working with specific clients. What happens when a helper does not have the appropriate skills to working with a culturally diverse client? Most likely, the client leaves the helping relationship prematurely, feels discouraged and dissatisfied with the helping process, and/or has little success in meeting his or her goals (see Box 8.2).

| **BOX 8.1** | **Lack of Knowledge (Blackbirds Sitting in a Tree)** |

A White female elementary school teacher in the United States posed a math problem to her class one day. "Suppose there are four blackbirds sitting in a tree. You take a slingshot and shoot one of them. How many are left?" A White student answered quickly, "That's easy. One subtracted from four is three." An African immigrant youth then answered with equal confidence, "Zero." The teacher chuckled at the latter response and stated that the first student was right and that, perhaps, the second student should study more math. From that day forth, the African student seemed to withdraw from class activities and seldom spoke to other students or the teacher....

If the teacher had pursued the African student's reasons for arriving at the answer zero, she might have heard the following: "If you shoot one bird, the others will fly away." Nigerian educators often use this story to illustrate differences in world views between United States and African cultures. The Nigerians contend that the group is more important than the individual, that survival of all depends on interrelationships among the parts.... (from Sue, 1992, pp. 7–8)

| BOX 8.2 | **Lack of Skills** |

A female [Asian] client complained about all kinds of physical problems such as feeling dizzy, having a loss of appetite, an inability to complete household chores, and insomnia. She asked the therapist if her problem could be due to "nerves." The therapist suspected depression since these are some of the physical manifestations of the disorder and asked the client if she felt depressed and sad. At this point, the client paused and looked confused. She finally stated that she feels very ill and that these physical problems are making her sad. Her perspective is that it was natural for her to feel sad when sick. As the therapist followed up by attempting to determine if there was a family history of depression, the client displayed even more discomfort and defensiveness. Although the client never directly contradicted the therapist, she did not return for the following session. (Tsui & Schultz as cited in Sue & Sue, 2008, p. 366)

If this helper had the appropriate knowledge and skills, he would have known that for Asian clients the mind and body are inseparable, and physical complaints are a common and acceptable means of expressing emotional problems. An appropriate response to this client would have been to focus on the somatic complaints and suggest physical treatments prior to working on emotional problems. (Sue & Sue, 2008)

As you can see in Box 8.2, there is a close connection between our beliefs about culturally diverse clients, our knowledge regarding such clients, and our effective use of skills.

In short, helpers who have a clear understanding of self, especially their own cultural identity, are able to develop healthy attitudes and beliefs, can gain the needed knowledge base to work with diverse clients, and can implement the appropriate skills for clients who are culturally different (see http://www.counseling.org/Resources/Competencies/Multcultural_Competencies.pdf for a copy of the Multicultural Counseling Competencies).

The RESPECTFUL Model

D'Andrea and Daniels (2005) suggest that in gaining cultural competence, professionals should adopt the **RESPECTFUL Model** of helping, which highlights ten factors that helpers should explore in trying to obtain a good understanding of their clients:

R—Religious/spiritual identity

E—Economic class background

S—Sexual identity

P—Psychological development

E—Ethnic/racial background

C—Chronological disposition

T—Trauma and other threats to personal well-being

F—Family history

U—Unique physical characteristics

L—Language and location of residence (p. 37)

D'Andrea and Daniels suggest that by addressing each of the above dimensions with clients, helpers can better understand the varying factors which impact client development, increasingly work in a more holistic fashion with clients, and be able to develop effective strategies when working with clients.

Tripartite Model of Personal Identity

Sue & Sue (2008) suggest that we should be aware of three spheres of our clients' lives (see Figure 8.3). They suggest that the *individual level* represents our clients' unique genetics and distinctive experiences. The *group level* in many ways reminds us of the RESPECTFUL model in that it reflects a wide range of factors that come to make up the unique world of the client. The *universal level,* they point out, comprises those shared experiences that come to define all of us as human and include "(a) biological and physical similarities, (b) common life experiences (birth, death, love, sadness, etc.), (c) self-awareness, and (d) the ability to use symbols such as language" (p. 39).

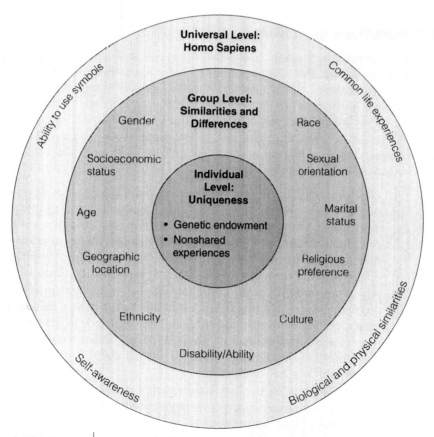

Figure 8.3 | The Tripartite Model of Personal Identity

Source: Sue, D. W., & Sue, D. (2008). *Counseling the culturally diverse: Theory and practice* (5th ed.). New York: Wiley, p. 38.

The **Tripartite model** is helpful because not only does it define a number of factors that human service professionals can target to better understand their clients (the group level) but also offers us a model for understanding how the client may be unique from us and similar to us.

GUIDELINES FOR WORKING WITH DIVERSE CLIENTS

Once the helper has gained an understanding of what is necessary to gain cultural competence, he or she is positioned to work with clients from many diverse cultures. Based on the Multicultural Counseling Competencies model, hopefully you have and will continue to have the attitudes and beliefs to work effectively with a wide range of clients. Next, you need the knowledge about these groups, including some of their unique qualities and traits. This, you gain from other classes, continuing education seminars, and through readings. The following, however, offers you some basic strategies when working with a wide range of clients.

The Role of Culture/Race in the Helping Relationship

Collectively, individuals from different racial and ethnic groups make up a large percentage of this country and include approximately 48.4 million (15.8%) Latinos/Latinas, 41.8 million (13.6%) African-Americans, 16 million (4.0%) Asians, 5.0 million (1.6%) American Indians and Alaska Natives, and 1.1 million (<1.1%) Native Hawaiian and other Pacific Islander (U.S. Census Bureau, 2009a). Although cultural differences are great among these groups, there are some broad suggestions that one can make when working with individuals from these cultures (McAuliffe, 2008; Sue & Sue, 2008):

1. *Have the right attitudes and beliefs, gain knowledge, and learn skills.* Be prepared to work with clients with varying cultural heritages by embracing the appropriate knowledge, skills, and beliefs prior to meeting with them.

2. *Encourage clients to speak their own language.* Make an effort to know meaningful expressions of your client's language. When language becomes a significant barrier, refer to a helper who speaks the client's language.

3. *Assess the cultural identity of the client.* Try to understand the client's racial/cultural identity. Do they consider themselves part of a certain group? Sometimes, clients see themselves differently than their helper views them. For example, a client who has acculturated and has little identification with his or her culture of origin is very different from a client from the same culture of origin who is a new immigrant.

4. *Check the accuracy of your interpretation of the client's nonverbals.* Don't assume that nonverbal communication is consistent across cultures. Ask the client about his or her nonverbals when in doubt.

5. *Make use of alternate modes of communication.* Use appropriate alternative modes of communication, such as acting, drawing, music, storytelling, collage making, and so forth, to draw out clients who are reticent to talk or have communication problems.

6. *Assess the impact of sociopolitical issues on the client.* Examine how social and political issues affect your client and make a decision about whether advocacy of client concerns can be helpful to the client's presenting problems.
7. *Encourage clients to bring in culturally significant and personally relevant items.* Have clients bring in items to help you better understand them and their culture (e.g., books, photographs, articles of significance, culturally meaningful items).
8. *Vary the helping environment.* When appropriate, explore alternative helping environments to ease the client into the helping relationship (e.g., take a walk, have a cup of coffee at a quiet restaurant, initially meet your client at his or her home).

The Role of Religion in the Helping Relationship

The religious makeup of America has shifted dramatically since 1960 (Newport, 2009), and today there are close to 79 religious groups, each having over 60,000 members (Lindner, 2009). About one-fourth of Americans identify as Roman Catholic and about one-half as Protestant; however, the word *Protestant* is used less frequently these days because people have a tendency to lump together the many religious beliefs the word encompasses. In addition, smaller numbers of Americans identify as Muslim, Jewish, Buddhist, Hindu, Unitarian, as well as a number of other religions (Kosmin & Keysar, 2008). With 83% of Americans claiming a religious affiliation and 88% saying that religious activities are important in their lives (Exploring Religious America, 2002), it is clear that helpers must understand the diversity of religious beliefs in America. With religion being the road to peace for many but the reason of conflict for some (see cartoon), a client's religious background and current religious beliefs may hold the key to understanding the underlying values

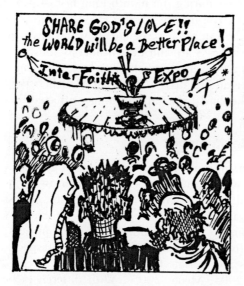 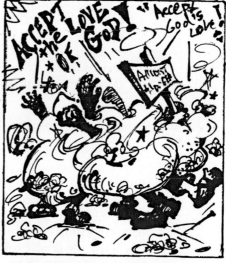

D. Baggarly

that motivate him or her. Some pointers to keep in mind concerning religion and the helping relationship include the following:

1. *Have the right attitudes and beliefs, gain knowledge, and learn skills.* Be prepared to work with clients of different religions by embracing the appropriate knowledge, skills, and beliefs prior to meeting with them.

2. *Determine the client's religious background early in the helping relationship.* To assist in treatment planning, know the client's religious affiliation. Be sensitive to any client who may resist discussion of his or her religious background.

3. *Ask the client how important religion is in his or her life.* Assess the part religion plays in a client's life to assist in goal setting and treatment planning. Do not assume that clients know much about their religion because they present themselves as deeply religious, or know little because they are not religious.

4. *Assess the client's level of faith development.* Low-stage faith development clients are dualistic, concrete, and work better with structure. High-stage clients are complex thinkers, value a variety of different kinds of faith experiences, and are comfortable with abstractions and self-reflection. Assessing the faith development of your clients will assist you in treatment planning (see Fowler, 1981/1995).

5. *Don't make false assumptions.* Don't stereotype (e.g., the helper who assumes all Jews keep kosher homes). Don't project (e.g., the helper who is Christian and assumes that people of all faiths are born with original sin).

6. *Become familiar with your client's religious beliefs and important holidays and traditions.* Learn about your client's religion to show respect and understanding and to not embarrass yourself (e.g., a Muslim would not want to be offered food before sunset during the month-long fast of Ramadan).

7. *Understand that religion can deeply affect a client on many levels, including unconscious ones.* Understand that some clients who deny a religious affiliation (e.g., "lapsed Catholics") are still driven unconsciously by the basic tenets of the religious beliefs they were originally taught (e.g., clients may continue to feel guilt over certain issues related to the religious beliefs they were taught, despite the fact that they insist they are no longer affected by their religion).

The Role of Gender in the Helping Relationship

Whether working with a man or a woman, knowledge of gender biases can allow a helper to be effective at what some have called **gender-aware helping** (Good & Brooks, 2005; Good, Gilbert, & Scher, 1990; Seem & Johnson, 1998). This perspective views gender as central to helping, views problems within a societal context, encourages helpers to actively address gender injustices, encourages the development of collaborative and equal relationships, and respects the client's right to choose the gender roles appropriate for himself or herself regardless of their political correctness (Kees, 2005; Mejia, 2005). With differences between men and women being great (see Table 8.1), it is important that we separately describe how to work with women in the helping relationship and how to work with men in the helping relationship.

Table 8.1 | Some Common Differences Between Men and Women

- Women are more nurturing, more compassionate, more relational, less focused on "doing" and more on "being" in relationships.

- Women have more difficulty expressing anger than men.

- Women struggle more with self-esteem and depression than men.

- Women earn less money for doing the same work as men.

- Job opportunities and advancement are fewer for women.

- Women are more frequently sexually harassed on the job and at other places.

- Women are physically abused by their spouses or partners at alarming rates.

- Single and divorced women and their children live below poverty level at alarming rates.

- Assumptions about the abilities of girls and women may prevent females from realizing their potential.

- Women tend to be more comfortable with expression of sad feelings, intimacy, and nurturing behavior and less comfortable with the expression of anger and assertive behavior.

- Women tend to be more socially compassionate and hold more traditional moral values.

- Women, on average, tend to be less comfortable in competitive situations.

- Women are more frequently misdiagnosed than men when seeking mental health services.

- Women are sometimes torn between their roles as nurturer and child-care provider and their place in the world of paid work.

- Nearly all cases of complaints made against therapists for sexual exploitation are from women complaining about male therapists.

- Women have unique biological problems (e.g., premenstrual syndrome, breast cancer, pregnancy, ovarian cysts, ovarian cancer).

- Men tend to seek counseling less frequently than women and have a more negative attitude toward the helping process.

- Men are more restrictive emotionally, less communicative, less affectionate, and less comfortable with sad feelings, collaboration, self-disclosure, and intimacy.

- Men tend to be more comfortable with angry feelings, aggression, and competitiveness.

- Men are sometimes ostracized for expressing feelings, especially those considered to be traditionally feminine feelings, and yet criticized for not being more sensitive.

- Men are criticized for being too controlling and self-reliant and made to feel inadequate if they do not take control.

- Men are socialized to be more aggressive and individualistic and are thus more prone to accidents, suicide, early death through wars, and acts of violence.

- Men are encouraged to be competitive and controlling (take charge), and yet these very behaviors lead to increased stress and are likely to play a factor in the shorter life expectancy of men in comparison with women.

- Men are socialized to not be engaged in child rearing and yet are criticized for being distant fathers.

- Men have unique biological problems (e.g., prostate cancer, prostatitis, higher rates of stress-related diseases, and testicular cancer).

- Men are placed in a position of being in charge of others, which sometimes results in the oppression of women. Such oppression not only harms women but harms men's psyches as well.

- Men commit the vast majority of crimes, and a particularly high percentage of violent crimes.

- Men have higher rates of substance abuse.

Women in the Helping Relationship   Several authors have suggested that women have special issues to address that are related to the development of their female identity and oppression they face in society. Using some of their ideas, the following offers some guidelines for assisting women through the helping relationship (American Psychological Association, 2007; Brown & Bryan, 2007; Brown, Weber, & Ali, 2008; Kees, 2005):

1. *Have the right attitudes and beliefs, gain knowledge, and learn skills.* Be prepared to work with women by embracing the appropriate knowledge, skills, and beliefs prior to meeting with them.

2. *Assure that the helping approach you use has been adapted for women.* Some approaches to helping are sexist. Take an inventory of your approach to ensure that it is effective with women.

3. *Establish a relationship, give up your power, and demystify the helping process.* Recognize the importance that power plays in all relationships and attempt to equalize the helper-client relationship. This can be done by downplaying the "expert" role, encouraging women to trust themselves, and practicing self-disclosure (particularly important with female helpers, but male helpers should be much more tentative with self-disclosure and be particularly careful not to sexualize the relationship).

4. *Identify social/political issues related to client problem(s) and use them to set goals.* Help women understand the nature of the problem within its sociocultural context and help them see how the unique dynamics of women tend to cause them to internalize these issues. For instance, it is common for abused women to blame themselves for the abuse. Help them see that they are not responsible for the abuse and help them set goals to break free of the abuse.

5. *Validate and legitimize a woman's angry feelings toward her predicament.* As women begin to recognize how they have been victimized, helpers should assist them in combating feelings of powerlessness, helplessness, and low self-esteem and help them identify their strengths.

6. *Actively promote healing through learning about women's issues.* Helpers should encourage women to learn more about women's issues. This can be done by providing written materials to women, suggesting seminars for them to attend, and offering a list of women's groups or women's organizations that support women's issues.

7. *Provide a safe environment to express feelings as clients begin to form connections with other women.* As women begin to gain clarity regarding their situation, they will see how society's objectification of women has led to fear and competition among women. This newfound knowledge will lead to a desire to have deeper, more meaningful connections with other women. Helpers should consider the possibility of providing a women's support group at this point in the helping relationship.

8. *Provide a safe environment to help women understand their anger toward men.* As women increasingly see that a male-dominated society has led to the objectification of women, they will begin to express increasing anger toward men. Helpers can assist clients in understanding the difference between anger at a man and anger at a male-dominated system. Slowly, women will see that some men can also be trusted.

9. *Help clients deal with conflicting feelings between traditional and newfound values.* As women increasingly get in touch with newfound feminist beliefs, they will become torn between those beliefs and values that do not seem congruent with those beliefs (e.g., wanting to stay home to raise their children). Helpers should validate these contradictory feelings, acknowledge the confusion, and assist clients to fully explore their belief systems.

10. *Facilitate integration of the client's new identity.* Helpers can assist clients in integrating their newfound feminist beliefs with their personal beliefs, even those personal beliefs that may not seem to be traditionally feminist. Clients are able to feel strength in their own identity development and no longer need to rely on an external belief system.

11. *Say goodbye.* As women increasingly feel comfortable with their newfound identities, it is time to let them go and experience their new selves in the world.

Men in the Helping Relationship

Researchers began tracking the "feminization" of mental health care more than a generation ago, when women started to outnumber men in fields like psychology and counseling. Today the takeover is almost complete. (Carey, 2011, para. 4)

Like women, a number of authors have offered ideas that can be incorporated into a set of guidelines when working with male clients. And with so many more female helpers than males, it is important that all helpers understand these guidelines (Berger, Levant, McMillan, Kelleher, & Sellers, 2005; Good & Brooks, 2005; Greer, 2005; McCarthy & Holliday, 2004; Mejia, 2005; Wexler, 2009):

1. *Have the right attitudes and beliefs, gain knowledge, and learn skills.* Embrace the appropriate knowledge, skills, and beliefs prior to meeting with a male client.

2. *Accept men where they are, as this will help build trust.* Men, who are often initially very defensive, will work hard on their issues once they can trust their helper.

3. *Don't push men to express what may be considered "softer feelings."* Don't push a man to express feelings, as you may push him out of the helping relationship. Men tend to be uncomfortable with certain feelings (e.g., deep sadness, feelings of incompetence, feelings of inadequacy, feelings of closeness), but more at ease with "thinking things through," problem solving, and expressing some feelings, such as anger and pride (see Box 8.3).

4. *Early on in therapy, validate the man's feelings.* Validate whatever feelings a man expresses, and remember that in order to protect their egos, men may initially blame others and society for their problems.

5. *Validate the man's view of how he has been constrained by male sex-role stereotypes.* Help to build trust by validating a man's sense of being constrained by sex-role stereotypes (e.g., he must work particularly hard for his family).

6. *Develop goals.* Collaborate with men and develop goals together. Men like structure and a sense of goal directedness, even if the plan is changed later on.

BOX 8.3 | Reinforcement of Stereotypes

Close your eyes for a moment and imagine a person running into a burning apartment building to save the lives of children. Stay focused on that image, and let it sink in. Now, close your eyes again and imagine six-month-old snuggling and being taken care of by their parent. The parent makes "google" sounds to get the attention of the infant and show the infant love. Imagine this in your mind's eye.

If you imagined a man running into the building and a woman snuggling with her child, you are probably like many Americans. Our imaginations reinforce our stereotypes. And we tend to see nurturing as a compassionate behavior and running into a building to save lives as a brave behavior. Both are important and perhaps reflect societal stereotypes of gender specific behaviors. But, in reality, can't we all be nurturing parents and brave heroes? In the helping relationship, men may present with some traditional male behaviors, but are capable of expressing many feelings—if given the time!

---

7. *Begin to discuss developmental issues.* Introduce male developmental issues so a man can quickly examine concerns that may be impinging upon him (e.g., having children, midlife crises, retirement) (Levinson, 1978).

8. *Slowly encourage the expression of new feelings.* As you reinforce the expression of newfound feelings, men will begin to feel comfortable sharing what are considered to be more feminine feelings (e.g., tears, caring, feelings of intimacy).

9. *Explore underlying issues and reinforce new ways of understanding the world.* Explore underlying issues as they emerge (e.g., childhood issues, feelings of inadequacy, father–son issues).

10. *Explore behavioral change.* As insights emerge, encourage men to try out new behaviors.

11. *Encourage the integration of new feelings, new ways of thinking, and new behaviors.*

12. *Encourage new male relationships.* Encourage new male friendships in which the client can express his feelings while maintaining his maleness (e.g., men's group).

13. *Say goodbye.* Allow men to experience their newfound self, so be able to say goodbye and end the helping relationship.

Gay, Bisexual, and Lesbian Individuals in the Helping Relationship

Current research suggests that sexual orientation is determined very early in life, is most likely related to biological and genetic factors, may be influenced by sociological factors, and has little, if anything, to do with choice (Saravi, 2007). Unfortunately, despite the fact that the mental health professional associations have depathologized sexual orientation, 48% of Americans continue to believe that being gay or lesbian is morally wrong (Saad, 2008). Although other polls show mixed views about homosexuality (Gallup, 2010; Saad, 2006), stereotypes concerning gays and lesbians continue to flourish even though most gays and lesbians do not fit them. A number of important points regarding gay, bisexual, and lesbian individuals have been highlighted by many authors, some of which are summarized here (e.g., Pope, 2008; Sue & Sue, 2008; Szymanski, 2008):

1. *Have the right attitudes and beliefs, gain knowledge, and learn skills.* Be prepared to work with gay, lesbian, and bisexual clients by embracing the appropriate knowledge, skills, and beliefs prior to meeting with them.

2. *Have a gay, lesbian, and bisexual friendly office.* Make sure that your intake forms are gay, lesbian, and bisexual friendly. Some helpers may choose to have literature in their office that promotes a gay friendly atmosphere. Others may just want to assure that there are no heterosexist materials in the office.

3. *Help gays, lesbians, and bisexuals understand and combat societal forms of oppression.* Oppression and discrimination of gays, lesbians, and bisexuals is rampant throughout American culture, and it is important that gays, lesbians, and bisexuals understand how it affects them, what they can do to combat it, and how they can gain a sense of empowerment despite it.

4. *Adopt an affirmative and nonheterosexist attitude.* The importance of adopting an attitude that affirms your client's right to his or her sexuality cannot be stressed enough, as so many individuals (including helpers!) have embedded biases and stereotypes about gays and lesbians.

5. *Don't jump to conclusions about lifestyle.* There is no "one" gay, lesbian, or bisexual lifestyle, and helpers should not jump to conclusions about how their clients live out their sexuality.

6. *Understand the differences among people who are gay, lesbian, and bisexual.* Although lumped together here, and often confused as embodying many of the same characteristics, there are great differences among gay, lesbian, and bisexual individuals. For instance, bisexuals are often ostracized by heterosexuals and sometimes by gays and lesbians. Moreover, identity development for gays, lesbians, and bisexuals is considerably different.

7. *Know community resources that might be useful to gay men, lesbian women, and bisexual individuals.*

8. *Know identity issues.* Be familiar with the identity development of gays, lesbians, and bisexuals, especially as it relates to the coming-out process (e.g., Morrow, 2004; Szymnaski, 2008).

9. *Understand the complexity of sexuality.* People express sexuality in different ways. Gay and bisexual men, for instance, may be more sexual than some lesbians. Also, the expression of sexuality in men and women sometimes differs, with women being more focused on relationship issues.

10. *Understand the idiosyncrasies of religious views of homosexuality.* Some religions view being gay, lesbian, or bisexual as sinful, while others are accepting of different sexual orientations. Also, how an individual adheres to the beliefs of his or her religious sect can vary dramatically. For instance, one Catholic might view his being gay as sinful, while another might see it as being normal.

11. *Recognize the importance of addressing unique issues that some gays, lesbians, and bisexuals may face.* Although the research is mixed, there is some evidence

that gays and bisexual men may face a higher rate of substance abuse and sexually transmitted diseases and that lesbians may face a higher rate of domestic violence, sexual abuse, and substance abuse. Know the prevalence of these and other issues within the specific population and the unique ways of treating them.

The Homeless and the Poor in the Helping Relationship

With over 700,000 people being homeless in America on any particular day and about 3.5 million experiencing homelessness in a given year, homelessness in America is a national crisis (National Coalition for the Homeless, 2009). In past years, being poor did not necessarily mean one was at greater risk of being homeless, but today, being poor is often one step away from not having a roof over one's head. The number of poor Americans is about 40 million, a little over 13% of the population, and 19% of all children today live in poverty (U.S. Census Bureau, 2009b). In addition, poverty in the United States continues to be associated with race (see Figure 8.4).

Some unique points that should be considered when working with the homeless and the poor include the following (Chinman, Bailey, Frey, & Rowe, 2001; Lum, 2009; Steinhaus, Harley, & Rogers, 2004; Substance Abuse and Mental Health Services Administration, 2010):

1. *Have the right attitudes and beliefs, gain knowledge, and learn skills.* Be prepared to work with the homeless and the poor by embracing the appropriate knowledge, skills, and beliefs prior to meeting with them.
2. *Focus on social issues.* Help clients obtain basic needs such as food and housing, as opposed to working on intrapsychic issues.
3. *Know the client's racial/ethnic/cultural background.* Be educated about the cultural heritage of clients, because a disproportionate number of the homeless and the poor come from diverse racial/ethnic/cultural groups.
4. *Be knowledgeable about health risks.* Be aware that the homeless and the poor are at much greater risk of developing AIDS, tuberculosis, and other diseases,

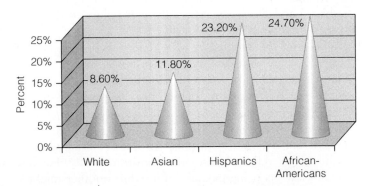

Figure 8.4 | Percentage of Individuals Below Poverty Levels as a Function of Race

and be able to do a basic medical screening and have referral sources available.

5. *Be prepared to deal with multiple issues.* Be prepared to deal with mental illness, chemical dependence, and other unique problems, because as much as 50% of the homeless are struggling with these problems.

6. *Know about developmental delays and be prepared to refer.* Know how to identify developmental delays and have potential referral sources, because homeless and poor children are much more likely to have delayed language and social skills, be abused, and have delayed motor development.

7. *Know psychological effects.* Be prepared to deal with the client's feelings of despair, depression, and hopelessness as a result of being poor and/or homeless.

8. *Know resources.* Be aware of the vast number of resources available in your community and make referrals when appropriate.

9. *Be an advocate and stay committed.* Because the homeless and the poor are often dealing with multiple issues, and because a high percentage of them have mental illness, advocating for their unique concerns and being committed to them is particularly important as this gives them the message that you are truly there for them.

Older Persons in the Helping Relationship

In 1900, 4% of the U.S. population was over 65 years of age, by 1960 it was 9%; today it's about 13%, and it is estimated that by 2030 it will be close to 20% (U.S. Census Bureau, 2003, 2008b). With these changing demographics, there has been an increased focus on treatment for and care of older persons. Older persons have a number of problems and concerns that need to be addressed in the helping relationship (Goodman, Schlossberg, & Anderson, 2006; Lum, 2009; Myers & Harper, 2004; Schwiebert, Myers, & Dice, 2000). The following are some guidelines for working effectively with older clients:

1. *Have the right attitudes and beliefs, gain knowledge, and learn skills.* The helper's stereotypes and biases may affect their prognosis of clients from this population. Be prepared to work with older clients by embracing the appropriate knowledge, skills, and beliefs prior to meeting with them.

2. *Adapt your helping style.* Adapt your style to fit the needs of the older client. For instance, for the older person who has difficulty hearing, the helper may use journal writing or art therapy. For clients who are not ambulatory, the helper may need to see the client in his or her home. In addition, know that certain interventions, such as group and life review, seem particularly advantageous with older persons if used appropriately.

3. *Build a trusting relationship.* Spend time building a trusting relationship. Remember that older persons tend to be less trustful of helpers, having grown up in a generation when such relationships were far less common.

4. *Be knowledgeable about issues many older persons face.* There are a number of issues that seem more prevalent within the geriatric population, including

loss and grief, depression, elder abuse, sleep disturbance, health concerns, identity issues, substance abuse, dementia, and others. Be knowledgeable of and assess for these issues.

5. *Know about possible and probable health changes.* Be aware of the many potential health problems common to older persons and have readily available referral sources. Predictable changes in health can lead to depression and concern about the future. Unpredictable changes in health can lead to loss of income and a myriad of emotional problems.

6. *Have empathy for changes in interpersonal relationships.* Changes in relationships may result from such things as retirement; the death of spouses, partners, and friends; changes in one's health status that prevent visits to and/or from friends; and relocations, such as to a retirement community, retirement home, or nursing home.

7. *Know about physical and psychological causes of sexual dysfunction.* Be aware of the possible physical and psychological causes of sexual dysfunction in older persons. As individuals age, it is fairly common for both men and women to have changes in their sexual functioning. Remember that regardless of our age, we are always sexual beings.

8. *Involve the client's family and friends.* As social networks change, it may become important to involve family and friends in treatment planning. Families and friends can offer great support to older persons.

With an increasing number of older persons in the United States, it is likely that more mental health providers who are trained in gerontology will be needed. Unfortunately, until recently training in this important area has been hard to find, and helpers have tended to avoid this specialization (Clawson, Henderson, Schweiger, & Collins, 2008; Stickle & Onedera, 2006). Perhaps it's time for the helping professions to place more emphasis on this important area.

HIV-Positive Individuals in the Helping Relationship

Today, over 1 million people in the United States are living with HIV, and about one in five of them don't know it (Centers for Disease Control and Prevention, 2010). It is also estimated that about 56,000 new cases of HIV arise each year, about 18,000 individuals die of the disease each year, and that close to 600,000 Americans have died since the disease was first identified. Unfortunately, AIDS continues to spread in this country, and worldwide an estimated 33 million children and adults are living with HIV (UNAIDS, 2010). A number of challenges face the helper who works with an individual who is HIV positive or who has AIDS. Some points to consider when working with an individual who is HIV positive include the following:

1. *Have the right attitudes and beliefs, gain knowledge, and learn skills.* Be prepared to work with HIV-positive individuals by embracing the appropriate knowledge, skills, and beliefs prior to meeting with them.

2. *Know the cultural background of the client.* Keep in mind that HIV-positive individuals are found in all cultures, races, and ethnic groups. Helpers need to remember that a client's background (e.g., culture, race, religion, gender) may change how the helper works with him or her.

3. *Know about the disease and combat myths.* Knowledge helps fight fear. Armed with knowledge, helpers can become advocates for the HIV-positive person.

4. *Be prepared to take on uncommon roles.* Realize that the helper may need to be an advocate, a caretaker, and a resource person for the client, roles in which the helper has not always been comfortable.

5. *Be prepared to deal with unique treatment issues.* Be prepared to deal with unique problems, including feelings about the loss of income from the loss of work or the high cost of medical treatment, depression and hopelessness concerning uncertain health, changes in interpersonal relationships when others discover the client is HIV positive (rejection, pity, fear, and so forth), and the probability that the client will have friends and loved ones who are HIV positive or have died of AIDS if he or she is from a high-risk group.

6. *Deal with your own feelings about mortality.* Be able to deal effectively with your own feelings about a client's health and mortality issues and how those feelings may raise issues concerning your own mortality.

7. *Understand the legal and ethical implications of working with individuals who may pose a risk to others or may be considering end-of-life decisions.*

8. *Offer a "strength-based" approach to treatment.* Help clients focus on what is positive in their lives and the possibilities that exist for them instead of focusing on diagnosis and the dread of the disease.

The Chronically Mentally Ill in the Helping Relationship

With 26% of Americans being diagnosed with a mental disorder every year (see Figure 8.5), almost all human service professionals will be working with some individuals who are struggling with such a disorder. Unfortunately, many of the chronically mentally ill find themselves on the streets and homeless, with some sources stating that as many as 26% of all homeless people may have severe psychiatric problems (Substance Abuse and Mental Health Services Administration, 2010). Helpers who will be working with the chronically mentally ill will need to understand psychiatric disorders, psychotropic medications, and the unique needs of the chronically mentally ill, such as dealing with homelessness, continual transitions, difficulty with employment, and dependent family relationships. The following treatment guidelines are focused on working with such individuals (Garske, 2009; Lum, 2009; Walsh, 2000; Wong, 2006):

1. *Have the right attitudes and beliefs, gain knowledge, and learn skills.* Be prepared to work with the mentally ill by embracing the appropriate knowledge, skills, and beliefs prior to meeting with them.

2. *Help the client understand his or her mental illness.* Fully inform clients with up-to-date knowledge about their mental illness. Many do not have an understanding of their illness, the course of the illness, and the best methods of treatment.

3. *Help the client work through feelings concerning his or her mental illness.* Mental illness continues to be stigmatized in society, and clients are often

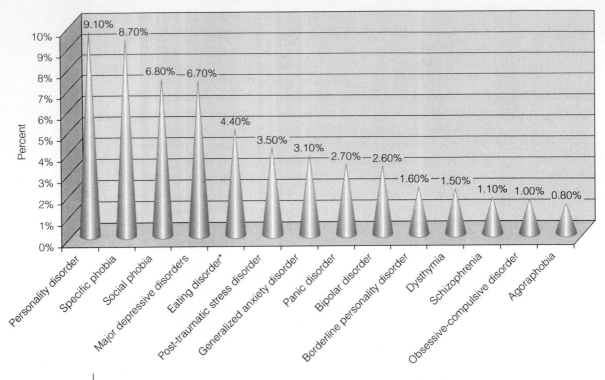

Figure 8.5 | Percentage of Adults with Select Mental Disorders Per Year

*Percentage of eating disorders are over a lifetime.
Source: National Institute of Mental Health (2008). *The numbers count: Mental disorders in America*. Retrieved from http://wwwapps.nimh.nih.gov/hcalth/publications/the-numbers-count-mental-disorders-in-america.shtml

embarrassed about their disorder. Support groups and a nonjudgmental attitude can go a long way in normalizing the view clients have of themselves.

4. *Ensure attendance.* Increase the chances of clients seeing a helper by calling the day before, having a relative or close friend assist the client in coming to your agency, or having helpers develop specific strategies to help clients make their appointments (e.g., putting Xs on a calendar). Clients will miss appointments due to denial about their illness, embarrassment about seeing a helper, problems remembering, or not caring.

5. *Assure compliance with medication.* Be vigilant about encouraging clients to continue to take their medication and assess its functionality. Clients will discontinue medication due to forgetfulness, denial about the illness, the false belief that they will not have a relapse because they feel better (the medication is working), and because the medication is not helpful for the particular client or the dosage is too small or too large.

6. *Assure accurate diagnosis.* Accurately diagnose clients to ensure proper treatment planning and the appropriate choice of medication. Accurate diagnosis

can be assured through testing, clinical interviews, interviews with significant others, and appropriate use of supervision.

7. *Reevaluate the client's treatment plan and do not give up.* Be committed to working with clients and reevaluate treatment plans as often as is necessary. The mentally ill are some of the most difficult clients to work with. Progress, if any, is slow, and it is easy to become discouraged.

8. *Involve the client's family.* Ensure adequate family involvement and have the family understand the implications of the client's diagnosis. Families can offer great support to clients with mental illness and can be a window into the client's psyche.

9. *Know resources.* Have a working knowledge of resources, as the mentally ill are often involved or need to become involved with many other resources in the community (e.g., Social Security disability, housing authority, support groups).

Individuals with Disabilities in the Helping Relationship

According to the census, approximately 54.4 million Americans had a disability (18.7%). And, of all Americans, for those 6 years and older, about 4.1 needed personal assistance with daily living; for those 15 years old and older, 3.4% had a problem seeing, 3.4% had hearing problems, 11.9% had difficulty walking, 8.2% had difficulty moving parts of their upper body, and 7.0% had cognitive, mental, or emotional impairments (U.S. Census Bureau, 2008a). In addition, you are more likely to have a disability if you live in the South, are poor, and are a minority. As federal laws have increasingly supported the right to services for individuals with disabilities, the helper has taken an increasingly active role in the treatment and rehabilitation of such individuals (Livneh & Antonak, 2005; Lum, 2009; Smart, 2009). Some treatment guidelines for working with the individual who has a disability include the following:

1. *Have the right attitudes and beliefs, gain knowledge, and learn skills.* Be prepared to work with clients who have a disability by embracing the appropriate knowledge, skills, and beliefs prior to meeting with clients.

2. *Have knowledge of the many disabling conditions.* To be effective, a helper should understand the physical and emotional consequences of the disability of the client.

3. *Help clients know their disabilities.* Inform clients of their disabilities, the probable course of treatment, and the prognosis. Such knowledge allows them to be fully involved in the helping process.

4. *Assist the client through the grieving process.* Help clients pass through stages of grief as they deal with their loss and move toward acceptance. Similar to the stages of bereavement (Kubler-Ross & Kessler, 2005), it is usual for a client to experience denial, anger, negotiation, resignation, and acceptance.

5. *Know referral resources.* Be aware of potential resources in the community (e.g., physicians, social services, physical therapists, experts on pain management, vocational rehabilitation). Individuals with disabilities often have a myriad of needs.

6. *Know the law and inform your client of the law.* Know the law to ensure that clients are receiving all necessary services and not being discriminated against. In addition, clients often feel empowered when they know their rights.

7. *Be prepared to do, or refer for, vocational/career counseling.* Be ready to either do career counseling or refer a client to a career counselor. Often, when faced with a disability, clients are also faced with making a career transition.

8. *Include the family.* Whenever possible and reasonable, include the client's family in the treatment process, as they can offer support, assist in long-term treatment planning, and help with the client's emotional needs.

9. *Be an advocate.* Advocate for clients by knowing the law, fighting for clients' rights, and assisting clients in fighting for their own rights. Individuals with disabilities are faced with prejudice and discrimination.

10. *Empower your clients.* Avoid being sympathetic and having low expectations, and listen to and support your client. Assume your client knows what is best for him or her.

ETHICAL, PROFESSIONAL, AND LEGAL ISSUES: MAKING WISE ETHICAL DECISIONS

Although our ethical code was cited in Chapter 7 as addressing a number of important issues when doing cross-cultural helping, others suggest that the use of codes alone can be problematic as they tend to "reflect the dominant culture's values at the expense of minority values" (Ridley, Liddle, Hill, & Li, 2001, p. 187). In addition, some helpers rigidly adhere to codes, which can negate the deeply reflective process that is sometimes needed when faced with difficult ethical dilemmas. Therefore, some suggest that rather than using ethical codes, it would be more advantageous to consider the moral underpinnings of codes, such as admonitions to respect the autonomy of the client, do no harm to others, promote the good of society, act in a fair manner, and maintain trust (Kitchener, 1984). However, others suggest that relying on moral admonitions may be based on particular values that may not be cross-culturally relevant. For instance, how one person defines the good of society may be drastically different from how another person defines it—or how another culture defines it.

Clearly, ethical decision making is complex. On the one hand, we must be careful when using the ethical guidelines, as they might hold some inherent bias and can be used in an absolutist and dualistic fashion. On the other hand, using a moral model may also be biased. At the very least, when making ethical decisions we must make careful, wise decisions based on all of the evidence. Such wise decisions often involve a deeply self-reflective process as well as the attainment of as much knowledge as possible of the situation at hand.

THE EFFECTIVE HUMAN SERVICE PROFESSIONAL: TRAINING CULTURALLY COMPETENT PROFESSIONALS

Although it has caught on quickly, the training of culturally competent helpers is relatively new. Training programs quickly need to adopt new methods of training to ensure that their students leave their programs culturally competent. There are many ways this can be done (Neukrug & Milliken, 2008):

1. *Weaving:* Weaving multicultural training throughout a program
2. *Course:* Offering a separate course on social and cultural issues
3. *Immersion:* Requiring one or more immersion activities where students are asked to participate in a culture/group which is new to them and diverse
4. *Supervision:* Providing supervision that focuses on cross-cultural issues
5. *Cases:* Using case studies in classes to highlight cross-cultural issues
6. *Dilemmas:* Providing dilemma discussions that gently push students into examining challenging problems a minority client might face
7. *Role-plays:* Conducting role-plays to watch and practice cross-cultural helping
8. *Group:* Providing group experiences that enable students to discuss their heritages and cultural affiliations
9. *Journaling:* Writing down thoughts in a journal as a way of revealing perceived threatening experiences relative to cross-cultural helping that a student might not reveal verbally
10. *Reading:* Reading about cross-cultural concerns and discussing the readings in class

Learning, however, is a lifelong process. When you leave your program, new theories will be developed and new strategies formed to work with clients from nondominant groups. In addition, it is hoped that your life experiences will reveal new awareness about yourself relative to cross-cultural helping. The culturally competent helper is always eager to learn about new theories and strategies and willing to grow personally in new ways. As you enter the human service profession, it is our hope that you will continually want to learn more about cross-cultural helping.

SUMMARY

This chapter began by stressing how America has changed over the last few decades in that it now has a great ethnic/cultural mix, a wide range of religions, changing sex roles, and changing attitudes toward a number of groups that have been historically discriminated against. This chapter then offered three models to help human service professionals work with this increasingly diverse population.

First, we examined the Multicultural Counseling Competencies model that suggests specific ways that all human service professionals should develop if they are to become culturally competent. This model suggests that all human services professionals should have the right attitudes and beliefs, knowledge, and skills, as applied in three areas: the helper's awareness of the client's world view, the helper's awareness of his or her own cultural values, and the helper's ability at using culturally appropriate intervention strategies. This was followed by the RESPECTFUL model which highlighted ten factors which helpers should attend to in their helping relationships. The last model, the Tripartite model, suggests that the human service professional should be aware of the individual, the group, and the universal spheres of our clients' lives.

A good portion of this chapter gave preliminary information as well as general guidelines about working with a wide range of groups that have been historically oppressed. These included cultural/racial groups; individuals from diverse religious backgrounds; men and women (gender-aware helping); gays, bisexuals, and lesbians; the homeless and the poor; older persons; individuals who are HIV positive; the chronically mentally ill; and individuals with disabilities.

When discussing ethical, professional, and legal issues, we noted that ethical codes can sometimes be suspect as they may reflect the dominant culture's values. On the other hand, it is also sometimes difficult to use moral models of decision making, as how they are interpreted may reflect our own cultural biases. We concluded the importance of making self-reflective and wise ethical decisions. This chapter ended with a discussion on the importance of keeping up, throughout our careers, with new ways of working with clients from nondominant groups.

Experiential Exercises

I. **Racist, Sexist, and Culturally Offensive Terms and Jokes**
    1. *Offensive Words:* Your instructor will ask all students to list every racist, sexist, or culturally offensive word or term they can think of. Write them on the board. Then, discuss the following:
        a. Why do people use these terms?
        b. How does each of us respond when we hear these terms?
        c. What responsibility does the human service professional have to combat the use of these terms?
        d. What responsibility does each of us have toward combating the use of these terms?
    2. *Offensive Jokes:* Your instructor will ask all students to anonymously write down racist, sexist, or culturally offensive jokes. Your instructor will then gather these and then discuss each of them with the class. Use the following questions as a guideline:
        a. Why do people say these jokes?
        b. What may be the origins of these jokes?
        c. How does each of us respond when we hear others say such jokes?
        d. What responsibility, if any, do we have to confront people who tell such jokes?
    3. *Garbage In, Garbage Out:* After you have finished items 1 and 2, take a piece of paper that has all of the terms and jokes on it and throw it out, symbolically getting rid of these offensive items. While throwing these papers out, the class should make a commitment to combat the use of such words, terms, and jokes by confronting those who use them.

II. **Gaining Knowledge About Some Select Groups**
    Interview an individual from one or more of the populations listed here, and ask the accompanying questions (and any other questions you think would be appropriate).
    1. *A Person from a Nondominant Group*
        a. When did you first realize that you were a person from a nondominant group (or a minority, person of color, person from a diverse group)?
        b. How did you feel you "fit in" to society when you realized you were not like the majority of people?

    c. Explain negative and positive experiences that you might attribute to being from a nondominant group.

    d. What prejudices have you experienced?

    e. What services have you been able to use due to your status as a "minority"?

    f. What are your thoughts about being given services that Whites cannot obtain?

    g. Overall, how do you think your ethnic/cultural group views a helping relationship?

    h. Would you, personally, see a helping professional? Why or why not?

2. *An Individual Who Has a Disability*

    a. How did you become disabled?

    b. What unique experiences have you had related to your disability?

    c. What prejudices have you experienced?

    d. What social services have you used?

    e. What social services would you like to have available?

    f. Is there anything you would like to have changed about your life related to your current status?

3. *A Poor Person and/or Homeless Person*

    a. How did you become homeless or poor?

    b. What unique experiences have you had related to your current life situation?

    c. What prejudices have you experienced?

    d. What social services have you used?

    e. What social services would you like to have available?

    f. How do you make it financially day to day?

    g. What financial resources are available to you?

4. *An Individual Who Is (or Was) Chemically Dependent*

    a. What led you to become chemically dependent?

    b. What drugs and/or alcohol do (have) you use(d)?

    c. What unique experiences have you had related to your substance abuse?

    d. What prejudices have you experienced?

    e. What social services have you used?

    f. What social services would you like to have available?

    g. How do you currently expect to handle your addiction to drugs and/or alcohol?

5. *An Individual Who Is HIV Positive*

    a. How did you become HIV positive?

    b. What unique experiences have you had related to being HIV positive?

    c. What prejudices have you experienced?

    d. What social services have you used?

    e. What social services would you like to have available?

    f. What societal changes would you like to see take place relative to your HIV-positive status?

6. *An Older Person*

    a. How do you feel about being an older person?

    b. What unique experiences have you had related to your age?

    c. What prejudices have you experienced?

       d. What social services have you used?
       e. What social services would you like to have available?
       f. What attitudes related to aging would you like to see changed in society?
   7. *An Individual Who Struggles with Mental Illness*
       a. When do you first remember having to deal with your mental health problems?
       b. What unique experiences have you had related to your mental illness?
       c. What prejudices have you experienced?
       d. What social services have you used?
       e. What social services would you like to have available?
       f. Has medication assisted you with your mental health problems?
       g. What changes in the mental health care delivery system would you like to see?

III. Identifying the Needs of Culturally Different Clients

The following is a list of select cultural groups. Some individuals from such groups have unique needs in the helping relationship that are related to their culture/ethnic background. Identify one or more of the groups listed, and discuss how you think the helping relationship might best work with individuals from that group. Feel free to add other groups to this list.

African-Americans	Latinos/Latinas	Asians
Native Americans	Fundamentalist	Men
Women	Gay men	Lesbians
Bisexuals	Older persons	The mentally ill
Individuals with disabilities	Homeless individuals	Poor individuals
Individuals who are HIV+	Transgendered persons	Atheist

IV. Examining the Main Values of the Helping Relationship

Column two of Table 8.2 lists the inherent values usually found in helping relationships in the United States. Thus, standard English is generally spoken, helpers usually believe that clients should take responsibility for themselves, and so forth. Take the cultural groups listed across the first row, or any other groups of your choice (simply place the name of the group in the top of column six), and compare the values usually found in the helping relationship to values you believe these cultural groups generally embrace. What differences do you notice? What can the helper do to make the helping relationship more amenable to the clients that you identified?

V. Ethical, Legal, and Professional Issues

In responding to these items, you may want to refer to the ACA's ethical code, which can be found in Appendix A.

   1. You realize when working with a client from Peru that the cross-cultural differences are making it difficult for you to be effective. Rather than referring the client, you decide to read more about your client's culture so you gain a better understanding of him. Is this ethical? Is this professional?

Table 8.2 | Focus of Helping Relationship and Focus of Specific Cultural Groups on Select Attributes

	Focus of Helping Relationship in United States	Latinos/Latinas	Muslims	Gay Men	Other?
Primary language	Standard English				
Locus of control/responsibility	High locus of control and responsibility				
Major values	Openness Intimacy Cause and effect Analytical Self-disclosure				
Mental and physical processes	Dichotomous Mind/body separation				
Gender focus	Nonsexist ideals stressed				
Focus on family	Nuclear family				
Religion	Generally neutral				

2. A White human service professional decides that he can best serve only White clients. He believes his biases are too great to overcome and that he has a "special niche" in offering workshops to White, well-to-do clients. Although he doesn't mind if a person of color shows up at this workshop, the way that he advertises tends to draw Whites. For instance, he sometimes puts an ad in the paper that states, "English speaking professional offers parenting workshop that addresses the concerns of upwardly mobile children and their parents." Is he acting ethically? Professionally? Legally?

3. When working with an Asian client who is not expressive of her feelings, a helper you know pressures the client to express feelings. The helper tells the client, "You can only get better if you express yourself." Is this helper acting ethically? Professionally? Do you have any responsibility in this case?

4. When offering a parenting workshop to individuals who are poor, you are challenged when you tell them that "hitting a child is never okay." They tell you that you are crazy and that sometimes a good spanking is the only thing that will get the child's attention. Do they have a point? What should you do?

5. A helper who is seeing a client who is HIV positive discovers that his client is having sex with others without revealing his HIV status. You tell him that you have a responsibility to report him to the police. Would this be ethical? Professional? Legal?

6. A colleague of yours is working with a Latina client who states there is little hope for happiness in her marriage. The client states that her husband's attitude toward her is constantly demeaning, but that there is little she can do. After all, she tells you that it is "out of her control" and in God's hands. Your colleague tells you that she is helping the client gain autonomy and to give up the notion of "fatialismo" or that fate controls one's life—a value held by some Latinos/Latinas. Is your colleague acting appropriately? Is there a better way for her to respond?

7. A professor of yours is a transsexual, and students in your class make jokes about him. What is your professional responsibility in this case? What thoughts do you have regarding your fellow students?

8. A helper, who is from a diverse culture, is seeing a client from the same culture. After the helping relationship has continued for a few months, the client says, "You can't help me—you're too rich to understand my circumstances." Could the client have a point? What are the pros and cons of the helper continuing to see the client? How should the helper proceed?

9. You discover that a colleague of yours has a patronizing attitude about his clients who have a disability. He often can be heard saying things like "Poor Joe, he's blind," or "It's a pity that a pretty girl like Joan is missing a leg." What, if any, responsibility do you have to confront your colleague?

10. Based on the lack of research that shows results and because he believes it is biased against gays and lesbians, a colleague of yours is against referring gay men for reparative therapy (counseling to convert a gay man to straight). One day, a gay man who is very depressed and upset about his sexuality asks this colleague for a referral to a reparative therapist. The colleague explains the lack of research and discusses with the client the positive and affirming aspects of being gay. The client begs for a referral, and the human service professional finally gives him one. Has the helper acted professionally? Ethically? Legally?

11. A colleague of yours identifies herself as a feminist. You know that when she works with some women, she actively encourages them to leave their husbands when she discovers the husband is verbally or physically abusive. Is she acting ethically? Should you do anything?

Research, Evaluation, and Assessment

CHAPTER CONTENTS

Research

Evaluation and Needs Assessment

Assessment and Testing

Ethical, Professional, and Legal Issues

The Effective Human Service Professional

Summary

Experiential Exercises

Walking down a street in Cincinnati one day a person came up to me and said, "Do you want to take a personality test?" I said, "Sure!" I was brought into a storefront office and spent about 30 minutes completing an inventory. When I finished, I was asked to wait a few minutes while they scored the instrument. Then, a person came into the room and said, "Well, you have a pretty good personality, and you're fairly bright, but if you read L. Ron Hubbard's book on Dianetics and become involved in Scientology, you will have a better personality and be even brighter." However, having taken course work in testing, I questioned whether the test truly measured personality and intelligence and the way in which the instrument was interpreted.

Ten years later, I'm walking down a street in Minneapolis, and a person comes up to me and says, "Do you want to take a personality test?" Well, now I realize that this person is trying to get me to be involved with Scientology. I say to him, "What evidence do you have that this test is statistically valid and reliable?" He assures me that it is. I say, "I would like some evidence," at which point he tells me that at the headquarters in New York, they have that information. I say to him, "I'll buy the book on Dianetics and read it after the information is sent to me." He agrees. I never hear from him again. The book is still sitting in my library.

A student of mine conducted a study on the relationship between the number of years of yoga meditation and self-actualizing values. She believed the more you meditated, the more self-actualized you would be. She went to an ashram (a yoga retreat center) and had a number of individuals fill out an instrument to measure how self-actualized they were; she then collected information from the same individuals on how long they had been meditating. After collecting her data and performing a statistical analysis, she found no relationship. Because she herself had meditated for years, she strongly felt that she would find such a relationship. Upon finding no relationship, she said to me, "There must be something wrong with this instrument or this research, because people who have meditated for years are clearly more self-actualized than those who have just started meditating." I suggested there was nothing wrong with the research or the instrument, but that perhaps she had a bias because of her own experiences with meditation. I explained that this does not mean that meditation does not affect people, but that in this one area, using this instrument, the evidence showed that no relationship existed. I told her that research is not how you feel something is but what you find something is. When she was able to see her own biases, she realized that perhaps I was right.

I am the "evaluator" for some of the programs in our department. Every year I have students take a number of surveys assessing a wide range of items. I assess if they have learned all of what they think they should have learned, if they felt good about their internship, if they thought their supervisor was knowledgeable and helpful, if faculty were good teachers, and on and on. It's rather involved. Many of the surveys are online, which makes it easier for students to access, and I save a few trees.

Testing, research, and evaluation, that's what this chapter is about, and that is something you will be involved with as a human service professional. Thus, this chapter will explore some of the major kinds of qualitative and quantitative research designs, examine types of program evaluation, and offer an overview of assessment procedures. Near the end of the chapter, we will review ethical, professional, and legal issues related to informed consent in research, program evaluation, and assessment techniques; the use of human subjects in research; and the proper use of testing data. This chapter will conclude with a discussion on how the information that we gain from research, program evaluation, and assessment is an evolving process that allows us to continually add new knowledge to the field.

RESEARCH

Conducting Research

The inquiry of truth, which is the love-making, or wooing of it, the knowledge of truth, which is the presence of it, and the belief of truth, which is the enjoying of it, is the sovereign good of human nature. (Sir Francis Bacon, 1597/1997)

Research answers the questions "Are our hunches about the world correct?" and "How might what we are doing affect the future?" Best and Kahn (2006) describe research as "the systematic and objective analysis and recording of controlled observations that may lead to the development of generalizations, principles or theories, resulting in prediction and possibly ultimate control of events" (p. 25). Research can be anything from counting the number of times a child acts out during the day, to surveying opinions of human service professionals, to performing a complex statistical analysis of a specific counseling approach when working with clients. Before conducting research, however, one must develop a hypothesis or research question.

The Hypothesis, the Research Question, and Literature Review

Kuhn (1962) said that new knowledge is built on former knowledge and shifts in our understanding of the world take place when former knowledge no longer explains current phenomena. In a sense, as Sir Francis Bacon said so eloquently, we are forever seeking the truth. In performing research, one of our first steps is to develop a **hypothesis** or **research question** in an effort to test propositions that are derived from theories and prior research (Leary, 2007; Sommer & Sommer, 2002). For us to come up with our hypothesis or question, we need to do a thorough **review of the literature.**

A review of the literature examines all the major research conducted in the area we are exploring. This is accomplished by conducting a search of professional publications, usually journal articles and books. Three particularly popular electronic databases through which one can search are **Educational Resources Information Center (ERIC), PsycINFO,** and **EBSCO** (databases are also valuable tools for papers). For instance, if I were interested in examining some aspect of the human services work environment, after accessing a database through my library, I would type in key descriptors, that is, major terms to be searched. In this case, key descriptors might include *jobs, human services, social services, careers,* and *occupations.* A list of abstracts would then be generated that contained all of the articles with one or more of these descriptors. After initially doing this, it is often necessary to refine the search by typing in additional descriptors. Eventually, I have a readable list of abstracts that I can review. After reviewing the abstracts, I decide which articles I want to fully read. These days, articles are often available electronically as a "full-text" article, online through your college library. Sometimes, however, you might have to go to the library to get hold of an article or order one through your interlibrary loan office of your library.

After reviewing the articles, I would begin to identify the variables I specifically wanted to examine in my research. A **variable** is "any characteristics or quality that differs in degree or kind and can be measured" (Sommer & Sommer, 2002, p. 85) (e.g., height, intelligence, self-esteem, job satisfaction). For instance, in my computer search I might have found a number of articles on job satisfaction (variable 1) of human service professionals who work at varying social service agencies (variable 2). I could then begin to formulate a research question or a hypothesis around these variables.

In guiding research, when variables are measured and used to distinguish *differences* between groups, hypotheses are generally developed; when variables are measured and used to examine *relationships* between groups, hypotheses *or* research questions are generated; and when variables are measured and used to *describe* current events or conditions, research questions are generated. In the preceding example, one hypothesis might be the following: "Human service professionals who work at mental health centers will be more satisfied than will those who work at child protective services" (note the comparison of groups, thus a hypothesis). On the other hand, a research question might be the following: "What roles and functions performed by human service professionals provide job satisfaction?"

Defining Quantitative and Qualitative Research Designs

Research designs can broadly be categorized as quantitative or qualitative in nature. **Quantitative research** assumes that there is an objective reality within which research questions can be formulated and scientific methods used to measure the probability that certain behaviors, values, or beliefs either cause or are related to other behaviors, values, or beliefs. **Qualitative research,** on the other hand, holds that there are multiple ways of viewing knowledge and that one can make sense of the world by immersing oneself in the research situation in an attempt to provide possible explanations for the problem being examined (Heppner, Wampold, & Kivlighan, 2008). Table 9.1 gives a summary of distinguishing features of qualitative and quantitative research.

Qualitative and quantitative research approach the analysis of research problems differently. Thus, it is not surprising that their designs vary dramatically. Whereas quantitative research attempts to reduce the problem to a few very specific variables that can be experimentally manipulated, the aim of qualitative research is to make sense out of the problem by analyzing it broadly within its naturally occurring context. Therefore, we will separately examine a few of the more popular quantitative and qualitative research designs while keeping in mind that some

Table 9.1 | Distinctions Between Quantitative and Qualitative Research

	Quantitative	Qualitative
Assumptions about knowledge	"Truth" is sought through research. Knowledge is used to develop hypotheses.	Reality is socially constructed and there are multiple realities. Knowledge emerges through research.
Research methods used	Mathematical, statistical, and logical. Hypothesis testing and attempt to find answer to research questions. Deductive process.	Philosophical and sociological. Multiple methods to understand research question. Immersion in task with goal to have knowledge emerge. Inductive process.
Biases and validity	Bias is problematic. Increased control of study to increase validity to reduce bias.	Bias is acknowledged. Reduced through the use of multiple methods of attaining data and examining results.
Goals and generalizability	To discover evidence and "truth" and generalize to larger audience.	To uncover information and describe findings in order to enlighten.
Researcher role	Detached, objective scientist.	Researcher is immersed in social situation and describes and interprets findings.

researchers combine these two approaches and use a **mixed methods** approach (Gall, Gall, & Borg, 2010).

Quantitative Research

Although there are many forms of quantitative research, four of the more popular types are **true experimental research, causal-comparative (ex post facto) research, correlational research,** and **survey research.**

True Experimental Research   In true experimental research, you manipulate variables to see what effect they have on the outcome you are examining. This type of research uses hypotheses and allows you to look at the causes of behavior. Usually, the variable being manipulated is called the **independent variable,** and the variable you are measuring is called the **dependent variable.** In addition, **random assignment** of subjects to treatment groups is almost always used. For instance, if I wanted to examine the effect of different kinds of multicultural counseling training, I could randomly assign students to three groups: one where no training took place, and two other groups that were provided different kinds of training in multicultural counseling. After the training was complete, I could measure how effectively the students learned multicultural counseling skills. However, in some cases random assignment is difficult, if not impossible to do (see Box 9.1). In these cases, we might decide to conduct some other, less rigorous type of study, such as is done in causal-comparative research.

Causal-Comparative (Ex Post Facto) Research   Because experimental research involves random assignment and the manipulation of variables, it is often impractical or impossible to implement (Heppner et al., 2008). Therefore, causal-comparative research, sometimes called ex post facto research, which allows one

---

BOX 9.1 | **Failed Attempt at True Experimental Research**

A colleague and I decided to conduct research on the effects of aerobic exercise on personality variables. After exploring the literature, we found possible links between such an exercise and the personality variables of self-actualization, depression, and anxiety. We approached our local YMCA, which was running a rather extensive aerobic exercise program, and the staff agreed to let us talk with individuals who were about to start their exercise program. They also agreed to let these people have eight weeks of free membership at the YMCA if half of them (randomly chosen) would not start aerobics for eight weeks. We found three instruments to measure our personality measures, with the intent of comparing, at the end of eight weeks, the group that started aerobics with the group that waited. We excitedly met with about 50 potential subjects for our study. We told them our plans, and they looked at us and said, "Are you kidding? We want to start our aerobic exercise now!"

Our good intentions were not going to sway these individuals who were ready to get going with their exercise. Unfortunately for us, we could not implement our study. Instead, we used a causal-comparative design, which would not be as powerful conducting true experimental research.

to examine variables of intact groups, is often employed. For instance, let's say I wanted to measure how satisfied 100 human service majors were at four different kinds of jobs (e.g., mental health, social services, unemployment, rehabilitation), 1 year after graduation. If this were a true experimental design, I would have to randomly assign 100 graduates to these four jobs, and then compare how satisfied they were at their various jobs 1 year later. Clearly, this would be impossible. However, I could compare job satisfaction of human service professionals 1 year after they have been hired at these four kinds of jobs. I would accomplish this by giving each intact group a scale that measured job satisfaction, and then I would examine statistical differences among the four groups. Because random assignment is not used, any differences found cannot be attributed solely to the type of job (e.g., perhaps people who have a tendency to be more satisfied pick certain jobs). Therefore, in this type of research, we cannot be assured that one variable causes another. However, this research can often give us a good sense of the relationship between variables.

Correlational Research   Two popular kinds of correlational research are **simple correlational studies**, which explore the relationship between two variables, and **predictive correlational studies**, which are used to predict scores on a variable from scores obtained from other variables. Correlational research uses **correlation coefficients** to show the strength of the relationship between two or more sets of scores. A correlation coefficient ranges from -1.0 to $+1.0$ and generally is reported in decimals of one-hundredths (see Figure 9.1). A positive correlation shows a tendency for two sets of scores to be related in the same direction. A negative correlation shows an inverse relationship between two sets of scores. For instance, if I were interested in the relationship between the ability to be empathic and dogmatic, I could obtain scores from one group of individuals on these two variables and correlate them. In this case, you would likely see a negative correlation, which would indicate that individuals who were more empathic tended to be less dogmatic and vice versa.

Generally, r is used to describe the strength of the relationship. For instance, if I found a correlation coefficient of .89 between height and weight, I would say $r = .89$. Or, if I found that grades in college had a mild negative correlation of $-.24$ with the number of hours per week spent in pursuing leisure activities, I would present the correlation as $r = -.24$. It should be stressed, however, that correlational studies do not show cause and effect because other, often unknown, variables may be responsible for the relationship between the two variables. For instance, in a study examining academic achievement, researchers found a high correlation between the number of bathrooms in the home and how well children did in school. Certainly, having more bathrooms does not cause higher academic achievement. Other factors are undoubtedly the cause. For instance, those

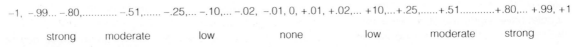

Figure 9.1 | The Range and Strength of Correlation Coefficients

individuals who have more bathrooms likely have more money and are probably more educated. Thus, other variables are the cause for this unlikely correlation.

Survey Research   In survey research, a questionnaire is designed to gather specific information from a target population. For instance, we might send a questionnaire to human service professionals in an effort to understand what variables might be related to level of job satisfaction at various types of human service jobs. In this case, we could examine many variables such as salary, number of years at the job, and educational level, and perhaps ask those surveyed to rate their job satisfaction. We could then use charts and graphs to illustrate the differences between the various jobs on these variables.

To illustrate the type of information one can obtain from surveys, Neukrug, Milliken, and Shoemaker (2001) completed a survey to determine if human service practitioners, educators, and students had ever seen a counselor, and for those who had, the kinds of characteristics they sought in a counselor. It was found that 75% had been in counseling, with women seeking counseling at higher rates than men and practitioners attended counseling at higher rates than educators or students. The researchers also found that the qualities most sought in choosing a counselor were competence, trustworthiness, warmth and caring, openness, and empathy, whereas research productivity, a reputation for being a therapist's therapist, and spiritual orientation were the least-rated qualities deemed important for choosing a counselor.

Although survey research can be interesting, it cannot tell us the underlying reasons for our results. For instance, in our research on counseling attendance, we were not able to determine why individuals attended counseling and if certain types of counseling were more beneficial than others. Therefore, survey research can be limiting, although sometimes intriguing.

Qualitative Research

As noted earlier, the approach to qualitative research varies dramatically from that used for quantitative research. Although there are a number of different kinds of qualitative research, three of the most popular types are **grounded theory, ethnographic research,** and **historical research.**

Grounded Theory   Developed by sociologists Glaser and Strass (Buckley, 2010; Houser, 2009), grounded theory is a process in which a broad research question is examined in a multitude of ways that eventually leads to the emergence of a theory. For instance, let's say I was interested in the research question: "How are helping skills developed in human service work?" I first would come up with a series of related questions that could be asked of human service professionals, such as:

- What skills were most important to you when you first started in this field?
- What skills have you discarded from your early work with clients?
- What skills have you adapted in your later work with clients?
- How have your skills evolved since you started in this field?
- What do you think has been most important in your skills development?

After coming up with questions, I would prepare to interview human service professionals. For instance, I might come up with "focus groups" of professionals who had been in the field for a determined amount of time (e.g., 10 years) and begin to seek their responses to the questions as well as additional questions that might emerge as the discussions unravel. This process would unfold through a series of steps, which include preparing, data collection, note taking, coding, and writing.

Preparing   This phase is when you reflect on your own biases and prepare to collect information from your participants. You are aware that meeting with individuals in and of itself will affect how they respond, and you attempt to be respectful, nonjudgmental, and a good listener.

Data Collection   This phase has to do with the process you use for obtaining your information. As noted, focus groups are often a common method of collecting data, although other methods can be used (e.g., examining writings of individuals, observing in naturalistic settings). When interviewing others, it is here that I would use my list of questions.

Note-Taking   Many grounded theorists do not take notes at all; instead, they rely on their memories to write down the most important elements after having collected information. However, others find no problem with note-taking or even recording the interviews. In either case, this process should be as nonintrusive as possible and should allow for participants to express their opinions.

Coding   **Coding** has to do with identifying common themes among the various conversations being listened to and giving them a code. This helps to organize the data you have collected. As individuals code, "core" categories will emerge that begin to point to broad themes evident in the data collection. Saturation of themes occurs when you realize that many individuals are referring to the same core themes. It is then that the process is nearing its end.

Writing   As the final themes emerge through the coding process, the researcher is ready to write up his or her findings. For instance, in examining how human service professionals develop their skills, I might find that such professionals pass through a series of stages in the development and refinement of their skills.

Ethnographic Research   *Ethnography* refers to the description (*graphy*) of human cultures (*ethno*). Sometimes called **cultural anthropology**, ethnographic research was made popular by **Margaret Mead,** who studied aboriginal youth in Samoa by immersing herself in their culture as she attempted to understand their lifestyle (Mead, 1961). Ethnographic research assumes that phenomena or events can best be understood within their cultural context. Take an event out of its context, and its meaning is likely to be interpreted from the context of the researcher rather than from its original social context. Ethnographers, therefore, seek to understand events by understanding the meanings that people place on them from within their natural contexts.

The first step in conducting ethnographic research is to identify the group to be studied and the general problem to be researched. Conducting a literature review

As a participant observer, Margaret Mead (1901–1978) gained a deep understanding of the culture she was observing by living with the people.

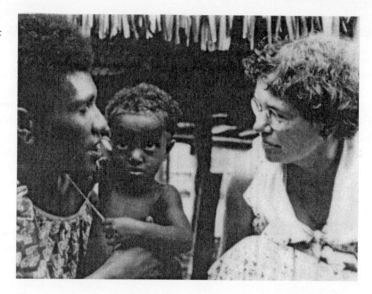

can help the researcher gain a better understanding of the culture or group being studied and assists in defining the purpose of the research and in developing research questions. Before entering the culture, the researcher should develop a plan for implementing his or her data collection methods, and then the researcher should decide on the best way to immerse himself or herself in the culture being explored. Three common methods used in ethnographic research are **observation, ethnographic interviews,** and collection of **documents** and **artifacts.**

Observation   Ethnographers will often observe a situation or phenomenon and describe, using extensive notes, what they view. Although sometimes qualitative researchers take nonengaged roles when observing, more often they become **participant observers.** In this kind of observation, the researcher may actually live and interact with the group and take notes about its interactions (Gall et al., 2010). However, it is important that the observer do not interfere with the natural process of the group. The observer should take scrupulous notes and carefully listen to the individuals being observed in an effort to obtain a rich appreciation for the ways in which the group constructs reality. It is particularly important that the observer record what role he or she has taken while observing and what effect, if any, observation may have had on the group being observed (see Box 9.2).

Ethnographic Interviews   Ethnographic interviews are a second popular qualitative method of collecting data from a culture or group. Such interviews involve asking open-ended questions as a method of understanding how the interviewees construct meaning. Interviews may be informal; guided, where questions are outlined in advance; or standardized, where the exact questions are determined before the interview, but the responses remain open-ended. As with participant observation, the interviewer must take scrupulous notes or record the interviews to obtain verbatim accounts of the conversations.

BOX 9.2 | Disruptive Observation of a Third-Grade Class

While working in New Hampshire, I was once asked to debrief a third-grade class that had just finished a trial period in which a young boy, who was paraplegic and had a severe intellectual disability, was mainstreamed into their classroom. During this trial period, a stream of observers from a local university had come into the students' classroom to assess their progress. Because this was not participant observation, the observers would sit in the back of the classroom and take notes about the interactions between the students. This information was supposed to be used later to decide whether it was beneficial to all involved to have the student with the disability mainstreamed.

When I met with the students, they clearly had adapted well to this young boy. Although the students seemed to have difficulty forming relationships with him, his presence seemed in no way to detract from their studies or from their other relationships in the classroom. However, almost without exception, the students noted that the constant stream of observers interfering with their daily schedule was quite annoying. Perhaps if participant observation had been employed, where an observer interacted and was seen as part of the classroom, the students would have responded differently.

Collection of Documents and Artifacts Artifacts are symbols of a culture or group that provide the researcher an understanding of the beliefs, values, and behaviors of the group. To understand the meaning an artifact holds, researchers need to know how the artifact was produced, where it came from, its age, how it was used, and who used it. Interpretation of the meaning of artifacts should be corroborated from observations and through interviews. Major categories of artifacts are personal documents, such as diaries, personal letters, and anecdotal records; official documents, such as internal and external papers and communications, records and personnel files, and statistical data; and objects that hold symbolic meaning of the culture (e.g., Native American headdresses) (McMillan & Schumacher, 2010).

Historical Research Historical research relies on the systematic collection of information in an effort to examine and understand past events from a contextual framework. When doing historical research, the researcher generally has a viewpoint and needs to go to the literature to support this viewpoint. Then, the researcher will begin to collect data to show that his or her viewpoint has validity. At any point, the researcher's point of view might change as he or she is influenced by the literature or by the sources of data obtained. Whenever possible, when collecting data for historical research, researchers use **primary sources,** or the original record, rather than **secondary sources,** which are documents or verbal information from sources that did not actually experience the event. Examples of primary sources include **oral histories, documents,** and **relics** (Gay, Mills, & Airasian, 2009; McMillan & Schumacher, 2010).

Oral Histories Oral histories are created when researchers directly interview an individual who participated in the event or observed the event in question.

Documents   Documents are records of events—such as letters, diaries, autobiographies, journals and magazines, films, recordings, paintings, and institutional records—that are generally housed in libraries or archival centers.

Relics   Relics are a variety of objects that can provide evidence about the event in question. Such things as books, maps, buildings, artifacts, and other objects are some examples of relics.

In conducting historical research, it is important that the researcher interpret information from within the historical frame that is being examined. This is often a long and tedious process. For instance, examine the historical research in Box 9.3, written by a friend of mine when examining the letters of St. Paul from the New Testament (see Lanci, 1997, 1999).

BOX 9.3 | Historical Research: A New Temple for Corinth*

My project began because I thought it might be interesting to take a new look at the letters of St. Paul. They have been extremely influential in the formation of Christianity, and yet they are rarely examined as artifacts of a world that existed 2,000 years ago, a world very different from our own. Today, Christians look at them as theological treatises, but Paul wrote them as letters of guidance to specific Christian communities with specific challenges and problems.

I took one letter (1 Corinthians) and one image he uses (the community as a temple) in one passage (Chapter 3, verses 16–17), and tried to see if traditional interpretations could be challenged by looking more closely at the actual historical and cultural context of the Corinthian people to whom Paul wrote. Traditionally, interpreters have assumed that Paul was spurning the Jewish temple in Jerusalem, the temple of his youth (since he was Jewish), and telling the Corinthian Christians that they were themselves the new temple of God. I knew this to be historically uncertain, since there was no external evidence that Paul ever turned his back on the Jerusalem temple. I wondered how else this text might be interpreted.

I began by studying the conventional ways that people interpret the target passage and discovered some basic flaws in their views. To do this, I studied other primary texts to discover what functions temples played in cities like Corinth. Some of these texts were inscriptions found at archaeological sites, including Corinth. Others were literary texts by Roman authors. In addition, I studied the archaeological remains of the temples of Corinth, visiting the site three times, talking with archaeologists and biblical scholars who were also studying Corinth.

What I found was that it is likely Paul was not referring to the Jerusalem temple, since his audience was Gentiles and there were plenty of other temples to which Paul could refer. And, I discovered that Paul was probably using the temple/community image to help the Corinthians understand who they were as a community, as opposed to attempting to get them to turn away from Jerusalem. Past interpretations have unfortunately been used to support anti-Semitic attitudes because some interpretations are that Paul rejected his Jewish faith in favor of a new Christian one. This new, and I believe more historically accurate, interpretation supports the notion that Paul never stopped being a Jew; he just changed from being a traditional observer of Judaism to a Jew who believed that Jesus was the Messiah and was expressive of the fullness of Judaism. This sort of Jewishness was not rejected by other Jews until about 30 years after Paul died.

*By John Lanci, Ph.D.

Examining Results

Once you have completed your literature review, set up your design, and performed your study, you are ready to analyze your results. Many statistical analyses can be used in examining your research. Separate courses in both research and statistics, however, would be needed to comprehend the complexity of analyses that can be performed in good research.

In quantitative research, when you are examining differences between groups or the relationship between groups, you can perform a number of analyses. Terms that you might see in the literature that examine group differences and relationships between groups include **t-tests, analysis of variance (ANOVA)**, and **correlations**. To decide if there is statistical significance between groups, you will see a **probability level** set, which indicates the probability that the results you found could be found by chance alone. For instance, much research will set its probability at the .05 level which means that the likelihood the results happened by chance is less than 5 out of 100. Or, put another way, your results are probably caused by the factors you are examining. In literature, this is reported as $p < .05$ (p = probability, $<$ = less than).

In the reporting of survey research, **descriptive statistics** are usually used. Descriptive statistics include **measures of central tendency** (mean, median, and mode), **measures of variability** (e.g., range, standard deviation), **percentages**, and **frequencies** (see the section on "Measures of Central Tendency and Measures of Variability" in this chapter). These statistics are often presented in charts, graphs, and tables. These formats allow you to examine the overall results of your data. Table 9.2, based on a survey by Neukrug, Milliken, and Shoemaker (2001), is an example of a table using descriptive statistics with percentages.

The ability to control extraneous variables is one way we can assess the **validity** of our results in quantitative research. Control of extraneous variables is built into some kinds of quantitative research more than other kinds (experimental research is highly controlled). However, no research can be totally controlled, and there may be some reason to question any research.

Table 9.2 | Attendance in Counseling by Member Type and by Gender of Members of the National Organization of Human Services

	Total in Counseling*	Individual (101)	Group (59)	Family (55)	Couple (30)	Other (18)
Educator (102)	77 (75.5%)	73 (71.6%)	28 (27.5%)	18 (17.6%)	30 (29.4%)	2 (2.0%)
Practitioner (59)	49 (83.1%)	47 (79.7%)	16 (27.1%)	7 (11.9%)	17 (28.8%)	1 (1.7%)
Undergrad (56)	38 (67.9%)	35 (62.5%)	16 (28.6%)	11 (19.6%)	17 (30.3%)	1 (1.8%)
Grad (31)	23 (74.2%)	21 (67.8%)	9 (29.0%)	7 (22.6%)	9 (29.9%)	0 (0%)
Other (18)	16 (88.9%)	16 (88.9%)	8 (44.4%)	5 (27.8%)	5 (27.8%)	0 (0%)
Males (43)	28 (65.1%)	27 (96.4%)	12 (27.9%)	5 (11.6%)	11 (25.6%)	1 (2.3%)
Females (163)	126 (70.3%)	118 (72.4%)	47 (28.8%)	35 (21.5%)	34 (20.8%)	3 (1.8%)
Total (206)	154 (74.8%)	145 (70.4%)	59 (28.6%)	40 (19.4%)	45 (21.8%)	4 (1.9%)

*Individuals may have identified themselves in more than one category (e.g., educator and practitioner). "Total" results eliminate duplications.

Qualitative data collection, particularly grounded theory and ethnographic research, relies on a process called **inductive analysis,** which means that patterns and categories emerge from data (McMillan & Schumacher, 2010). Thus, the researcher who is examining the data collected through the various methods mentioned looks through the information for patterns, ways of categorizing information, and ways of selecting important pieces of information. As this process continues, the researcher begins to see particular points emerge.

Ethnographic and grounded theory researchers classify their data by a process called coding which breaks down large pieces of data into smaller parts that seem to hold some meaning to the research question. For instance, if I were involved in a study to determine what problems at-risk high school students might have in a specific school, I might observe the youths; interview them; interview their teachers, school counselors, parents, and peers; and collect school records. I would then go through all these pieces of information and try to select patterns and themes that seem to emerge. By collecting data in multiple ways, I am **triangulating** the data, or increasing the validity of my results. Eventually, I would carefully review all the data and look for words, phrases, and ways of acting that seemed to be pointing in similar directions.

In all types of qualitative research, the researcher must go through a rigorous process of reviewing the data, synthesizing results, and drawing conclusions and generalizations. Sometimes, the researcher's original research question changes as he or she goes through the involved process of reviewing the literature and analyzing the sources. The results of the research are a product of a logical analysis of the materials obtained rather than a statistical analysis as we find in quantitative research. Finally, the researcher needs to **bracket,** or not get caught up in his or her point of view, and should be open to offering opinions that both support and contradict the ultimate findings.

The ability to provide reliable and valid results in qualitative research is based on whether the researcher was able to use multiple methods of gathering information and how well the researcher is able to record information accurately (Gall et al., 2010; McMillan & Schumacher, 2010). For instance, this could involve taking verbatim accounts when interviewing people, using precise and concrete descriptions, using multiple researchers to get many perspectives and to look for similar themes among researchers, mechanically recording data, using primary sources whenever possible, asking participants to make their own records and to match the researcher's understanding of events with participants' understanding of events, checking meanings with participants, and reviewing any data that seem atypical or discrepant.

Discussing the Results

Probably the most important aspect of research is the conclusions drawn from the study. Conclusions are based on the data and information collected, and it is at this point that researchers can present their theories about the meaning of the study results. Although such discussions allow for some leeway, researchers should not take giant leaps in an effort to present "the truth." For instance, in Table 9.2, one can easily see that a much larger number of individuals attended individual counseling compared with group, family, or couples counseling. However, any discussion about why this is the case should be worded carefully and tentatively because the researcher should not make major interpretive statements regarding the data.

Using Research in Human Service Work

Knowledge of basic research techniques is valuable for human service professionals for a number of reasons. First, such knowledge enables human service professionals to understand professional journal articles and to make conclusions concerning what might be the most effective interventions for their clients. Second, research can validate what we are doing, while at other times, it might suggest new ways of approaching client change (Lambert, 2004). Third, research might suggest new avenues to explore and is often the basis for future research. Finally, the use of basic research techniques can be valuable for program evaluation.

EVALUATION AND NEEDS ASSESSMENT

Whereas research tends to examine new paradigms to expand understanding and knowledge that can be applied to practice, evaluation and needs assessment techniques have to do with assessing and addressing gaps in existing systems to improve their worth and value (Houser, 2009; Leary, 2007; Royse, Thyer, & Padgett, 2006). Whereas evaluation informs us about how well we have done something (e.g., a workshop, conference, class), a needs assessment gives us information about what should be done.

Evaluation

Evaluations are conducted to determine if a program we have offered has been effective and what can be done to improve it (e.g., a workshop, conference, class). Two types of evaluation are **formative evaluation** and **summative evaluation.**

Formative Evaluation (Process Evaluation)   When presenting a program, workshop, or conference, assessing effectiveness through an ongoing evaluation process is important. Formative evaluation, sometimes called process evaluation, involves the assessment of a program during its implementation to gain feedback about how effective it has been and to allow for changes in the program as needed. The most basic way to conduct formative evaluation is to ask for verbal feedback from your audience. In this case, presenters need to be open to feedback, especially any negative criticism, and be willing to change their programs midway. A little less threatening, and sometimes more revealing, is to have participants write down reactions to the program while it is occurring. Doing this anonymously allows participants to express their feelings openly, without fear of repercussions. Along these same lines, participants can be asked to complete rating forms during the program, so researchers can obtain ongoing feedback. The advantage of rating forms is that you can easily collate the data and get a sense of how the whole group feels about aspects of the program. The disadvantage is that rating forms do not allow for feedback outside the questions being asked. To offset this, rating forms often include a section that requests written feedback.

Summative Evaluation (Outcome Evaluation)   Summative evaluation, sometimes called **outcome evaluation,** is used to show the efficacy of a program that has been completed in order to determine if it should be used in the future (e.g., a parenting workshop). Summative evaluations can also be used to show funding agencies and agency administrators that your program was effective. Summative evaluation is generally a more formal process than formative evaluation and often assesses a large segment of the people who have been involved with the program. It often involves the use of basic assessment procedures, such as rating scales and open-ended surveys. For instance, a few years back I received a federally funded grant to administer a program at a local school that would identify, assess, and intervene with students at risk for drug and alcohol abuse. In measuring its effectiveness, a couple of measures were employed. First, an objective test to measure knowledge obtained by the participants was developed and administered. Second, rating scales were used at the conclusion of the program to assess total program effectiveness (see Box 9.4).

Needs Assessment

A **needs assessment** is a process of determining and addressing needs or "gaps" between current conditions and desired conditions and are often used to improve an existing structure, such as an organization or some aspects of a community. Thus, if I wanted to address problematic issues for human services professionals at a social service agency, I could develop a broad-based needs assessment that asks helpers to respond to a wide range of questions about the workplace. Or, I might be interested in assessing child-care needs of parents within a certain community to help decide what kinds of services, if any, should be developed. Needs assessments can be conducted through mail surveys, online, or in any fashion where you can access your targeted population. Descriptive statistics are generally used when pulling together the results. After the information is collected and collated, a plan of action needs to be developed to address the identified needs.

BOX 9.4 | **Outcome Evaluation of a Drug and Alcohol Training Program: Program Evaluation (N = 202)**

Describe your reaction to each of the following statements in terms of the scale below:

| 1. Never | 3. Sometimes | 5. Always |
| 2. Seldom | 4. Usually | 6. Not applicable |

Program presenters	Mean	Standard Deviation
1. were well prepared.	4.7	.3
2. delivered material in a clear, organized manner.	4.7	.2
3. stimulated intellectual curiosity.	3.9	.5
4. showed respect for questions and opinions of participants.	4.6	.3
5. allowed for relevant discussion when appropriate.	4.7	.3
6. were concerned that participants understood them.	4.6	.2
7. were accessible for individual and group concerns.	4.6	.1
8. offered information applicable to one's field.	4.0	.5
9. presented in a comfortable, conducive environment.	4.4	.2
10. provided a beneficial, educational experience.	4.1	.6

The Human Service Professional and Program Evaluation

At some point in your career as a human service professional, you will be asked to run a program for your clients. It may be a self-esteem program, a job-awareness program, a parenting program, or simply a program that explains the services of your agency to your clients. Whatever program you run, you will want to receive feedback about its effectiveness. To improve the program while it is occurring or to improve it for the next time that it might be given, formative and summative evaluation measures should be undertaken. Program evaluation also has an important place in examining the effectiveness of job-related behaviors at your agency. A responsible agency is willing to look at the effectiveness of its employees and its programs. Such evaluation can greatly assist in understanding what works and what needs to be changed.

In these times of fiscal conservatism and of accountability of programs, evaluation of agencies has become extremely important. No longer can programs and agencies deliver services without some evidence that what they are doing is working. The use of evaluation techniques is an important step in the accountability process and assures the public and funding agencies that you are performing essential and effective services for your clients (Leary, 2007).

ASSESSMENT AND TESTING

Defining Assessment

Today, the term *assessment* includes a broad array of evaluative procedures that yield information about a person (Neukrug & Fawcett, 2010). Assessment consists of a wide variety of different kinds of procedures that can be broadly grouped under four areas: **ability testing, personality testing, informal assessment,** and the **clinical interview** (see Figure 9.2).

As a human service professional, you will be involved with assessment. You may be administering tests and will likely be called to interpret some assessment techniques. You may be asked to consult with clients, parents of clients, and other professionals about a client's assessment results. You may use tests in research and in evaluation, and you will read about assessment techniques in the professional literature. Assessment techniques have permeated many aspects of our society, and they are an intricate part of the work of the human service professional. Let's examine some of the different kinds of assessment techniques we may encounter.

Types of Assessment Techniques

Assessment of Ability   Although there are many kinds of **ability tests,** their overarching purpose is to measure aspects of the cognitive domain. Ability tests can be broadly categorized into **achievement testing,** which assesses what one has learned, and **aptitude testing,** which assesses what one is capable of learning (see Figure 9.3).

Achievement Tests (Survey Battery, Diagnostic, and Readiness)   Achievement tests include *survey battery tests, diagnostic tests,* and *readiness tests* (see Figure 9.3).

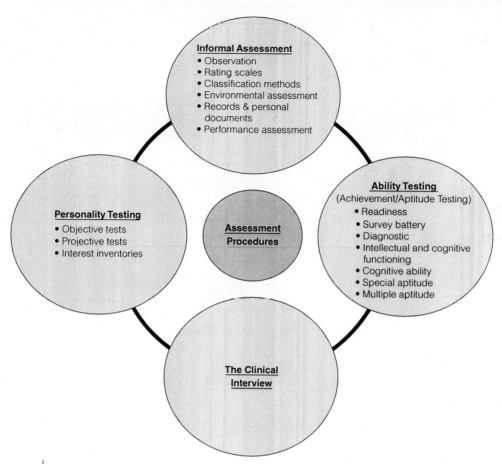

Figure 9.2 | Assessment Categories

Survey battery tests are used to measure general achievement and are commonly administered in the schools, usually to large groups of students. Probably you are familiar with these types of tests through your own education (e.g., *the Iowa Test of Basic Skills* and the *Stanford Achievement Test*). The uses of survey battery achievement tests are many and include assessment of a student's ability level, determination of teaching effectiveness, and examination of the general level of students' ability throughout a school or school system.

Diagnostic achievement tests, which are used to delve more deeply into areas of suspected learning problems, are often given one-to-one by an experienced examiner such as a school psychologist or learning disabilities specialist. Often these tests are recommended following the results of a survey battery achievement test and when, in consultation with parents and teachers, it seems probable that a student may have a learning disability. This means it is suspected that the student's ability is much lower in one or more specified areas than his or her average ability in other areas. Today, if an individual is found to have a learning disability, laws protect the child's right to education (see Box 9.5).

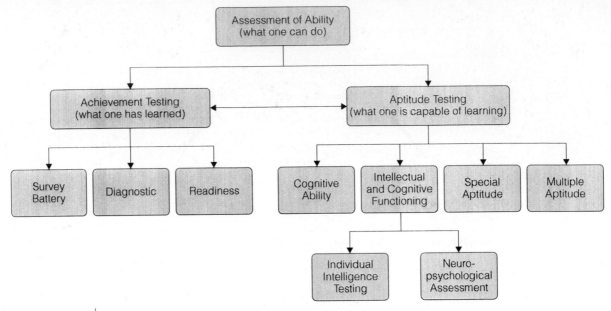

Figure 9.3 | Ability Testing (Tests in the Cognitive Domain)

Readiness tests are used to assess an individual's ability to move on to the next educational level. These days, readiness tests are mostly used to determine if a child is developmentally ready to move on to first grade, since kindergarten-age children develop at different rates.

Aptitude Tests   Four major kinds of aptitude tests include *tests of intellectual and cognitive functioning* (individual intelligence tests and neuropsychological assessment), *cognitive ability tests*, *special aptitude tests*, and *multiple aptitude tests* (see Figure 9.3).

Individual intelligence tests, which are given one-to-one to measure general intellectual ability, are administered by highly trained examiners, most often psychologists. These

---

BOX 9.5 | **PL 94-142 and the IDEA**

With the passage of **Public Law 94-142** (PL 94-142) in 1975 (Federal Register, 1977) as well as the more recent **Individuals with Disabilities Education Act (IDEA),** millions of children and young adults between the ages of 3 and 21 who were found to have a learning disability were assured the right to education within the **least restrictive environment.** These laws also asserted that any individual who was suspected of having one of many disabilities that interfere with learning had the right to be tested, at the school

system's expense, for the disability. Thus, diagnostic testing, usually administered by the school psychologist or learning disability specialist, became one of the main ways of determining who might be learning disabled. These laws also stated that a school team would review the testing, and other assessment information obtained, and that the student with the learning disability would be given an **Individual Education Plan (IEP)** that states which services would be offered to assist the student with his or her learning problem.

tests have a broad range of uses, such as helping to identify individuals who are learning disabled, developmentally delayed, intellectually disabled, or gifted. They can even be used as an indicator of personality characteristics and sometimes are a part of a broader neuropsychological assessment. Neuropsychological assessment is conducted when there is a suspected brain injury, such as from an accident or war injury. It assesses what aspect of brain functioning is impaired and what can be done to assist the person in the future.

Cognitive ability tests, which are often given in groups, are used to determine a student's overall capability in school or to predict how well an individual will do in school. Therefore, they are sometimes used for school placement and as predictors of ability in college (e.g., *ACTs* and *SATs*), graduate school (e.g., *GREs*), and professional schools (Neukrug & Fawcett, 2010; Stricker & Burton, 1996). These tests are one method of identifying students with a learning disability, as higher scores on a cognitive ability test as compared to an achievement test may indicate a deficit in the area assessed by the achievement test.

Special aptitude tests focus on measuring specific segments of ability (e.g., spatial ability, eye-hand coordination, mechanical ability) and are often used to predict the potential for success at specific jobs or training programs. For instance, one's aptitude on an eye-hand coordination test may be used to predict success at operating complex machinery in a factory, or a drawing test may be used to predict success in art school. Multiple aptitude tests, which measure a number of specific segments of ability, are used to understand an individual's aptitude on a broad range of abilities. Results of these tests can be used in occupational decision-making. Some examples of multiple aptitude tests include the *Differential Aptitude Test* (DAT), which is frequently used by high school counselors, and the *Armed Services Vocational Aptitude Battery* (ASVAB), which is given by the military for free in schools.

Although achievement testing measures what a person has learned and aptitude testing measures one's potential for learning, in point of fact, there is often much overlap between the two. This is why there is a two-headed arrow in Figure 9.3. For instance, one would be naive to assume that the SATs or the GREs are not measuring what one has learned. However, because they are both used to predict future performance, they are considered aptitude tests.

Personality Assessment   The assessment of personality includes measuring one's temperament, habits, likes, disposition, and nature (Neukrug & Fawcett, 2010). The most common kinds of **personality assessment** include *objective tests, projective techniques,* and *interest inventories* (see Figure 9.4).

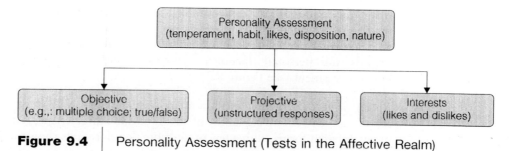

Figure 9.4 | Personality Assessment (Tests in the Affective Realm)

Objective Personality Tests Often given in a multiple-choice or true/false format, objective personality tests measure some aspect of personality. Thus we might find tests measuring anxiety, depression, psychosis, suicidal tendencies, eating disorders, marital satisfaction, and so on. Some of these tests, like the *Minnesota Multiphasic Personality Inventory-2* (MMPI-2), measure psychopathology and probably assess at least some aspects of one's temperament, or embedded personality styles. Others, like the *Myers-Briggs Type Indicator* (MBTI), measure common "normal" personality qualities that are more likely to change over time. Some uses of objective personality tests include deepening client insight, determining clinical diagnosis, making predictions about future behaviors, determining personality characteristics for the court (e.g., child custody, child molestation accusations), and screening applicants for sensitive jobs (e.g., working with children or nuclear arms).

Projective Techniques Projective techniques assess personality characteristics by having individuals respond to unstructured stimuli. Stimuli presented allow for a broad range of responses that represent conscious and unconscious needs, desires, likes, drives, and personal struggles. For instance, the *Rorschach* test, one of the most widely used projective tests, uses inkblots as stimuli to which the individual responds. After all the responses are collected, the examiner interprets their meaning. Other types of projective techniques include sentence completion, where a client is given a sentence stem (e.g., My mom is …) and the client completes it with the first thing that comes to mind; drawings, where the client is asked to make a specific drawing which is later interpreted (e.g., a drawing of the client's family all doing something together); and techniques in which the individual is asked to develop stories from pictures that are presented.

Interest Inventories Used to determine the likes and dislikes of a person as well as an individual's personality orientation toward the world of work, interest inventories are almost exclusively used in the career counseling process. These instruments are able to predict job satisfaction based on occupational fit. For instance, if, based on the results of an interest inventory, a person chooses a job that seems to match his or her personality type, then that person is more likely to be satisfied in that occupation than a person who does not have an occupational fit. Although many interest inventories exist, two of the more popular are the *Strong Interest Inventory* and the *Self-Directed Search* (SDS).

Informal Assessment Procedures Informal assessment instruments are generally developed by the individual who is going to be giving the procedure (e.g., helper, teacher) (Neukrug & Fawcett, 2010). Although they are often less valid than other kinds of instruments, they offer us an important and relatively easy method of examining a slice of behavior of an individual. Some of the more common informal procedures include rating scales, observation, classification systems, records and personal documents, environmental assessment, and performance-based assessment (see Figure 9.2).

Rating Scales Rating scales allow an individual to give a subjective rating of a behavior on a scale to obtain a quantity of an attitude or characteristic. Rating scales come in many different forms, with a few of the more popular kinds shown in Box 9.6.

BOX 9.6 | Rating Scales

The following are examples of four rating scales. Consider how you might use them.

Numerical Scale

With "0" being equal to the worst depression you ever had and a 10 being equal to the best you could possibly feel, can you tell me where on a scale of 0–10 you fall today?

| 1 | 2 | 3 | 4 | 5 | 6 | 7 | 8 | 9 | 10 |

Worst depression   Best I could feel

Semantic Differential Scale

Place an "X" on the line to represent how much of each quality you possess:

Sadness————————————————————————————————Happiness

| 1 | 2 | 3 | 4 | 5 | 6 | 7 | 8 |

Introverted————————————————————————————Extroverted

| 1 | 2 | 3 | 4 | 5 | 6 | 7 | 8 |

Anxious——————————————————————————————————Calm

| 1 | 2 | 3 | 4 | 5 | 6 | 7 | 8 |

Rank Order Scale

Please rank order your preferred method of doing counseling. Place a 1 next to the item that you most prefer, a 2 next to the item you second most prefer, and so on down to a 5 next to the item you prefer least.

_____ I prefer listening to clients and then reflecting back what I hear from them in order to facilitate client self-growth.

_____ I prefer advising clients and suggesting mechanisms for change.

_____ I prefer interpreting client behaviors in the hope that they will gain insight into themselves.

_____ I prefer helping clients identify which behaviors they would like to change.

_____ I prefer helping clients identify which thoughts are causing problematic behaviors and helping them to develop new ways of thinking about the world.

Likert-Type Scale

Indicate how strongly you agree or disagree with each of the following statements:

	Strongly disagree	Somewhat disagree	Neither Agree nor disagree	Somewhat agree	Strongly agree
It is fine to view a client's personal Web page (e.g., Facebook, LinkedIn, blog) without informing the client.	1	2	3	4	5
It is okay to tell your client you are attracted to him or her.	1	2	3	4	5
There is no problem in counseling a terminally ill client about end-of-life decisions, including suicide.	1	2	3	4	5

Observation Conducted by a professional who wishes to observe an individual (e.g., home social service aide observing a family), by significant others who have the opportunity to observe an individual in natural settings (e.g., parents observing a child at home), and even by a client who is asked to observe specific behaviors he or she is working on changing (e.g., eating habits), observation can offer an easy and important tool in understanding the individual.

Classification Systems In contrast to rating scales that tend to assess a quantity of specific attributes or characteristics, classification systems provide information about whether an individual has, or does not have, certain attributes or characteristics. Some of the more common classification systems include behavior or feeling word checklists (see Box 9.7). The kinds of classification methods that one can create are innumerable and are limited only by your imagination. For instance, one can come up with a classification method that asks clients to examine and choose items that represent their "irrational thoughts." Or, an older person might be asked to pick from a long list of physical barriers to living fully (difficulty getting out of the bath, problems seeing, etc.).

Environmental Assessment Environmental assessment includes collecting information about a client's home, school, or workplace usually through observation or self-reports (e.g., checklists). This form of appraisal is more systems oriented and naturalistic, and can be eye-opening because even when clients do not intentionally mislead their helpers, they will often present a distorted view based on their own inaccurate perceptions or because they are embarrassed about revealing some aspect of their lives (e.g., a person living in poverty might not want to reveal an unpleasant home situation).

BOX 9.7 | Behavior Checklist of Abusive Behaviors

Check those behaviors you have exhibited toward your partner and your partner has exhibited toward you.

	Exhibited by you to your partner	Exhibited by your partner to you
1. Hitting	————	————
2. Pulling hair	————	————
3. Throwing objects	————	————
4. Burning	————	————
5. Pinching	————	————
6. Choking	————	————
7. Slapping	————	————
8. Biting	————	————
9. Tying up	————	————
10. Hitting walls or other inanimate objects	————	————
11. Throwing objects with an intent to break them	————	————
12. Restraining or preventing from leaving	————	————

Records and Personal Documents   A number of common forms of records and personal documents are used to inquire about the client, including asking the client to write an *autobiography,* collecting *anecdotal information* (e.g., typical or atypical work behaviors in a personnel file), completing a *biographical inventory* (detailed picture of client from birth by conducting an involved interview or by having the client answer a series of questions on a checklist), examining *cumulative records* (e.g., school records), completing a *genogram,* or having the client write *journals* and/or keep *diaries* (e.g., sleep journal, where one writes down his or her dreams and explores patterns among the dreams).

Performance-Based Assessment   This kind of assessment evaluates an individual using a variety of informal assessment procedures that are based on real-world responsibilities that are not highly loaded for cognitive skills. These tests are used when large numbers of nondominant group individuals have been shown to do less well on a standardized test but as well on the actual performance for which the test is assessing (e.g., job performance). Thus, these performance-based tests, which predict as well as the standardized tests, are used in their place. For instance, rather than giving a highly loaded cognitive test that may predict well for Whites who want to become firefighters, but not predict well for some minority groups, individuals can be given a series of alternative procedures to assess how quickly they can respond to realistic situations they might actually face on the job as firefighters.

The Clinical Interview   The clinical interview, another assessment technique, allows the helper to obtain an in-depth understanding of the client through an unstructured or structured interview process. The **structured interview** allows the examinee to respond to a set of preestablished items verbally or in writing. This kind of interview allows for a broad assessment of client issues but sometimes does not allow for in-depth follow-up in one area. The **unstructured interview,** on the other hand, does not have a preestablished list of items or questions and client responses to helper inquiries establish the direction for follow-up questioning. Some professionals prefer using a **semi-structured interview,** which is a cross between the two kinds of interviewing techniques. The clinical interview serves a number of purposes (Neukrug & Fawcett, 2010). For instance, the interview

1. Sets a tone for the types of information that will be covered during the assessment process,
2. Allows the client to become desensitized to information that can be very intimate and personal,
3. Allows the helper to assess the nonverbal signals of the client while he or she is talking about sensitive information, thus giving the helper a sense of what might be important to focus upon,
4. Allows the helper to learn firsthand the problem areas of the client and place them in perspective, and
5. Gives the client and helper the opportunity to study each other's personality style to assure that they can work together.

Norm-Referenced, Criterion-Referenced, Standardized, and Nonstandardized Assessment

Generally, assessment techniques are either **norm-referenced** or **criterion-referenced**. In norm-referenced assessment, the individual can compare his or her score to the conglomerate scores of a peer or norm group, which often consist of a national representative sample of individuals. Many tests that are sold by national publishing companies are norm-referenced. In contrast, criterion-referenced assessment techniques are designed to assess specific learning goals of an individual. Achievement of these goals, as measured by a criterion-referenced procedure, shows mastery of the subject matter at hand. Oftentimes, criterion-referenced procedures are used with individuals who are learning disabled, because goals can be individualized for the student based on his or her specific learning problem.

Standardized assessment procedures are administered in the same manner and under the same conditions each time they are given. In contrast, **nonstandardized assessment** procedures are not necessarily given under the same conditions and in the same manner at each administration. Often, informal assessment procedures are nonstandardized. However, this is not a hard-and-fast rule (see Table 9.3).

An example of a standardized, norm-referenced test is the exam to become a Human Services—Board Certified Practitioner (HS—BCP) given by the Center for Credentialing and Education (CCE). To pass this exam, an individual has to reach a certain pass score as compared to the national sample of those who have taken the exam.

Table 9.3 | Comparison of Standardized, Nonstandardized, Norm-Referenced, and Criterion-Referenced Assessment

	Standardized	Nonstandardized
Norm-referenced	These assessment instruments must be given in the same manner and under the same conditions each time they're given. Often, they are highly researched objective instruments that are developed by publishing companies. Usually, large norm groups are available with which the individual can compare his or her results.	These assessment instruments may vary in how they are administered and generally are not as rigidly researched as the standardized tests. However, because of their informal nature, they may be more practical for the purpose for which they are being used. Scores that are later compared to a norm group should be viewed more tentatively than standardized tests.
Criterion-referenced	These instruments are given in a standard manner and have preset learning goals that are based on an individual's personal educational objectives. Often created by large publishing companies, individuals who take these tests generally have the ability to tackle their individualized learning goals and have their results compared to national norm groups.	These instruments are informally made, often by teachers, and are based on the teacher's knowledge of his or her students and the content area being tested. The teacher can develop an individualized test that has preset learning goals for each student. The informal nature of these instruments means that norm groups are rarely available for comparisons.

Examples of standardized, criterion-referenced assessment procedures include nationally made individual achievement tests, which are often given to learning disabled students. These tests are administered the same way each time, but a student takes only those parts of the test relevant to his or her individual learning goals as defined by a special education teacher. This test could additionally be norm-referenced if a comparison to a national norm group is desired and available.

Using a checklist to measure self-concept while observing a child in a class and then comparing the child's scores to those of a local norm group (e.g., students in the school) might be an example of a nonstandardized and norm-referenced test.

Finally, a behavioral aide that has developed targeted learning goals for students might create a nonstandardized, criterion-referenced assessment procedure. The aide, who is working with children with behavioral problems, might develop a set of procedures in which he or she can count specific behaviors related to problem behaviors of each child. After counting the behaviors, the aide would determine whether they have reached their targeted goals (the criterion).

Basic Test Statistics

Relativity of Scores   John receives a score of 47 on a test. How did he do? Jill receives a 95 on a different test. How did she do? If John's test score was 47 out of 50, he probably did pretty well. But, if 1,000 people take the test and everyone but John receives a score of 50 out of 50, we might view his test score a little differently. What about Jill's score? Is a score of 95 good? If the best possible score is 100, perhaps it is a good score. But what if the best possible score is 200, or 550, or 992? If 1,000 people take the test and Jill's score is the highest, we might say that she did well, at least compared with this group. But if her score is at the lower end of the group of scores, then comparatively she did not do well. To make things even more complicated, what if a high score represents more of an undesirable trait (e.g., cynicism or depression)? Then clearly, the higher Jill scores compared with her peer or norm group, the worse she has done comparatively. What's important here is the concept that scores on tests—particularly norm-referenced, standardized testing scores—are relative, and an individual's raw score makes sense only in its relative position to his or her group.

Measures of Central Tendency and Measures of Variability   When comparing an individual's test scores with the scores of his or her norm group, understanding **measures of central tendency** and **measures of variability** of the test is very important. Measures of central tendency include the *mean*, the average of all the scores; the *median*, the middle score representing the point where 50% of the examinees score above and 50% fall below; and the *mode*, the most frequent score. Two important measures of variability are the *range*, which represents the spread of scores from the highest to the lowest score, and the *standard deviation*, which represents how much, on average, scores vary from the mean. For instance, one test has a mean of 52 and a standard deviation of 20. This means that most scores (about 68%) on this test range between 32 and 72 (± 1 standard deviation, or $52 + 20$

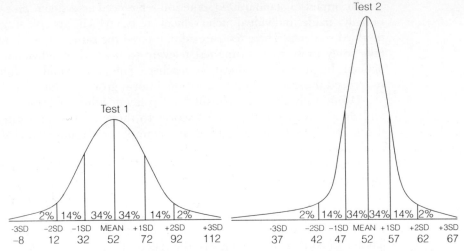

Figure 9.5 | Comparison of Normal Curves with Different Standard Deviations

and 52 − 20) (see Figure 9.5). Another group of scores also has a mean of 52, but this test has a standard deviation of 5. This means that most of the scores (about 68%) range between 47 and 57 (±1 standard deviation, or 52 + 5 and 52 − 5). Clearly, even though the two tests have the same mean, the range of scores around the mean varies considerably. An individual's score of 40 would be in the average range on the first test but well below average on the second test. If you know the measures of central tendency and the measures of variability of the group of scores, you can compare your scores to these measures.

Test Worthiness

Four qualities that are particularly important in establishing the worthiness of an assessment instrument are (1) **validity**, whether or not a test measures what it is supposed to measure; (2) **reliability**, how accurately or precisely a test measures a trait or ability; (3) **practicality**, the ease of administration and interpretation of the test; and (4) **cross-cultural fairness**, whether or not the test measures what it is supposed to measure for all subgroups to which the test is given (Neukrug & Fawcett, 2010). Let's take a closer look at these qualities that together are **called test worthiness.**

Validity   Test validity involves a systematic method of showing that a test measures what it purports to measure. A test's validity is a function of how it is created. To create a valid test, one should do a thorough analysis of the literature concerning the test content, consult with experts about the test content, compare the test with other tests of a similar nature, and more. Often, a statistical analysis is used to show test validity. Some of the more popular types of validity are *content validity, concurrent validity, predictive validity,* and *construct validity.* Validity is a statement about the test, not about the people taking the test.

Reliability   The second quality that is examined in determining the adequacy of an assessment instrument is reliability. Whereas validity is used to show that a test is measuring what it's supposed to measure, reliability examines the accuracy of test scores. If a test were reliable, one could assume that an individual's score would remain about the same even if that individual were to take the test a number of times (assuming the person did not change—that is, learn something new—between test administrations). As with validity, reliability measures the adequacy of the test and does not make a statement about the people taking the test. Some of the more common types of reliability are *internal consistency, split-half reliability, parallel forms reliability,* and *test-retest reliability.*

Practicality   Suppose I have a test that can accurately assess mental health diagnoses, but each administration costs $1,000. This test may be good at what it does, but the cost may be prohibitive. Or, suppose we have an instrument that can accurately measure learning disabilities but takes a school psychologist 2 days to administer. Cost and time are two aspects that we must struggle with when deciding whether a test is practical. Practicality includes issues related to the cost of testing, the ease of administration, the length of the test, and the ease of test interpretation. A test can have good validity and good reliability, be cross-culturally fair, yet not be a practical test to give.

Cross-Cultural Fairness of Tests

> Tests must be used in ways that, as far as possible, take advantage of the tremendous utility of test and other assessment data, while also facilitating optimal understanding and nurturance of a wide range of individual and cultural differences. (Walsh & Betz, 2001, p. 424)

The last quality important in determining the worthiness of a test is whether it is cross-culturally fair. Although it is impossible to eliminate all bias from tests, one should expect that the bias is small enough to allow for justifiable interpretations of any individual's score. When examining cultural bias, test publishers should have exhaustively reviewed the extent to which the content of a test has cultural bias. For those instruments that are used to predict future behavior, the test should be shown to be predictive for minority groups. This does not mean that it will predict in the same manner for all groups, but that the predictive validity of each subgroup was examined and that the test was shown to predict accurately for each subgroup (Anastasi, 1992; Anastasi & Urbina, 1997). In fact, the U.S. Supreme Court case of ***Griggs v. Duke Power Company*** (1971) asserted that tests used for hiring and advancement at work must show that they can predict job performance for all groups. Helpers need to be aware of bias in testing, ethical issues related to assessment and multiculturalism, and state and national laws related to the use of tests with minorities (see Box 9.8).

BOX 9.8 | **The Use of Intelligence Tests with Minorities: Confusion and Bedlam**

The use of intelligence tests with minorities has always been an area of controversy. Some states banned the use of intelligence tests in certain circumstances with some minority groups (Swenson, 1997). If intelligence tests are used with minority clients, the examiner needs to know the proper way to administer and score them.

The concern for bias in testing has gone so far, that if the situation weren't so serious, it would almost be comical. Take the case in California of Mary Amaya, who was concerned that one of her sons was being recommended for remedial courses he did not need. Amaya had an older son who was found not to need such assistance after he was tested. Amaya requested intelligence testing for her other son. However, since the incident with her first son, laws had been changed, and California decided that intelligence tests were culturally biased and thus banned their use for certain minority groups. Despite the fact that Amaya was requesting the use of an intelligence test, it was found that she had no legislative right to have it given to her son.

The Human Service Professional's Use of Assessment Techniques

> Qualified test users understand the measurement characteristics necessary to select good standardized tests, administer the tests according to specified procedures, assure accurate scoring, accurately interpret test scores for individuals and groups, and ensure productive applications of the results. (Association for Assessment in Counseling, 2003, p. 5)

The American Psychological Association (APA) adopted a three-tier system for establishing test user qualifications which most publishers use. Although the APA is currently reevaluating this system (Bartram, 2001), many test publishers continue to use it or similar versions (American Psychological Association, 1954). They state that associate- and bachelor-level individuals who have some knowledge of assessment and are thoroughly versed with the test manual can give a "Level A" test and, under some limited circumstances, a "Level B" test. For example, teachers can administer most survey battery achievement tests, and human service professionals can give some basic personality tests. Master's-level helping professionals who have taken a basic course in tests and measurement can administer "Level B" tests. However, they cannot administer tests that require additional training, such as most individual tests of intelligence, most projective tests, and many diagnostic tests. These "Level C" tests are reserved for those who have a minimum of a master's degree, a basic testing course, and advanced training in the specialized test (e.g., school psychologists, learning disabilities specialists, clinical and counseling psychologists, or master's-level therapists who have gained additional training).

Although the human service professional may not have the advanced training needed to administer many tests, it is common for a client of a human service professional to have taken some assessment instruments. For example, assessment instruments are commonly used in unemployment offices where vocational assessments help clients find jobs, at the community-based mental health center where assessment is useful for diagnosis and treatment, or at schools where assessment helps identify children with special needs as well as measures students' progress. Such techniques have become critical to the overall treatment process. Thus, it is important for the human service professional to have adequate knowledge of assessment instruments in order to understand their role in addressing client needs.

ETHICAL, PROFESSIONAL, AND LEGAL ISSUES

Informed Consent

Informed consent involves the client's right to know the purpose and nature of all aspects of client involvement with the helper. In reference to research and assessment procedures, clients have the right to know the general purposes of the research in which they are involved as well as how any assessment techniques they are taking are going to be used. Except in special cases (e.g., court referrals for testing), clients also have the right to refuse to take part in any assessment and research. Corey, Corey, and Callanan (2011) note that when a client is not fully informed, the helper is open to liability concerns. Most ethical guidelines speak directly to the issue of informed consent. For instance, the Ethical Standards of Human Service Professionals states,

> Human service professionals negotiate with clients the purpose, goals, and nature of
> the helping relationship prior to its onset as well as inform clients of the limitations of
> the proposed relationship. (See Appendix A, Statement 1)

Today, an increasing number of authors are recommending that clients sign informed consent forms indicating that they are fully aware of any therapeutic, assessment, or research procedures in which they are participating (Cottone & Tarvydas, 2007; Remley & Herlihy, 2010). With assessment procedures and research becoming more prevalent, the issue of informed consent has become paramount, especially in light of the liability-conscious society we live in.

Use of Human Subjects

Stanley Milgram's "shocking" research on obedience (1965, 1974) dramatically affected the way research has been conducted in the United States. Recruiting subjects through a local newspaper ad, he told them that they would be participating in research on the effects of punishment in learning. Assigning them to the role of teacher, he told the subjects that they would be administering an electrical shock to a learner every time the person did not complete a task properly. In actuality, the equipment was not hooked up, and the learner was an actor who would respond every time a "shock" was administered. As the experiment continued, the teacher was told to increase the voltage, and the learner, who initially was making mild grunting sounds following the shock, began to respond more strongly, eventually screaming. Despite the fact that many of the teachers objected to what they were doing, with prodding by the experimenter, 65% of the subjects ended up administering 450 pseudo-volts to the learner, enough to harm or kill a person had the equipment been hooked up. Although the results were interesting, Milgram's research was much criticized for its potential psychological harm to the participants.

As a result of this study, as well as other research that had the potential to cause psychological or even physical harm to subjects, many restraints have been placed on the types of research in which people can participate. In fact, research like Milgram's could not legally be done today, and restraints on research that might cause physical or psychological harm are now guided by ethical standards and by legislation. For instance, most ethical guidelines now limit the amount of deception allowed in the use of research. In addition, federal legislation now requires that all organizations that conduct research supported by federal funds have a human subjects committee or **Institutional Review Board** (IRB) whose purpose is to ensure that there is little or no risk to research participants. Today, many institutions have adopted human subjects committees even if they do not receive federal funds.

Proper Interpretation and Use of Test Data Because human service professionals are not experts in test administration and test interpretation, they must rely on those who are. However, effective human service professionals can use the results of test data in their work with clients. Therefore, they should carefully read the results of test reports and consult with experts in the field to understand how such data can best serve their clients. As noted earlier in this chapter, the proper use of test data involves sensitivity to clients, knowledge of informed consent, and awareness of the cultural biases that are inherent in some tests. Finally, human service professionals should understand that testing is one small aspect of a broader analysis of the individual that is called assessment. A test should never be used only to make predictions. If one test is helpful, two will be more helpful. And, if two tests are helpful, then two tests and a clinical interview will be even better! And, if two tests and a clinical interview are better, then what about interviewing others who know the individual being assessed? Whenever important decisions are being made, a careful assessment that is reliable, valid, and cross-culturally fair should be undertaken.

THE EFFECTIVE HUMAN SERVICE PROFESSIONAL: UNDERSTANDING THE CHANGING FACE OF RESEARCH, PROGRAM EVALUATION, AND ASSESSMENT

The main purpose of research, program evaluation, and assessment is to benefit our clients. Research can help us understand those interventions that are most effective with our clients; program evaluation can help us understand whether the programs we are offering benefit our clients; and assessment techniques can help clients better understand themselves. Research, as Kuhn (1962) notes, is an ever-evolving process that continually adds new knowledge to the field. Assessment procedures are always improving, giving us better insights into the clients with whom we work. And, because the evaluation process relies heavily on research and assessment techniques, it too is an evolving process. Effective human service professionals do not view research, evaluation, and assessment as a fearful or stagnant process. Instead, they understand that new research ideas, new assessment procedures, and new programs will be devised, and they are excited about such developments and smart enough to adapt the information obtained from this newly gained knowledge.

SUMMARY

In this chapter, we examined the nature and purpose of research, evaluation and needs assessment, and assessment and testing. Starting with research, we noted that it adds knowledge to our field and therefore helps us make wise decisions concerning how we can best conduct our work as human service professionals. We noted that in conducting research, one needs to do a literature review and come up with a hypothesis or research question. We suggested a number of databases one can use for conducting a literature review. We then went on to compare and contrast two broad categories of research: quantitative research and qualitative research.

Quantitative research, we stated, relies on controlled research designs and can be applied in a laboratory setting or in the field. Quantitative research tests hypotheses or clarifies research questions. Qualitative research is generally field research that relies on the researcher to carefully observe and describe phenomena and to interpret the phenomena within a social context. This kind of research bases itself on the research question.

We briefly reviewed four kinds of quantitative research, specifically examining true experimental research, causal-comparative (ex post facto) research, correlational research, and survey research. We also explored three kinds of qualitative research called grounded theory, ethnographic research, and historical research. We explained that in qualitative research, the researcher goes through a rigorous process of reviewing the data, synthesizing results, and drawing conclusions and generalizations. The researcher needs to be careful to avoid getting caught up in his or her point of view and should be open to offering opinions that both support and contradict the ultimate findings. In contrast, the quantitative method attempts to carefully control the study, and we noted a number of statistical analyses that might be used in helping the quantitative research develop conclusions and recommendations. Regardless of the type of research you are doing, certain steps must be followed in implementing research, including reviewing the

literature, developing a hypothesis or research question, designing the study, finding ways to analyze the data, and discussing the results.

The second major topic of this chapter was evaluation and needs assessment. We noted that whereas evaluation informs us about how well we have done something (e.g., a workshop, conference, class), a needs assessment gives us information about what should be done. In discussing evaluation, we noted that they are conducted to determine if a program we have offered has been effective and what can be done to improve it (e.g., a workshop, conference, class). We noted that formative evaluation takes place during the activity being measured, whereas summative evaluation takes place at the conclusion or after an activity has occurred. We pointed out that evaluation ensures that the services we are offering our clients are of high quality and that they can also be used to attest to the accountability of our programs.

Relative to needs assessment, we pointed out that such an assessment is a process of determining and addressing needs or "gaps" between current conditions and desired conditions and are often used to improve an existing structure, such as an organization or some aspects of a community. Some examples were given.

Assessment was our third major topic in this chapter. We first noted that testing was a subset of the larger category called assessment. We then identified and defined a number of assessment categories, including ability testing, such as survey battery tests, diagnostic tests, and readiness tests; aptitude testing, such as intellectual and cognitive functioning (intelligence tests and neuropsychological assessment), cognitive ability tests, special aptitude and multiple aptitude tests; personality tests, such as objective tests, projective tests, and interest inventories; informal assessment procedures, including observation, rating scales, classification systems, environmental assessment, records and personal documents, performance-based assessment; and the clinical interview, which can be structured or nonstructured. We also discussed the difference between standardized and nonstandardized testing and norm-referenced and criterion-referenced testing, and gave examples of assessment procedures in each of these areas.

Relative to testing, we next discussed test worthiness, which refers to four qualities that should be examined in determining whether a test should be used: validity, reliability, practicality, and cross-cultural fairness. We also discussed the importance of understanding the concepts of measures of central tendency and measures of variability in the interpretation of tests. We noted that although human service professionals do not have the training to give many of the more in-depth tests, they will be constantly exposed to test reports and test data. Therefore, it is important to be in close consultation with supervisors and experts in test administration.

Relative to ethical, professional, and legal issues, we noted that whether one is conducting research or using assessment procedures, it is important to fully inform our clients of the purpose and nature of their involvement. We noted that clients have a right to informed consent concerning all aspects of their treatment. We also noted for ethical adherence, one should have a human subjects committee, and if receiving federal funds, an Institutional Review Board review the proposed research. We next pointed out the importance of the proper interpretation of test information and noted that it is generally better to use a number of assessment procedures when making decisions about clients.

Finally, whether human service professionals are involved in research, the evaluation process, or assessment, we noted that it is important that these processes are seen as evolving. In other words, as research, evaluation, and assessment techniques are refined, effective human service professionals must be willing to examine and adapt the new knowledge gained from them in ways that will benefit their clients.

Experiential Exercises

I. **Critiquing a Journal Article**

Obtain a research article from a human service journal and, using the following criteria, critique the article.

1. Have the authors used quantitative or qualitative research methods?
2. What kind of quantitative (e.g., true experimental, causal-comparative, correlational, survey) or qualitative (e.g., historical, ethnographic) methods have been used?
3. Was the hypothesis or research question based on an adequate literature review?
4. What results were found?
5. What are the implications of the results for the human service professional?
6. What future research might arise out of this research?
7. Generally, what did you think of the article?

II. **Designing a Research Study**

Have the instructor divide the class into groups of four or five students. Each group is to design a research study concerning the effectiveness of human service professionals with their clients. Each group is to design one of the following types of studies: a true experimental study, a causal-comparative study, a correlational study, a survey study, a grounded theory study, a historical research study, or an ethnographic study. In designing your study, make sure you address the following issues:

1. Literature review
2. Hypothesis or research question
3. Research design

4. Results
5. Discussion

III. Developing Evaluation Instruments

In small groups or as a class, develop a formative and a summative evaluation instrument for your class.

IV. Evaluating an Evaluation Form

1. Evaluating an Evaluation Form—Part 1

   Most colleges and universities have some form of course evaluation that is completed at the end of the semester. Obtain a copy of the evaluation form that is used at your college, and discuss any positive and negative aspects of that form.

2. Evaluating an Evaluation Form—Part 2

   Visit a local social service agency, and see whether the agency has any evaluation forms that are used to assess client satisfaction, the effectiveness of programs, or the overall effectiveness of the agency. Share these instruments in class.

V. Sharing Experiences with Testing

In class, discuss any positive or negative experiences you have had relative to taking a test.

VI. Advantages and Disadvantages of Testing

In small groups, discuss the following issues, pick a spokesperson, and report back to the class. Have the instructor write on the board the advantages and disadvantages that are noted by the groups.

1. The advantages and disadvantages of the SATs
2. The advantages and disadvantages of individual intelligence testing
3. The advantages and disadvantages of personality assessment
4. The advantages and disadvantages of using assessment techniques with clients.

VII. Using Tests with Clients

Refer to the different types of assessment procedures listed in this chapter, and discuss how they might be used for each of the following scenarios:

1. Johnny is a 12-year-old child in seventh grade. His grades have always been average, but recently his math scores have dropped considerably. In addition, he tells you that he found out not long ago that his parents are getting divorced.
2. William is 35 years old and recently separated. A few months following the separation, his wife accused him of molesting their four-year-old child. He vehemently denies this accusation and states that she is "just saying those things in order to gain custody."
3. Judy is applying for a high-security job with the CIA. Following a background check, as a matter of course, they give her a number of assessment instruments.
4. Juanita is in lower management at a major computer firm. Her supervisor is thinking of recommending her for a promotion. Her new job would involve making quick decisions, and it requires a stable personality.

5. Jason is considering changing careers. He is not sure what career options are open for him and is unclear about what he likes to do. He is also unclear about what he is good at.

VIII. Evaluating the Passion Test

Using the following "Passion Test," discuss the following:

1. How might you show that this test is or is not valid?
2. How might you show that the test is or is not reliable?
3. Are any of the test questions cross-culturally biased? Explain.
4. What assumptions does this test make about men, women, and sexual orientation?

The Passion Test

Using the following response choices, answer each item:

a. very true   b. somewhat true   c. a little bit true   d. not at all true

_____ 1. I like to have romantic dinners.

_____ 2. I think Beyonce or Ryan Gosling is very hot.

_____ 3. I like to have flowers sent to me.

_____ 4. I prefer spicy food to bland food.

_____ 5. I would like to spend a week on the Riviera.

_____ 6. To me, romance is all in the head.

_____ 7. I make love at least once a day.

_____ 8. I would rather have a steamy conversation than have sex.

_____ 9. I believe that passion is related to how much a person cares about you.

_____ 10. I exercise at least three times a week.

IX. Ethical and Professional Vignettes (Discuss the ethics of the following scenarios)

1. Recently, there has been some research on the effectiveness of various drugs to combat HIV. To test if there is any effect, a drug company obtains permission to randomly assign individuals who have tested HIV positive to two groups. One group will get a new drug, and the second group will get a placebo (a sugar pill). Individuals do not know to which group they belong. Is this ethical? Professional? Legal?

2. Based on the available research, a human service professional who works at a 30-day rehabilitation center for chemically dependent individuals develops a program on confrontation and humiliation. Although individuals can theoretically leave at any time, in this program, those who do not admit to their addictions and those who do not begin to make major changes in their lives are heavily confronted by the whole group, are forced to shave their heads, and during "social time" are made to sit in their rooms and think about their lives. Is this ethical? Professional? Legal?

3. To become more familiar with a local community religious group, a human service professional decides to become a participant observer and spends a week with the community at their retreat center. Part of their ritual is to

smoke marijuana during their meditation times. Following the week at the center, he reports them to the local law enforcement agency for the illegal use of drugs. Is this ethical? Professional? Legal?

4. After receiving negative feedback concerning a workshop on communicating with teenagers, a human service professional decides, "They really didn't want to learn how to communicate with their kids. I simply won't do workshops on this topic for 'those people' anymore." Is this reasonable? Ethical? Professional?

5. During the taking of some routine tests for promotion, it is discovered that, based on the results of the tests, there is a high probability that one of the employees is abusing drugs and is a pathological liar. The firm decides not to promote him and instead fires him. Is this ethical? Professional? Legal?

6. An African-American mother is concerned that her child may have an attention deficit disorder. She goes to the teacher who supports her concerns, and they go to the assistant principal, requesting testing for a possible learning problem. The mother asks if the child could be given an individual intelligence test that can screen for such problems, and the assistant principal states, "Those tests have been banned for minority students because of concerns about cross-cultural bias." The mother states that she will give her permission for such testing, but the assistant principal says, "I'm sorry, we'll have to make do with some other tests and observation." Is this ethical? Professional? Legal?

7. A test that has not been researched to show that it is, or is not, predictive for the success of minority graduate students in social work is used as part of the program's admission process. When challenged on this, the head of the program states that the test has not been proven to be biased and that the program does have other criteria that it uses for admission. Is this ethical? Professional? Legal?

8. A social worker with no training in career development is giving interest inventories as she counsels individuals for career issues. Can she do this? Is this ethical? Professional? Legal? If this social worker were a colleague of yours, what, if anything, would you do?

A Look to the Future: Trends in the Functions and Roles of the Human Service Professional

CHAPTER CONTENTS

A student of mine asked a question in class that I thought I had answered a number of times. She asked it on a day when I had a cold and was not feeling well, and I remember responding somewhat belligerently by saying something like "I've answered this question four times before!" After class, I saw that she looked angry, so I asked her what was going on. She stated, "I thought you were condescending toward me, and it makes me feel like not asking any more questions." I realized she was right, and I apologized. I also knew that sometimes I get like that. I try my best to be accepting of students, but I know that sometimes I just "lose it." This student reminded me again that I still have issues to work on. Change for me is not easy, and when I think of my clients attempting to make change and having difficulty, I try to remember that in certain areas of my life I, too, have difficulty.

I sometimes joke with my colleagues about the trends in the titles of conferences that have been held within recent years. Every conference seems to have a theme like "Human Services in the Twenty-First Century and Beyond," "Transformation of the Human Service Profession," "The New Millennium and Beyond: Change in Human Services," and "Change, Metamorphosis, and Trends for the Future." No question, change is on people's minds. Some workshops at these conferences are exciting because they present new, cutting-edge information about innovative ways to work with clients and systems. However, I find that more often than not, the changes they are talking about are implemented very slowly. The tendency to maintain the status quo is great, whether it be within ourselves, in our families, in social systems, or in organizations.

Despite the tendency to keep things the way they are, there is some inner sense in all of us that change keeps us alive. This chapter will look at some of the changes that will likely take place in the human services. Some will assuredly take place, and others may fall by the wayside. For instance, we will explore current trends in working with some special populations including the incarcerated, their families, and the victims of crime; those who are HIV positive; the homeless and the poor; older people; individuals who are chronically mentally ill; individuals with disabilities; and individuals at risk for chemical dependence. Next, we will focus on how our future in the human services will be affected by a greater emphasis on the following standards in the profession: program accreditation, credentialing, ethical standards, and the Skill Standards.

As this chapter continues, we will explore how technology has affected, and will continue to affect, our work as human service professionals. With crisis and disasters facing our country and the world, we will next examine how training in crisis, disaster, and trauma counseling will become important. Then, we will focus on how human service professionals will continue to have a positive, developmental, and primary prevention emphasis when working with clients.

Changes in managed health care and the role of the human service professional in managed health will be the next area discussed. A related issue, the role of human services in medicine, will then be looked at. Social justice, advocacy, and multicultural counseling, areas that have already been described in the book in some detail, will then be highlighted as a continuing critical aspect of the human services in the twenty-first century. An increasing international perspective will then be described. How stress, cynicism, and burnout will affect the work of the human service professional and what he or she can do about it will be discussed next. This will lead into the importance of human service professionals focusing on their own wellness. This chapter will conclude with a discussion about the significance of continuing education and how the effective human service professional is positive, forward-looking, and desirous of change.

TRENDS IN CLIENT POPULATIONS

Touched on in Chapters 7 and 8, the human service professional will increasingly find himself or herself working with a number of unique groups of individuals. These include people who are incarcerated, their families, and the victims of crime; those who are HIV positive; the homeless and the poor; older people; individuals who are chronically mentally ill; people with disabilities; and individuals at risk for chemical dependence. Let's take a brief look at why these groups will be so important in the future.

The Incarcerated, Their Families, and the Victims of Crime

In the United States today, there are about 2.3 million Americans in jail or prison and close to 5 million on probation or parole—over 3% of all U.S. adult residents—and of these, an extremely large number are minority males (Bureau of Justice Statistics, 2010; Gleissner, 2010). With most prisoners being undereducated, abused as children, abusers of drugs and alcohol, and coming from dysfunctional families, the need for social services is paramount. As a result, human service professionals will find themselves providing a wide range of mental health services for those who are incarcerated, their families, and those who are the victims of crime (Gater, 2011; Haynes, 2011). With the many needs of these clients, a multisystem approach that addresses this broad range of services will need to be implemented (Hershenson et al., 2003; Hicks-Coolick & Millsap, 2001). Unless there is a drastic reduction in crime in the United States, many human service professionals will find themselves working within the criminal justice system well into the twenty-first century.

Families and friends of the incarcerated, victims of crime, and our communities are all affected by crime and its aftermath.

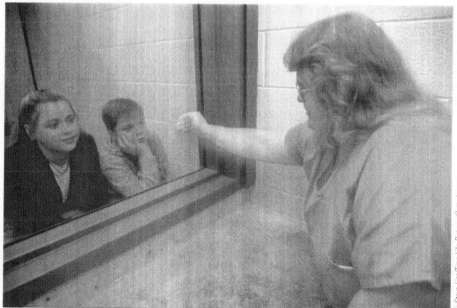

© Steve Liss/Time Life Pictures/Getty Images

Individuals Who Are HIV Positive

> An energized HIV-prevention movement, marching hand in hand with the movement to make access to treatment universal, is a goal truly worth the effort it will take. (Piot, Bartos, Larson, Zewdie, & Mane, 2008, p. 857)

It is now estimated that over 1 million people in the United States are HIV positive; and, since AIDS was first identified, more than half a million Americans have died of the disease (Centers for Disease Control and Prevention, 2010). AIDS continues to spread in this country and worldwide, with approximately 33 million children and adults being HIV positive or having AIDS (UNAIDS, 2010). With 10% of the world's population and 64% of the world's cases of AIDS, sub-Saharan Africa has been most affected by the AIDS epidemic. However, clearly there is no immunity from the epidemic as the disease continues to spread around the world. With early identification and treatment of HIV being a key to a longer and healthier life (Centers for Disease Control and Prevention, 2007), it is clear that human service professionals can and will play a vital role in helping to identify those who may be HIV positive and in offering counseling and supportive services to HIV-positive individuals and their families. It is also critical that human service professionals are on the forefront of advocating for increased testing and for cheap and widespread use of anti-AIDS drugs for individuals in this country and throughout the world. In addition, with sexual activity with an HIV-positive individual being potentially life-threatening, human service professionals may very well be challenged with ethical dilemmas concerning protecting confidentiality with their client versus complying with the duty to warn those who may be unwittingly exposed to the virus (Wong-Wylie, 2003; Yarhouse, 2003).

Magic Johnson has an upbeat attitude and finds ways of helping the under-privileged despite his HIV-positive status

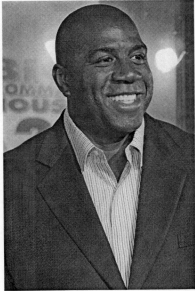

Lucas Jackson/Reuter/CORBIS

The Homeless and the Poor

> Now we can walk on the moon and thousands of dying people cannot walk to a cup of food or clean drinking water. (Dykeman, 1997, pp. 3–4)

It is estimated that as many as 3 million Americans may be homeless in any one year, including 1.3 million children (National Law Center on Homelessness & Poverty, 2010), and despite a considerable increase in the homeless population over the past 15 years, resources to serve these individuals have remained minimal. In recent years, the faces of the homeless have changed dramatically and now include children who have run away from home, single-parent families, intact families who have no place to live, poor single men and women, and the deinstitutionalized mentally ill (see Box 10.1).

In past years being poor did not necessarily mean one was at greater risk of being homeless, but today it is often one step away from not having a roof over one's head. The number of poor Americans is 40 million, or about 13% of the population (U.S. Census Bureau, 2009b). In addition, a staggering 19% of all children in the United States live in poverty. Also, poverty is associated with race, as 24.7% of African-Americans, 23.2% of Hispanics, 11.8% of Asians or Pacific Islanders, and 8.6% of Whites live below the poverty level (see Figure 8.4 from Chapter 8).

BOX 10.1 | **An Interview with Al**

Al is a 41-year-old homeless man in Norfolk, Virginia. Although raised in New York City, he and his family of origin now live in Norfolk. Having some college credits and growing up with modest means, he notes, "My dad grew up in the Depression. I never thought that I would be in this situation." He goes on to state that suddenly becoming homeless can happen to anybody. Until recently, Al was staying with his parents, adopted sister, and her three children. However, after his father had a mild stroke, he felt that he was a burden on his family, so he took to the streets. He states that he believes things have become much worse during the past 10 years and notes that he made more money as a teenager than he does now.

Although Al is homeless, he usually has a roof over his head at night. Generally, he stays at one of the local church shelters or at the Union Mission. Every morning Al goes to a temporary job-placement service with the hope of finding work. Al states that obtaining food is usually not a problem because local religious groups and shelters provide some food daily. Al has a 23-year-old daughter and 4-year-old twin boys. He says, "It hurts that I don't have a job—hurts that I can't support them."

Al believes that about one-third of homeless people would work if employment were available, that some of the homeless are those who have been institutionalized for mental illness and are probably incapable of working, and that some of the homeless have developed attitudes from years of hopelessness. He says the street term for such people is "ate up." Being on the streets, according to Al, has a domino effect. A homeless person has few resources, no nice clothes, no place to keep personal things and records, and little hope. The result: Pulling oneself out of the situation is difficult. Al, however, seems to keep a positive attitude and states, "Sometimes I slip into a blue funk, but I don't lose hope." He says that keeping a positive attitude is like playing mental volleyball, where he keeps going back and forth between being in a funk and feeling okay.

The negative results of homelessness and poverty include a wide range of educational, social, psychological, and physical problems (American Psychological Association, 2011b). And, although the *McKinney Act* of 1987 provides mental health services, substance abuse treatment, outreach services, emergency food and shelter, housing, health care, education, job training, and child care, the outlook for this segment of society seems bleak (U.S. Department of Housing and Urban Development, 2011). The human service professional of the future will undoubtedly be faced with individuals who are poor, homeless, and destitute and they must have the knowledge and skills to work with this population.

Older People

With increased longevity and decreased birthrates, the population of older persons is steadily rising, and by the year 2030, it will be close to 20% (U.S. Census Bureau, 2003, 2008b). And, as America has become increasingly diverse, so has our aging population. As the population of individuals over 65 years old continues to rise, so does their need for increased social services in such areas as income assistance, health care, housing, employment, leisure activities, and environmental assistance (e.g., large-print books) (Clubok, 2001; Russell-Miller, 2001; Stickle & Onedera, 2006) (see Box 10.2). It is therefore not surprising that across the country

Many of the homeless in America have little hope for the future.

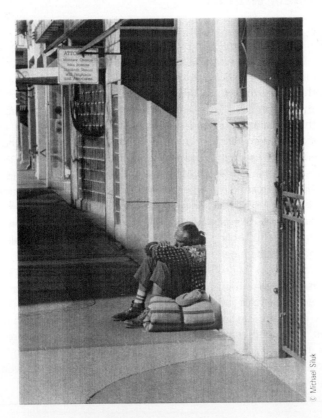

© Michael Siluk

BOX 10.2 | Needs of Older Americans

In an effort to understand some of the needs of older Americans, I visited a local community center that had organized senior services. These included meals at reduced prices, educational activities such as guest speakers on a variety of topics, and social activities such as movies and trips to local theater productions. At the center, I had lunch with Irving, Lasard, Izzi, Jeanette, Max, Joe, and some other senior citizens; their average age was about 80 years old. We had an informal discussion about a number of issues facing older Americans. Although there was some debate concerning the amount of federal subsidies that

should be given to seniors, some of their major issues seemed clear. For instance, all felt that seniors are entitled to safe and secure housing, good medical care, transportation, healthy meals, and federal assistance in the delivery and implementation of these programs. Most of the group felt that they had spent a lifetime working hard and now deserved something in return. Finally, it was clear that many of these seniors were dealing with losses of spouses, friends, and relatives in their lives. This psychological component was clearly not being attended to by any of the available services.

we have seen an increase in day treatment programs for the elderly at community mental health centers, long-term care facilities such as nursing homes, housing settings that are specifically geared toward older persons, foster care settings for the older persons, senior centers, and programs for older persons offered through religious organizations and social service agencies. Unfortunately, older persons have a high percentage of mental health needs yet attend counseling at lower rates than others (Myers & Harper, 2004). With the growing number of older persons in the United States, along with more programs to serve this population, more human service professionals will be needed to work with this population in the years to come.

Seniors at a community center discuss some of the problems they face in older age. Jewish Community Center of Tidewater, Norfolk, VA

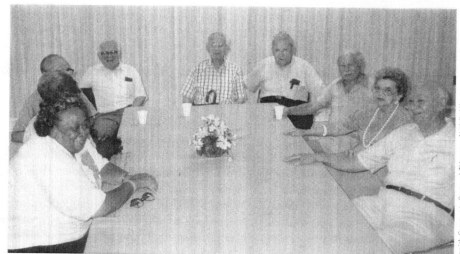

Jewish Community Center of Tidewater, Norfolk, VA

Individuals Who Are Chronically Mentally Ill

In 1955 there were 560,000 inpatients in psychiatric hospitals in the United States, and by 1995 this figure had fallen to 69,000 (Burger, 2011). Although there has been a great reduction in inpatient hospitalizations over the years, it is not the result of a dramatic improvement in the mental health of Americans, but the consequence of a number of important events since the 1950s. In fact, although there are fewer individuals who are now hospitalized for psychiatric problems, today there are over 8,000 centers that offer some form of mental health services (Manta, 2011). The reasons for the reduction in inpatient care yet concurrent increase in services are many.

First, the development of new psychotropic medications, such as **antipsychotics** (e.g., Haldol, Thorazine, Risperidone), **antidepressants** (e.g., Prozac, Zoloft, Elavil), and **anti-anxiety agents** (e.g., Valium, Tranxene, Xanax), has made the management of severe emotional conditions possible outside the inpatient setting. Second, the passage of the **Community Mental Health Centers Act** of 1963 funded the establishment of mental health centers and made it possible for many of those with severe emotional problems to obtain outpatient mental health services for free or at low cost (Burger, 2011). Third, the proliferation of social service programs introduced through the **Great Society** initiatives of the Johnson presidency created a myriad of social service agencies, many of which service the multiple needs of the chronically mentally ill. Finally, in 1975, the U.S. Supreme Court decision ***Donaldson v. O'Connor*** stated that a person who is not dangerous to self or others could not be confined in a psychiatric hospital against his or her will (Box 10.3). This case and others were instrumental in the eventual **deinstitutionalization** of mental patients. One result of these events is the proliferation of services for the mentally disabled—services often staffed by human service professionals. As a result of all of these changes, the human service professional of the future will be intimately involved in providing social services for individuals who are chronically mentally ill.

Individuals with Disabilities

As noted in Chapter 8, about 19% of Americans over the age of 5 have a disability which are mostly in one or more of the following areas: sight; hearing;

BOX 10.3	***Donaldson v. O'Connor:*** **The Deinstitutionalization of Mental Patients**

In 1975, the U.S. Supreme Court decided a case that dramatically affected the status of mental hospitals in the United States. Kenneth Donaldson, who had been committed to a state mental hospital in Florida and confined against his will for 15 years, sued the hospital superintendent, Dr. J. B. O'Connor. Despite this, the hospital refused to release Donaldson, stating that he was still mentally ill. The U.S. Supreme Court unanimously upheld lower court decisions, stating that the hospital could not hold him against his will if he was not in danger of harming himself or others. This decision led to the large-scale release of hundreds of thousands of individuals across the country who had been confined in mental hospitals against their wills and who were not a danger to self or others.

walking; moving the upper body; cognitive, mental or emotional; or other (U.S. Census Bureau, 2008a). In addition, you are more likely to have a disability if you live in the South, are poor, and belong to a minority group.

Although illegal, individuals with disabilities continue to be discriminated against in a variety of ways, such as being denied jobs or educational opportunities or by not being given access to business and recreational facilities. But, as disturbing as the above are, perhaps the worst mistreatment of people with disabilities is the reaction many get from others. Many individuals with disabilities are feared, ignored, stared at, infantilized, treated as intellectually inferior, accused of faking their disability, or pitied.

A number of federal laws have had an impact on the ability of individuals with disabilities to receive services. For instance, the *Education for All Handicapped Children Act* of 1975 (**PL 94-142**) and the subsequent *Individuals with Disabilities Education Act* (**IDEA**) assure the right to an education within the least restrictive environment for all children who are identified as having a disability that interferes with learning. Also, the *Rehabilitation Act* of 1973 assures access to vocational rehabilitation services for adults with disabilities who are in need of employment. The *Americans with Disabilities Act* of 1992 updated these laws and assures that qualified individuals with disabilities could not be discriminated against in job application procedures, hiring, firing, advancement, compensation, fringe benefits, job training, and other terms, conditions, and privileges (U.S. Department of Labor, n.d.).

As new medical procedures make it possible for individuals to live with disabling and chronic health conditions, we may see an increase in the number of individuals with disabilities. This will result in additional needed services for these individuals, services in which we may find the human service professional taking an increasingly active role. Finally, let us remember that we are all only temporarily able-bodied.

Despite being born with cerebral palsy and later having an accident that resulted in quadriplegia, Lisa Lyons obtained her master's degree in counseling.

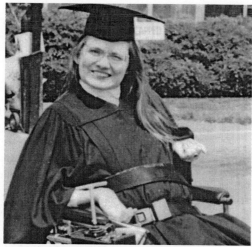

Courtesy Lisa Lyons

Individuals at Risk for Chemical Dependence

The substance abuse statistics in the United States are staggering (U.S. Department of Health and Human Services, 2010). For instance, for individuals aged 12 and older, in 2009 the following was found:

- 3.9 million (1.5%) were dependent on or abused illicit drugs
- 19.3 million (7.6%) were dependent on or abused alcohol or illicit drugs
- 15.4 million (6.1%) were dependent on or abused alcohol
- 21.8 million (8.7%) were actively using illicit drugs
- 131 million (51.9%) drank alcohol
- 17.2 million (6.8%) were heavy drinkers
- 60 million (23.7 %) had participated in binge drinking once or more in the past 30 days
- 4.3 million (1.7%) had received treatment for a substance abuse problem

Drug and alcohol abuse today can be found in the inner cities and in middle-class America. It not only affects the users but has a great impact on family members and on society (Woititz, 2002). There is little question that substance abuse is related to many of the problems facing our nation, including violent crime, problems on the job, and changing morals. Thus, the widespread abuse of substances, unfortunately, provides an array of places for mental health professionals to work, including hospital detoxification (detox) units, halfway houses, and drug and alcohol treatment centers (U.S. Department of Health and Human Services, 2009).

STANDARDS IN THE PROFESSION

Thus, standards are a mark of the maturity of a profession and offer a benchmark of excellences to which individuals and programs should adhere. (Milliken & Neukrug, 2010, p. 5)

Standards raise a profession to its highest level. Four standards that have taken prominence in the human services recently, and will likely be crucial in the decades to come, are program accreditation, credentialing, ethical standards, and the Skill Standards. Although these standards were discussed in detail in Chapters 1 and 2, here we will briefly highlight their importance for the future.

Program Accreditation

A major thrust of the **Council for Standards in Human Service Education** (CSHSE) is to provide an **accreditation** process for human service programs (CSHSE, n.d.; Kincaid & Andresen, 2010). Discussed in Chapter 2, accreditation is the mechanism that ensures that programs meet minimum competence and share similar curriculum and values as they train human service professionals. It also helps to delimit the professional identity of the human service professional. Accreditation in human services is relatively new; however, it will likely become increasingly important, if not essential, for human service programs of the future. One advantage of having graduates from an accredited program is that such graduates are waived some or all of the requirement of work experience when applying to take the exam to become a **Human Services—Board Certified Practitioner (HS—BCP)** (see Chapter 2 for a more involved discussion of accreditation).

Credentialing

As noted in Chapter 2, after years of discussion, the **Center for Credentialing and Education (CCE)**, in consultation with the **National Organization for Human Services (NOHS)** and **CSHSE**, developed a credentialing process for a human service professional to become a **Human Services—Board Certified Practitioner (HS—BCP)**. This certification allows those who hold a technical-level, associate-level, bachelor-level, or master-level degree in human services or a related degree to become certified (Hinkle & O'Brien, 2010). With close to 2,000 individuals quickly becoming certified since the process started in 2008, this credential has clearly become popular. Such a credential shows that human service professionals have obtained minimum competence in their field and is a mark of the maturity of the profession. If you would like additional information about this important milestone in the field of human services, see "Credentialing in the Human Services" in Chapter 2 or go to http://www.cce-global.org/HSBCP.

Ethical Standards

The development of the **Ethical Standards of Human Service Professionals**, which were approved in 1995 (see Appendix A), was a necessary step in the growth of the human service profession. Ethical standards are an important mark of a profession and indicate that there is a unique body of knowledge to which standards can be applied (see Chapter 2). More recently, CCE created a separate ethical code that is shorter but focused more on limiting infractions of human service professionals (Wark, 2010). Currently, the Ethical Standards are in the beginning stages of a revision, and if you are interested in assisting with that process, contact the board of NOHS and let them know! Additional information about ethics and the ethical code can be found in Chapter 2.

Skill Standards

During the 1990s, competencies for human service professionals and the skills needed to implement them were established through a national effort that included feedback from educators and practitioners (Taylor, Bradley, & Warren, 1996). The **Skill Standards** "define the competencies used by direct service workers in a wide variety of service contexts in community settings across the nation. Designed to be relevant to diverse direct service roles (residential, vocational, therapeutic, etc.), the standards are based upon a nationally validated job analysis involving a wide variety of human service workers, consumers, providers and educators." (NOHS, 2009b, para. 2). These standards have been critical in the development of accreditation standards and in the credentialing process. The new millennium will clearly see a more highly qualified human service professional as a result of these standards. See Chapter 2 for more information on the Skill Standards.

TECHNOLOGY IN HUMAN SERVICE WORK

With the vast majority of Americans owning a computer and having Internet access, the world has quickly changed, especially when we consider that only 20% of households had a computer in 1992, only 19% had Internet access in 1998, and PCs started mass production in the 1980s (U.S. Department of Commerce, 2000). Human service and other mental health professionals have quickly adapted to this new way of working by applying technology in a variety of ways, including the following (Kincaid, 2004a; Layne & Hohenshil, 2005; Rockinson-Szapkiw & Silvey, 2010):

1. A wide range of case management activities (e.g., managing caseloads, documentation and record keeping, billing, marketing)
2. The training of helping professionals (e.g., on-line supervision, wikis and discussion groups for shared learning, distance learning, webinars)
3. For clinical assessment and diagnosis (e.g., testing and assessment on the computer)
4. In communication (Listservs, e-mail, twitters, Facebook, etc.)
5. For online counseling and helping

Technology has become so pervasive, it is now being included as an important aspect of the ethical codes of some helping professions, and a recommendation has been made to include technology in the NOHS ethical standards revision (American Counseling Association, 2005; Kincaid, 2004b). Finally, one of the most controversial topics relative to counseling is conducting counseling and supportive work on the Internet. Such practices raise concerns around informed consent, confidentiality, legitimacy, and credentialing and will need to be continually discussed as technology becomes increasingly used and more complex.

CRISIS, DISASTER, AND TRAUMA TRAINING

The horror of hurricane Katrina and the attack on the twin towers taught us that as a country, our readiness to react to a disaster was not particularly good and that many human service professionals were not adequately prepared to conduct **crisis, disaster**, and **trauma counseling**. Thus, there has been particular push in recent years to have helpers trained appropriately to work with crises, disasters, and with individuals in trauma. As human service professionals have often been part of the first responder teams in disaster and crisis situations, ensuring that they are adequately trained in this important area will become increasingly important. With professionals needing specialized skills in these areas, in the future, we will likely see CSHSE accreditation standards addressing this important curriculum area (see Box 10.4).

A DEVELOPMENTAL AND PRIMARY PREVENTION EMPHASIS

The mental health professions have increasingly highlighted the importance of understanding the developmental level of the client, and this is likely to continue in the upcoming years. Such a focus views problems as a function of **developmental tasks** or milestones and a natural part of the life process (see Chapter 5). Framing problems in this light depathologizes clients because they become viewed as having

BOX 10.4	**Crisis Counseling Principles**

Training in crisis, disaster, and trauma counseling takes specialized skills. The **Federal Emergency Management Agency** (**FEMA**) has identified some key principles for the crisis counselor which need to be expanded upon when working with clients who have experienced crises and disasters. Their Crisis Counseling Program (CCP) is:

- *Strengths Based*—CCP services promote resilience, empowerment, and recovery.
- *Anonymous*—Crisis counselors do not classify, label, or diagnose people; no records or case files are kept.

- *Outreach Oriented*—Crisis counselors deliver services in the communities rather than wait for survivors to seek their assistance.
- *Conducted in Nontraditional Settings*—Crisis counselors make contact in homes and communities, not in clinical or office settings.
- *Designed to Strengthen Existing Community Support Systems*—The CCP supplements, but does not supplant or replace, existing community systems. (FEMA, n.d.; Key Principles section)

---

not yet completed certain stages of development instead of having embedded, "nonfixable" problems within.

There is a natural marriage between knowledge of development and **primary prevention** activities because if we are knowledgeable about what is likely to occur developmentally, we can prepare activities and workshops to ease individuals through stages in their lives (see *Journal of Primary Prevention*). This contrasts with **secondary prevention**, which focuses on the control of nonsevere mental health problems, and **tertiary prevention**, which concentrates on the control of serious mental health problems (Burger, 2011; Gladding & Newsome, 2010). Examine the continuum of Figure 10.1, and compare it with the focus of the human service professional as delineated in Table 1.2. Clearly, primary prevention fits naturally with the existing focus and training of the human service professional.

During this century, human service professionals will increasingly be asked to do something that is second nature to them—primary prevention. No doubt, the human service professional will be seen as an expert in wellness and prevention programs.

	Primary	Secondary	Tertiary	
Short term	→	→	→	Long term
Modifying behavior	→	→	→	Personality reconstruction
Wellness focus	→	→	→	Focus on pathology
Before problem occurs	→	→	→	After problem occurs
Preventive	→	→	→	Restorative

Figure 10.1 | Comparison of the Focus of Helpers Who Provide Primary, Secondary, or Tertiary Prevention

MANAGED HEALTH CARE

As a mechanism to reduce health care costs, in the 1960s **managed health care** was introduced into the United States. Then, in 1973, the *Health Maintenance Organization Act* was passed by Congress with its major focus being the expansion of health maintenance organizations and related programs (Preferred Provider Organizations [PPOs]; Employee Assistance Programs [EAPs]) in an effort to reduce costs associated with health care. Over the years, part of this reduction has included the overseeing of mental health services and the development of primary prevention activities to prevent illness. It is here that human service professionals have seen possibilities for employment. Overseeing of cost is sometimes provided by individuals with a degree in human services or a related field. Also, these individuals sometimes conduct primary prevention activities. It is likely that such employment will continue to expand as we move into the twenty-first century and as we continue to try and find ways to reduce costs of the health care system.

MEDICINE AND HUMAN SERVICES

As those in the medical professions become more comfortable working with those in the mental health professions, and as the helping professions become increasingly trained to work with those in the medical field, mental health professionals will be found working side-by-side with medical professionals (Bodenhorn & Lawson, 2003; Lees, 2011; Madson, Loignon, & Lane, 2009; Neukrug, 2001; Pence, 2008). Increasingly, mental health professionals will be found doing such things as the following:

- Counseling individuals and their families about the results of genetic testing
- Counseling individuals and their families about the progression of a disease
- Providing preventive and health education workshops for individuals
- Working with doctors' patients to foster motivation for prevention and treatment
- Being a referral source for counseling and related activities
- Being an advocate for the patients of medical professionals

If human service professionals are to work side-by-side with medical professionals, they will need to be well versed on the medical aspects of diseases and disabilities, be well trained in procedures that work with such populations, and know the ethical concerns related to them. Clearly, this century will bring some new challenges to those human service professionals who may work in this important area.

SOCIAL JUSTICE, ADVOCACY, AND MULTICULTURAL COUNSELING

The fact that two chapters in this book have been dedicated to these important topics reflects their ever-growing importance in human services. It seems clear that as human service professionals are called to work with an increasingly diverse population, they will need to have the attitudes and beliefs, knowledge, and skills to do so competently. And, as agencies increasingly focus on providing a multicultural environment in their attitude, in the people whom they employ, and in the types of clients they attract, human service students best be prepared for this work environment. Increasingly, you will see human service training programs infusing into their curriculum and/or offering separate courses on social justice, advocacy, and multicultural counseling (Neukrug & Milliken, 2008). Clearly, the human service professional of the twenty-first century will have to be a culturally competent professional.

INTERNATIONAL PERSPECTIVES

The world has become much smaller. Today, information is received, instantaneously, from all parts of the globe, and we are increasingly sharing resources, culture, and ideas. However, great differences continue to differentiate us. As human service professionals, we can help bridge these gaps by taking on a global perspective. Such a perspective might mean educating ourselves on international perspectives, learning from one another about how to implement social service programs, and sharing resources (Gray, 2005). As the richest country in the world, perhaps we have more to share in resources than do others, but we still have much we can learn from others. As we move into the twenty-first century, we are likely to see more of a focus on understanding human services from a global perspective.

STRESS, CYNICISM, AND BURNOUT

Human service professionals often witness the saddest side of humanity, such as when they work with clients who are homeless, hungry, or dealing with a recent loss. As a result of this difficult work, some human service professionals develop what has recently been called **compassion fatigue/vicarious traumatization syndrome** (Adams, Figley, & Boscarino, 2008; Sommer, 2008). No wonder many human service professionals who are poorly paid continually deal with high-stress situations, and receive minimal reinforcement for their work, eventually choose to change careers. Unfortunately, stress, cynicism, and burnout are likely to continue to be major concerns of human service professionals in the decades to come.

Hans Selye (1956, 1974), one of the leading researchers on stress, stated that stress is an adaptive response to a changing situation. **Stress** therefore can be seen as a healthy response that enables a person to handle new or highly charged situations (Pritts et al., 2000). However, too much stress has been associated with a myriad of psychological states as well as a wide range of physical illnesses (Chopra, 2009; Weil, 2009). To address these concerns, human service professionals will have to take a holistic look at themselves by attending to their psychological, physical, and spiritual health (see next section).

WELLNESS

Listed in Chapter 1 as one of the eight important characteristics of the effective helper, embracing a wellness perspective is crucial to alleviating stress, preventing cynicism, avoiding burnout, and lessening the possibility of conducting impaired work with our clients. Embracing such a perspective takes a deliberate and diligent effort, and although there are many methods of examining our own wellness, Myers and Sweeney (2008) offer one model that was described in Chapter 1. This model of the **Indivisible Self** suggests that we should focus on five factors when reviewing our own wellness: the creative self, the coping self, the social self, the essential self, and the physical self (see Box 10.5). You are encouraged to reread the section in Chapter 1 on embracing a wellness perspective and completing Exercise VIII if you have not done so already.

Finally, Carl Whitaker (1976) suggests a number of ways to keep oneself healthy. Noting his points and adding a few thoughts of my own, consider doing the following in your life:

1. Place yourself as a priority.
2. Learn how to love.
3. Listen to your impulses.
4. Listen to your inner voice, and listen to others.
5. Enjoy your significant other more than anyone else.
6. Fracture role structures and challenge authority.
7. Challenge yourself—you're not always right.
8. Build long-term relationships so you feel safe and grounded enough to express your feelings.
9. Act "crazy" and whimsical.
10. Face the fact that you must continue to grow and change until you die.

| **BOX 10.5** | **Summary of the Five Factors of the Indivisible Self** |

Creative Self

Open-mindedness, creativity, curiosity, sense of mastery and competence, ability to laugh at oneself, sense of humor about life, ability to express and being in touch with feelings.

Coping Self

Having satisfactory leisure time, being able to deal with stress, feeling a sense of self-acceptance, being real with self and others, absence of irrational beliefs, seeing reality in an accurate way.

Social Self

Having connections with others; being able to trust and have empathy for others; being able to maintain an intimate, trusting relationship with self-disclosure; accepting others unconditionally.

Essential Self

Having a belief in something beyond self (e.g., higher power; God, etc.); having a purpose in life; being optimistic and hopeful; practicing prayer, meditation, or worship; having a sense of moral values; being satisfied with one's gender; being satisfied with one's culture; taking care of one's wellness through preventive activities.

Physical Self (Nutrition and Exercise)

Having a healthy diet, maintaining a reasonable weight, being active physically in order to keep in good shape.

ETHICAL, PROFESSIONAL, AND LEGAL ISSUES: CONTINUING EDUCATION

Education never ends. Although you may work hard to obtain a degree, being effective throughout your career as a human service professional will require on-going learning. Once you are in the field, you will find that there are gaps in your education—things that were not stressed that seem essential for you to know at work. Therefore, obtaining continuing education beyond your degree is crucial. You can accomplish this through a variety of means. By joining the appropriate professional associations, you will be eligible to participate in workshops that keep you current regarding the most recent advances in the field. You can take additional coursework, perhaps to earn an advanced degree. Sometimes agencies will offer staff development workshops aimed at increasing skills in areas deemed important. Increasingly, credentialing boards are requiring continuing education to maintain professional credentials. This ensures that the professional is continuing to learn and that he or she can offer the best services possible to his or her clients.

THE EFFECTIVE HUMAN SERVICE PROFESSIONAL: ANXIOUS ABOUT CHANGE, DESIROUS OF CHANGE, HOPEFUL

As noted at varying points in this text, change is often not an easy process. It usually requires giving up an old system and accommodating to a new way of viewing the world. However, effective human service professionals, even though they may be anxious about the future, want to take on new challenges, are committed to their profession, and look at change as crucial to their own process of living and critical to the evolution of the profession (Evenson & Holloway, 2003). Human service professionals who are stressed, burnt out, cynical, and stagnant do little for themselves, probably provide poor services to their clients, and generally are not involved in positive ways with professional associations. On the other hand, human service professionals who are positive, forward-looking, and desirous of change are probably the people who work best with their clients and offer the most to the future of the field.

Who is the effective human service professional? It's my friend Bob, who attends workshops, has a positive attitude toward the future, takes care of himself by going to aerobics and meditating, and always has a positive attitude toward his clients. It's Rivers, who is encouraging of all people he meets, is a person you always want to hug, is warm, is caring, and is a great listener. It's Maggie, who is always willing to take a stand, an advocate for the underprivileged, and a person who is able to love. And it's Steve, who is a leader of others, is willing to confront his colleagues, even those to whom he is close, is constantly working on self-growth, and is always thinking about what he can do differently in the future. And it's you. Within yourself is the potential to be caring, loving, reflective, energized, an advocate, a risk taker, a leader, and a doer!

SUMMARY

This chapter focused on the future. In it, we examined some possible changes in the roles of the human service professional and discussed some of the client populations with whom the human service professional will most likely work in the upcoming years. These included the incarcerated, their families, and the victims of crime; those who are HIV positive; the homeless and the poor; older people; individuals who are chronically mentally ill; individuals with disabilities; and individuals at risk for chemical dependence. We then went on to discuss how the future will bring a greater focus on a number of standards in the profession, including program accreditation, credentialing, ethical standards, and the Skill Standards.

As this chapter continued, we discussed the role that technology is now playing in the work of the human professional and anticipated changes, related to technology, in the future. We then discussed how human service professionals will need to be better trained in crisis, disaster, and trauma counseling. We also noted the importance of human service professionals maintaining a positive outlook with their clients and having a developmental and primary prevention emphasis.

Changes in managed health care and the role of the human service professional in managed health was next discussed, and we noted that managed health might be an area that provides additional employment for human service professionals. We also looked at how human service professionals may increasingly work closely with those in the medical professions.

As this chapter continued, we noted that social justice, advocacy, and multicultural counseling, areas that were focused on in detail in this text, will continue to be important in the twenty-first century. We also noted that we will likely see an increasing international perspective in human services.

How stress, cynicism, and burnout will affect the work of the human service professional and the importance of addressing it was next examined in this chapter, and this led into a natural discussion on the importance of wellness by human service professionals. This chapter concluded with a discussion on the importance of continuing education in your future and how the effective human service professional is positive, forward-looking, and desirous of change.

Experiential Exercises

I. Interview a Person from a Special Population

Interview an individual in one or more of the following special populations, and ask the accompanying questions (and any other questions you think would be appropriate).

1. A Person Who Is Incarcerated
   a. Why were you incarcerated?
   b. What's it like for you to be in jail (or prison)?
   c. Do you believe you had a fair trial?
   d. What prejudices have you experienced?
   e. What social services have you used?
   f. What social services would you like to have available?
   g. Is there anything you would like to have changed about your life related to your current status?
2. A Person Who Has Been Victimized by Crime
   a. What is the nature of your victimization? (What happened to you?)
   b. What's it like being a victim of crime?

    c. Have you experienced any unusual reactions or prejudices from people as a result of your victimization?

    d. What social services have you used?

    e. What social services would you like to have available?

    f. What changes in society, including the social service system, would you like to see related to those who are victims of crime?

3. For any of the following individuals, see Exericse II of the "Experiential Exercise" in the back of Chapter 8:

    a. An individual with a disability

    b. A poor person and/or homeless person

    c. A person who is (or was) chemically dependent

    d. An individual who is HIV positive

    e. An individual who struggles with mental illness

II. Standards of Practice

Discuss, in small groups, why the following standards are likely to become more important.

1. Program accreditation
2. Credentialing
3. Ethical Standards
4. Skill Standards

III. Changes in Technology

1. *E-mail:* In small groups, discuss how e-mail has changed the way the helping professions offer services.

2. *Social Networking:* On your own, do a search for Listservs, twitters, and Facebook pages in the helping professions. Share your lists in class.

3. *Computers at Work:* For the following items, discuss how computers have changed the way that human service professionals conduct work.

    a. Client assessment

    b. Diagnosis

    c. Billing

    d. Note taking and case report writing

    e. Supervision

4. *Clients, Informed Consent, and Counseling Online:* The following describes a number of ethical issues related to technology and informed consent taken verbatim from the ethical code of the American Counseling Association (ACA, 2005, Standard, A.12.g). For each of the statements, on your own or in small groups, discuss how you would ensure adherence to the guidelines.

    "1. Address issues related to the difficulty of maintaining the confidentiality of electronically transmitted communications.

    2. Inform clients of all colleagues, supervisors, and employees, such as Informational Technology (IT) administrators, who might have authorized or unauthorized access to electronic transmissions.

    3. Urge clients to be aware of all authorized or unauthorized users including fellow employees who have access to any technology clients may use in the counseling process.

4. Inform clients of pertinent legal rights and limitations governing the practice of a profession over state lines or international boundaries.

5. Use encrypted Web sites and e-mail communications to help ensure confidentiality when possible.

6. When the use of encryption is not possible, counselors notify clients of this fact and limit electronic transmissions to general communications that are not client specific.

7. Inform clients if and for how long archival storage of transaction records is maintained.

8. Discuss the possibility of technology failure and alternate methods of service delivery.

9. Inform clients of emergency procedures, such as calling 911 or a local crisis hotline, when the counselor is not available.

10. Discuss time zone differences, local customs, and cultural or language differences that might impact service delivery.

11. Inform clients when technology-assisted distance counseling services are not covered by insurance."

5. *Technology and Ethical Standards for Human Service Professionals:* Now that you've examined some of the ethical concerns relative to technology that face human service professionals, in small groups, come up with your own ethical guidelines relative to technology and human service work. Address each of the following issues:

   a. Confidentiality and counseling online

   b. Security of records

   c. Viewing client social network pages without informing them (e.g., Facebook, blog, Web page)

   d. Having open access of your social network pages

   e. Obtaining informed consent from clients

   f. Addressing issues of imminent danger (e.g., client suicide or homicide)

6. *Professional Association Web Pages:* Your instructor will divide the class into small groups and ask each group to take one or more of the following professional organizations and examine its Web page. After the pages have been reviewed by the groups, report your findings to the class.

   a. American Association of Marriage & Family Therapy (AAMFT): www.aamft.org

   b. American Counseling Association (ACA): www.counseling.org

   c. American Psychological Association (APA): www.psych.org

   d. American Psychiatric Association (APA): www.apa.org

   e. American Psychiatric Nurses Association (APNA): www.apna.org

   f. Center for Credentialing and Education (CCE): www.cce-global.org /credentials-offered/hsbcp

   g. Counsel for Standards in Human Service Education (CSHSE): www.cshse.org

   h. National Association of Social Workers (NASW): www.nasw.org

   i. National Organization for Human Services (NOHS): www.nationalhumanservices.org

IV. Crisis, Disaster, and Trauma Training

1. What specific skills do you think you will need to have to be adequately trained in crisis, disaster, and trauma counseling?
2. What unique ethical dilemmas might you face as a helper who works with those in crisis, those who have faced disaster, and those facing a traumatic event?
3. How might crisis, disaster, and trauma counseling affect your ability to cope in the world?

V. Developmental Emphasis and Primary Prevention Emphasis

For each of the following theories, develop a primary prevention activity that could assist an individual through any stage of the theory (you may want to refer back to Chapter 5 for assistance).

1. Piaget's Theory of Cognitive Development
2. Kohlberg's and/or Gilligan's Theory of Moral Development
3. Erikson's Theory of Psychosocial Development
4. Kegan's Constructive Development Model

VI. Health Maintenance Organizations (HMOs), Preferred Provider Organizations (PPOs), and Employee Assistance Programs (EAPs)

In small groups, research an HMO, a PPO, an EAP, or a traditional health insurance plan. Compare and contrast these mental health delivery systems based on the following features:

1. What services are offered by each?
2. Does an individual need to go through a primary care physician to receive services?
3. Is preventive care covered?
4. How is specialty care dealt with?
5. Are mental health services covered?
6. What are the limitations of mental health services?
7. What is the payment for services, if any?
8. What are the job opportunities for an individual who has a degree in human services?

VII. Medicine and Human Services

1. In small groups, discuss the mental health implications for an individual who is faced with the following medical problems:
   a. An individual who is waiting for an organ transplant and will die if it is not received.
   b. An individual who might have the gene for a debilitating disease and has the opportunity, through genetic testing, to discover if he or she has the disease.
   c. An individual who carries a gene for a debilitating disease and is considering having a child.
   d. An individual who refuses medical treatment for himself or herself because of religious beliefs.
   e. An individual who refuses medical treatment for his or her child because of religious beliefs.

2. What are the implications for the families of the individuals noted in item 1?

3. What are the ethical, professional, and legal implications of working with the individuals noted in item 1?

VIII. Social Justice, Advocacy, and Multicultural Counseling

Answer the following questions concerning these topics:

1. What changes do you foresee in the future of the human service profession if, as predicted, these areas continue to be prominent in the field?

2. What are some positive and negative aspects to having same-culture helpers work with same-culture clients?

3. How do you think you will be personally affected by a more diverse group of human service professionals?

4. How might you go about creating a diversity-friendly atmosphere at an agency in which you work?

5. How might your role as an advocate for your client interfere or enhance your helping relationship with that client?

IX. International Perspectives

1. As a homework assignment, your instructor will assign different students in class to research the following:

a. the varying kinds of human service credentials available in specified countries from around the world.

b. the varying kinds of human service degrees available in specified countries from around the world.

c. varying kinds of human service agencies available in specified countries from around the world.

2. In class, discuss the results of the research conducted in item 1.

a. What are the similarities and differences of credentialing, degrees, and agencies?

b. What can other cultures learn from us?

c. What can we learn from other cultures?

X. Dealing with Stress and Burnout

1. Discuss the various ways that you deal with stress and burnout.

2. Are your ways of dealing with stress working for you?

3. Are there other ways that you might find to deal effectively with your stress?

4. What would you do if you noticed a colleague of yours was burnt out and was working poorly with clients?

5. What would you do if you were burnt out and were working poorly with clients?

XI. Wellness

1. If you have not done so, complete Exercise VIII in Chapter 1.

2. Make a list of ways that you harm yourself psychologically, physically, and/or spiritually. Share that list in small groups.

3. Make a list of ways that you take care of yourself. Share that list in small groups.

XII. Ethical and Professional Vignettes

Review the following vignettes and discuss in class. When appropriate, refer to the Ethical Standards in Appendix A.

1. A colleague tells you that he is working with an individual who just discovered that she carries the gene for a fatal disease. Although she will not get the disease, any child of hers has a 50% chance of developing the disease. She has told your colleague that she has decided to "have my tubes tied and not tell my husband." What ethical, professional, or legal obligation, if any, does your colleague have?

2. A classmate tells you that she sells flower extracts to clients to help them heal. She states this is the "wave of the future." Is this ethical? Professional? Legal? Is this reasonable? What, if anything, should you do?

3. A colleague of yours, who has a bachelor's degree in human services, decides to set up her own Web page where individuals can ask personal questions to which she will reply by e-mail. Is this ethical? Professional? Legal?

4. A colleague of yours, who has a degree in human services, decides to set up an online counseling Web page that uses instant messaging. Individuals can instant message (IM) the professional and have live counseling sessions through this process. Is this ethical? Professional? Legal?

5. You are aware that a colleague is no longer effective with his clients because he is burnt out. He does not realize this. What is your responsibility to the colleague? To his clients?

6. A colleague refuses to become involved in any professional associations, read any journals, or keep up with any advances in the field. She states, "I do what has been shown to be tried and true." Does she have a point? Is what she's doing ethical? Professional? What is your responsibility in this situation?

7. A faculty member at your school never acknowledges differences in clients as a function of cultural background. When a student notes this in class, her only response is, "Every helping relationship is a cross-cultural one, so why should I discuss any one culture in particular?" Does she have a point? Do you have any responsibility in this situation?

8. Your human service program is not approved by CSHSE. Do you have a responsibility to advocate for approval? Why or why not?

9. A colleague of yours often uses ethical guidelines from a related social service profession when the Ethical Standards of Human Service Professionals does not offer guidance in the direction he anticipates. Is this ethical? Professional?

10. A colleague offers a primary prevention workshop on avoiding the use of drugs and alcohol. Your colleague used to take drugs and drink heavily but has not taken any coursework or workshops in this area, nor has she read the literature on substance abuse. She notes, "I have my own experience; that's why I can do this workshop." Is this ethical? Legal? Professional?

11. You have decided to take a job with an HMO despite fiercely disliking the way the company does business. However, they are offering you a good salary, and you will be able to run psychoeducational workshops for adolescents and adults. Is it a good idea for you take the job? Why or why not?

Your Future in the Human Services

CHAPTER CONTENTS

Since you took a course that used this book, you probably have a strong interest in the human service profession, and you may be considering obtaining a job in human services or advancing in the field if you are already working in it. This afterword will give you additional ideas about your potential future in the human services. It will start by examining job trends and potential earnings in human services. Next, it will give you an opportunity to explore and reflect on your own career path and see if it fits the human service profession. Then, it will identify some important items to consider when applying to graduate school or to a job. How to develop an effective résumé will then be discussed as well as the increasing importance of having a portfolio. We will then examine ways of obtaining jobs and offer specific resources you can use to help you locate graduate schools. The afterword will conclude with a short discussion on being chosen or being denied your favorite job or graduate program.

TRENDS IN JOBS AND EARNINGS

Based on the *Occupational Outlook Handbook (OOH)*, by the year 2018 there are expected to be 431,500 jobs in human services, a 23% increase from 10 years earlier (U.S. Department of Labor, 2010–2011c). In fact, by 2018 the number of social and human service assistants is projected to grow much faster than the average for all occupations, ranking it among the most rapidly growing occupations. Average salaries tend to range between $25,000 and $35,000, although this varies considerably based on area in the country, experience, and education. In addition, those who remain in the field and obtain advanced degrees can often do quite well, earning up to $100,000 or more, especially if one moves into administration.

Today, approximately, one in four human service professionals is employed by state and local governments, and well over half are employed in health care and in social assistance industries. Many jobs will likely arise from the need to replace workers who advance, retire, or leave jobs in these areas. Some of the many job titles that human service professionals might find themselves applying for include "human service worker, case management aide, social work assistant, community support worker, mental health aide, community outreach worker, life skills counselor, social services aide, youth worker, psychological aide, client advocate, or gerontology aide" ((U.S. Department of Labor, 2010–2011d, Nature of Work section, para. 1), Nature of Work section, para. 1). So, these are some of the basics about possible employment, now you must ask yourself: "Is this field for me?"

CHOOSING A CAREER IN THE HUMAN SERVICES

Some of you are 100% sure that the human service field is the career for you. You may already be working in the field, or you may be considering what kind of job you want to obtain. Additionally, some of you may be considering graduate school. If this describes you, you may want to skip this section and move right along to the section entitled "Select Items to Consider When Choosing a Graduate Program or Finding a Job" (although the suggestions that follow can also be used with clients who are seeking career counseling).

Are You "Fit" for Human Services?

After reading this text, you should have a good sense of whether you are the person who embraces many of the characteristics of the effective human service professional as noted in Chapter 1. However, you may still be wondering, "Is this something I really *want* to do?" One additional way to decide if this field is right for you is to examine job characteristics of the human service occupations and see if they "ring true" for you. You can do this by going to the *OOH* (see http://www.bls.gov/oco/) or to **O*NET Online** (see http://www.onetonline.org/), two government-sponsored sites that give you a wealth of information about hundreds of jobs, many of which are in the social services. In addition, you might want to examine your interests to see if there is a fit between your personality type and the work environment of the human service field (see Activity 1).

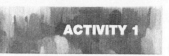

ACTIVITY 1 | # Understanding Your Holland Code

The **Holland Code** has been used extensively to assist in matching one's personality type (interests) with occupations. You can informally determine your Holland Code by reading their descriptions in Appendix B and rank ordering your first three choices from the definitions of the six codes. For instance, I am a "SIA." Your first three choices, in rank order, is your code! An even more valid way would be to have your instructor have you take one of the established interest inventories, such as the **Self-Directed Search** (Holland, 1994) or the **Strong Interest Inventory** (CPP, 2009).

After you have determined your code, read the section in Appendix B entitled *Understanding Your Code*. In addition, you might want to go to O*NET Online (http://www.onetonline.org/) and put in occupations like "human services" and/or "counselor." If you scroll down to "interests," it will tell you what the Holland Code is for the specific job you are looking at. Then consider how close your occupational code is to the one you clicked on. Although you do not need to have the same code as the job you picked, there is some research that indicates the more your code is like the job code, the greater the likelihood that you will be satisfied at the job in question.

After you have finished comparing your code to specific occupations, find students with similar codes, and discuss the following:

1. What personality factors do you share in common?

2. What similar occupational interests do you share?

3. How does knowledge of your code confirm or question your decision to be a human service professional?

4. How might you use the Holland Codes when working with clients?

Choosing a Career: A Self-Analysis

If you feel in sync with the characteristics of effective human service professionals as listed in Chapter 1, and if the job characteristics noted in the *OOH* and O*NET Online "ring true" for you, and if there seems to be a "fit" between your Holland Code and Holland Codes in specific jobs in the human services, then you are probably a good candidate for the human service profession. However, one final and important step is to do a self-analysis. A number of factors affect our career decision-making process and awareness of them can help us make smart choices about our future career path.

a. *Early childhood:* Reflect upon and assess how early childhood issues affected your propensity toward certain careers. For example, I was always a "sensitive" child and this made me a more natural human service professional as I tend to be sensitive to the plight of others.

b. *Socioeconomic issues:* Assess how salary expectations will affect your status in the human service field. Will you make "enough" to feel satisfied? Will you make enough to support your family, should you have one?

c. *Parents' career development:* Assess how your parents' career development affected your aspirations. For instance, if your parents were "career military" and had aspirations for you to do the same, are you okay with going in a different path and possibly disappointing them?

d. *Emotional problems:* Assess how emotional problems could interfere with work in the human services. Is there unfinished business in your life that would make it difficult to work in some human service jobs? For example, if you were abused as a child, can you work with those who abuse?

e. *Situational issues:* Assess situational issues that could interfere with career decision making. For instance, what is the job availability of human service occupations in your area?

f. *Developmental level:* Assess your developmental level; that is, where in the career process are you? Whereas some individuals may just want "any job" in human services, others may be looking to "settle into" a career path.

g. *Worldview and beliefs about self:* Assess your worldview relative to human services. What does this career path mean to you? Does it fit your sense of what you want to do in the world?

You can see that a thorough career assessment can be a rather lengthy process. Examining one's "fit," looking at job characteristics, and reflecting on self is not done simply. However, using such a process can help ensure that you are making the right decision (see Afterword, Box 1).

BOX 1 | **Your Client's Career Choices**

Like our own decision regarding entering the human services, clients have similar decisions regarding their career paths. You can help them by having them go through the following steps:

Step 1: Take a career assessment inventory that assesses their Holland Code or related interests to see which jobs they might fit into nicely.

Step 2: Review O*NET Online and the *OOH*, and begin to examine potential jobs.

Step 3: Using "a through g" from this section, have your clients do a self-analysis just as you did.

Step 4: Have clients create a list of potential jobs.

Step 5: Have clients gather more information about the potential jobs (the Internet, informational interviews, books).

Step 6: Have clients begin to crystallize their choices and apply for jobs.

SELECT ITEMS TO CONSIDER WHEN CHOOSING A GRADUATE PROGRAM OR FINDING A JOB

Although this section is geared toward human services, even if you are considering another profession, you will find the general ideas presented here helpful.

Despite the fact that there are dozens of items to consider when selecting a graduate program or finding a job, the following pinpoints some critical elements. For instance, when making an informed decision about going on to graduate school, one should probably consider the following:

1. Whether or not the program is accredited
2. The kinds of specialties and degrees offered
3. The philosophical orientation of the program
4. Entry requirements
5. The size of the program and university
6. Faculty-student ratios
7. Diversity of the student body and of the faculty
8. The cost and number of available scholarships
9. Location
10. Job placement possibilities

Similarly, the job seeker should know the following:

1. The minimum credentials needed for the job
2. Specific requirements necessary to fulfill the job
3. The philosophical orientation of the setting
4. The number and type of clients one is expected to see
5. Other job roles and functions
6. Salary
7. Diversity of co-workers
8. Possibilities for job advancement

THE APPLICATION PROCESS

Having sat on selection committees for graduate programs and at human service agencies in both the public and private sectors, I have been amazed at the number of applicants who miss the basics in their application process. The following represent some items one should address when completing such applications:

1. Complete all necessary forms, and meet all application deadlines.
2. Make sure you address *each item* asked of you in the graduate application or in the job advertisement.
3. Do not submit cookie-cutter applications to different jobs or different graduate schools. Make sure that your application "speaks to" the school or job to which you are applying.
4. Take and be prepared for any necessary tests (e.g., GREs for graduate schools, personality tests for some jobs).
5. Write a great essay or statement of philosophy.
6. Find out if an interview is required, and prepare for it.
7. Find out about faculty members' research or be knowledgeable about your employer's background, and find an opportunity to ask questions about what they have accomplished.

8. Provide a well-written résumé.
9. Consider submitting a portfolio.
10. Use spell check, and check your grammar.
11. Be positive, focused, and prepared.
12. Don't be negative or cynical.

THE RÉSUMÉ

Some programs and most potential employers will ask you to submit a résumé. Good résumés present a well-rounded picture of who you are, so it's usually a good idea to submit one even if it is not asked for. Some general guidelines when developing your résumé include the following:

1. Make it readable, attractive, grammatically correct, and to the point.
2. Do not use gender bias words or phrases.
3. Do not be overly concerned about length. There has been a tendency in recent years to keep résumés under two pages. I don't agree. Whatever you decide the length of your résumé needs to be, make sure it is not hard on the eyes of the reader.
4. Do not make the résumé too wordy or too chaotic.
5. Tailor your résumé to the requirements of the program or job being pursued.
6. Do not add detail that could have you eliminated from the selection process. For instance, sometimes individuals include a career goal that is at odds with the goals of the program or the job at hand.
7. Do not sell yourself short. For example, I have seen many individuals not list jobs they have had because they were not in the human services field. Don't forget that all experience is good experience and that jobs have transferrable skills.
8. Brag about yourself, but don't sound narcissistic.

For a more detailed look at résumés, get a good book on résumé writing, such as *Amazing Résumés* (Bright & Earl, 2009) or *Best Résumés for College Students and New Grads* (Kursmark, 2001). In addition, today, there are some great Web sites to help you build a terrific résumé.

THE PORTFOLIO

In addition to a résumé, a portfolio may increase your chances of being admitted to graduate school or obtaining a job (Cobia, 2005). Portfolios include materials that demonstrate the ability of the student/professional and may include such items as a résumé, transcripts or videos of the applicant's work with clients (clients' identities are hidden), supervisor's assessment of the applicant's work, a paper that highlights the applicant's view of human nature, examples of how to build a multicultural work environment, a statement about the applicant's approach to working with clients, a major paper, and more. Although portfolios have, in the past, been a "paper" project, today's portfolios are often placed on a CD or online (Willis & Wilkie, 2009).

FINDING A JOB/LOCATING A GRADUATE PROGRAM

You're ready to find a job or apply to a program. So where do you look? There are some specific ways to increase your chances of obtaining your dream job and places you can contact to find the graduate program of your choice. The following section provides some resources to help you find a job or apply to graduate school.

Finding a Job

There are a number of things you can do to increase your chances of finding a job. Some of these include networking, going on informational interviews, responding to ads in professional publications, interviewing at national conferences, using the services of college and university job placement services, and more.

Networking   You've finished your training and now are ready to find a job. What do you do? Well, if you wanted to get a head start on the process, you would have joined your local, state, and national professional associations prior to finishing your training. Networking in this manner is one of the most widely used and best methods of obtaining a job. When people see you and are impressed with you, you have gained a foot in the door. And sometimes, you even get a job offered on the spot (see Afterword, Box 2)!

Going on Informational Interviews   You have your résumé and have developed a portfolio; you're networked; you look good and sound good—now what do you do? Well, you've probably identified a few different types of jobs in the human services field. Now it's time to find some people who have these jobs and go on informational interviews. These interviews will allow you to get a closer look at exactly what people do and will help you make a decision regarding whether or not you really want to pursue a particular job. In fact, sometimes people will let you shadow them on the job, and sometimes informational interviews can lead you to a specific job opening.

Responding to Ads in Professional Publications   Today, there are a number of professional publications that list jobs locally, statewide, and nationally. An active local or statewide human services association may have a job bank and may list jobs in its newsletter. The *Link*, NOHS's newsletter, periodically lists jobs, and

BOX 2	Afterword

Randy was a former student of mine who was enthusiastic about the human services field. He joined his professional associations, he worked with me on research, and he participated in professional activities whenever possible. Because Randy was so involved, he had the opportunity to co-present a workshop with me at a state professional association conference. His enthusiasm and knowledge so impressed one of the participants, that at the end of one workshop, she offered him a job—right there.

Counseling Today, ACA's monthly periodical, lists a variety of counseling-related jobs throughout the country. So does the APA newspaper, *The Monitor*. Similarly, the *Chronicle of Higher Education* lists jobs nationally, although many are for those with advanced degrees.

Interviewing at National Conferences Some of the larger national conferences will offer a process whereby individuals who are looking for jobs can interview with a prospective employer at the conference.

College and University Job Placement Services Job placement services and career management centers at colleges and universities will often have a listing of local community agencies that can be helpful when conducting a job search. Sometimes these placement services will have job listings and offer job fairs that are relevant for graduate students in counseling.

Other Job-Finding Methods Remember the tried-and-true methods for finding jobs—such as applying directly to an employer, responding to a newspaper ad, contacting a private or state employment agency, and placing an ad in a professional journal. These methods sometimes do work!

Locating a Graduate Program

A number of resources are available to assist potential graduate students in locating a graduate school. Some of these include the following:

- *Master's programs in social work:*
  Council on Social Work Education
  1725 Duke St., Suite 500
  Alexandria, VA 22314
  Phone: 703-683-8080
  Web site: http://www.cswe.org/Accreditation.aspx
  Related associations: Council on Social Work Education (www.cswe.org)
  National Association of Social Workers (www.naswdc.org)

- *Master's and doctoral programs in counseling:*
  Master's in school counseling, clinical mental health counseling, college counseling, substance abuse counseling, couples and family counseling
  Doctorate in counselor education and supervision

  1. *Council for Accreditation of Counseling and Related Educational Programs*
  1001 North Fairfax Street, Suite 510
  Alexandria, VA 22314
  Phone: 703-535-5990
  Web site: www.cacrep.org
  Related association: American Counseling Association (www.counseling.org)

2. *Counselor Preparation: Programs, Faculty, Trends* (13th. ed.) (2011).

Authors: Schweiger, W. K., Henderson, D. A., McCaskill, K., Clawson, T. W., & Collins, D. R.

Routledge, c/o Taylor & Francis, Inc.

7625 Empire Drive

Florence, KY 41042-2919

Phone: 800-634-7064

Web site: http://www.routledge.com/

E-mail: orders@taylorandfrancis.com

- *Doctoral programs in counseling and clinical psychology:*

  American Psychological Association (APA)

  750 First Street NE

  Washington, DC 20002

  Graduate and Postdoctoral Education

  Phone: 202-336-5979

  Web site: www.apa.org/education/grad/index.aspx

  Related association: American Psychological Association (www.apa.org)

- *Master's programs in rehabilitation counseling:*

  National Council on Rehabilitation Education

  Dr. Charles Arokiasamy, Chief Operating Officer

  California State University, Fresno

  5005 N. Maple Ave, M/S ED 3

  Fresno, CA 93740

  Phone: 559-906-0787

  E-mail: charlesa@csufresno.edu

  Web site: www.rehabeducators.org/directory.html

  Related associations: American Rehabilitation Counseling Association (www.arcaweb.org)

  National Rehabilitation Counseling Association (http://nrca-net.org)

- *Master's programs in marriage and family therapy:*

  Commission on Accreditation for Marriage and Family Therapy Education

  112 South Alfred Street

  Alexandria, VA 22314-3061

  Phone: 703-838-9808

  Web site: www.aamft.org (click "Education and Training" and "Accreditation")

  Related association: American Association for Marriage and Family Therapy (www.aamft.org)

- *Clinical pastoral programs:*

    Association for Clinical Pastoral Education, Inc.

    1549 Clairmont Road, Suite 103

    Decatur, GA 30033

    Phone: 404-320-1472

    Web site: www.acpe.edu

- *Master's programs in art therapy:*

    American Art Therapy Association

    225 North Fairfax Street

    Alexandria, VA 22314

    Phone: 888-290-0878

    Web site: http://www.americanarttherapyassociation.org/aata-educational
    -programs.html

    Related association: American Art Therapy Association (www.arttherapy.org)

BEING CHOSEN, BEING DENIED

Human service educators avoid saying a person is "rejected" from a program or a job, suggesting instead that the individual was denied admission or given other opportunities. Nevertheless, most people who are not admitted to their first-choice school or not offered their dream job often do feel rejected. If you are denied admission or not offered a desired job, ask for feedback about your application and/or the interview process. Although it is sometimes hard not to take a denial personally, this can be an opportunity to discover what you can do to improve your application. Once you know what was amiss, you can increase the chances of obtaining your chosen graduate program or job.

SUMMARY

This afterword began by examining job trends and potential earnings in human services, noting that there will be a steady and solid growth of jobs in the human services in the upcoming years. It then offered some potential job areas to consider when seeking employment. Next, we have suggested ways of considering whether the human services field is the correct occupational path for you. For instance, it was suggested that you assess whether you embrace the qualities of the effective human service professional listed in Chapter 1 (relationship building, empathy, genuineness, acceptance, cognitive complexity, embracing a wellness perspective, competence, and cross-cultural sensitivity). Then, it presented information on the Holland Code and gave you ways to assess whether your code "fit" the human services. Also, it provided you with a number of areas in which you might want to do a self-analysis to decide if this is the correct field for you (e.g., examining early childhood, socioeconomic issues, parents' career development, emotional problems, situational issues, developmental level, and worldview).

In considering a graduate program or in finding a job, a number of items were discussed, and it was suggested that the professional should reflect on each of these prior to deciding where to apply. Some items to address during the actual application process were then discussed. How to develop a good essay and the importance of having a portfolio were next examined. Finally, specific ways to find a job (e.g., networking, informational interviews, responding to ads in professional publications, interviewing at national conferences, placement centers, and other "tried-and-true" methods) were discussed, and this was followed by a listing of specific books and Web sites you can use to find more information about graduate schools. The afterword concluded with a short discussion on what it means to be denied a job or not be accepted to a specific graduate school.

Ethical Standards of Human Service Professionals

PREAMBLE

Human services is a profession developing in response to and in anticipation of the direction of human needs and human problems in the late twentieth century. Characterized particularly by an appreciation of human beings in all of their diversity, human services offers assistance to its clients within the context of their community and environment. Human service professionals and those who educate them, regardless of whether they are students, faculty or practitioners, promote and encourage the unique values and characteristics of human services. In so doing human service professionals and educators uphold the integrity and ethics of the profession, partake in constructive criticism of the profession, promote client and community well-being, and enhance their own professional growth.

The ethical guidelines presented are a set of standards of conduct which the human service professionals and educators consider in ethical and professional decision making. It is hoped that these guidelines will be of assistance when human service professionals and educators are challenged by difficult ethical dilemmas. Although ethical codes are not legal documents, they may be used to assist in the adjudication of issues related to ethical human service behavior.

SECTION I—STANDARDS FOR HUMAN SERVICE PROFESSIONALS

Human service professionals function in many ways and carry out many roles. They enter into professional-client relationships with individuals, families, groups, and communities who are all referred to as *clients* in these standards. Among their roles are caregiver, case manager, broker, teacher/educator, behavior changer, consultant, outreach professional, mobilizer, advocate, community planner, community change organizer, evaluator and administrator (SREB, 1969). The following standards are written with these multifaceted roles in mind.

The Human Service Professional's Responsibility to Clients

Statement 1   Human service professionals negotiate with clients the purpose, goals, and nature of the helping relationship prior to its onset as well as inform clients of the limitations of the proposed relationship.

Statement 2   Human service professionals respect the integrity and welfare of the client at all times. Each client is treated with respect, acceptance and dignity.

Statement 3   Human service professionals protect the client's right to privacy and confidentiality except when such confidentiality would cause harm to the client or others, when agency guidelines state otherwise, or under other stated conditions (e.g., local, state, or federal laws). Professionals inform clients of the limits of confidentiality prior to the onset of the helping relationship.

Statement 4   If it is suspected that danger or harm may occur to the client or to others as a result of a client's behavior, the human service professional acts in an appropriate and professional manner to protect the safety of those individuals. This may involve seeking consultation, supervision, and/or breaking the confidentiality of the relationship.

Statement 5   Human service professionals protect the integrity, safety, and security of client records. All written client information that is shared with other professionals, except in the course of professional supervision, must have the client's prior written consent.

Statement 6   Human service professionals are aware that in their relationships with clients power and status are unequal. Therefore they recognize that dual or multiple relationships may increase the risk of harm to, or exploitation of, clients, and may impair their professional judgment. However, in some communities and situations it may not be feasible to avoid social or other nonprofessional contact with clients. Human service professionals support the trust implicit in the helping relationship by avoiding dual relationships that may impair professional judgment, increase the risk of harm to clients or lead to exploitation.

Statement 7   Sexual relationships with current clients are not considered to be in the best interest of the client and are prohibited. Sexual relationships with previous clients are considered dual relationships and are addressed in Statement 6 (above).

Statement 8   The client's right to self-determination is protected by human service professionals. They recognize the client's right to receive or refuse services.

Statement 9   Human service professionals recognize and build on client strengths.

The Human Service Professional's Responsibility to the Community and Society

Statement 10   Human service professionals are aware of local, state, and federal laws. They advocate for change in regulations and statutes when such legislation conflicts with ethical guidelines and/or client rights. Where laws are harmful to individuals, groups or communities, human service professionals consider the conflict between the values of obeying the law and the values of serving people and may decide to initiate social action.

Statement 11   Human service professionals keep informed about current social issues as they affect the client and the community. They share that information with clients, groups and community as part of their work.

Statement 12   Human service professionals understand the complex interaction between individuals, their families, the communities in which they live, and society.

Statement 13   Human service professionals act as advocates in addressing unmet client and community needs. Human service professionals provide a mechanism for identifying unmet client needs, calling attention to these needs, and assisting in planning and mobilizing to advocate for those needs at the local community level.

Statement 14   Human service professionals represent their qualifications to the public accurately.

Statement 15   Human service professionals describe the effectiveness of programs, treatments, and/or techniques accurately.

Statement 16   Human service professionals advocate for the rights of all members of society, particularly those who are members of minorities and groups at which discriminatory practices have historically been directed.

Statement 17   Human service professionals provide services without discrimination or preference based on age, ethnicity, culture, race, disability, gender, religion, sexual orientation or socioeconomic status.

Statement 18   Human service professionals are knowledgeable about the cultures and communities within which they practice. They are aware of multiculturalism in society and its impact on the community as well as individuals within the community. They respect individuals and groups, their cultures and beliefs.

Statement 19   Human service professionals are aware of their own cultural backgrounds, beliefs, and values, recognizing the potential for impact on their relationships with others.

Statement 20   Human service professionals are aware of sociopolitical issues that differentially affect clients from diverse backgrounds.

Statement 21   Human service professionals seek the training, experience, education and supervision necessary to ensure their effectiveness in working with culturally diverse client populations.

The Human Service Professional's Responsibility to Colleagues

Statement 22   Human service professionals avoid duplicating another professional's helping relationship with a client. They consult with other professionals who are assisting the client in a different type of relationship when it is in the best interest of the client to do so.

Statement 23   When a human service professional has a conflict with a colleague, he or she first seeks out the colleague in an attempt to manage the problem. If necessary, the professional then seeks the assistance of supervisors, consultants or other professionals in efforts to manage the problem.

Statement 24   Human service professionals respond appropriately to unethical behavior of colleagues. Usually this means initially talking directly with the colleague and, if no resolution is forthcoming, reporting the colleague's behavior to supervisory or administrative staff and/or to the professional organization(s) to which the colleague belongs.

Statement 25   All consultations between human service professionals are kept confidential unless to do so would result in harm to clients or communities.

The Human Service Professional's Responsibility to the Profession

Statement 26   Human service professionals know the limit and scope of their professional knowledge and offer services only within their knowledge and skill base.

Statement 27   Human service professionals seek appropriate consultation and supervision to assist in decision-making when there are legal, ethical or other dilemmas.

Statement 28   Human service professionals act with integrity, honesty, genuineness, and objectivity.

Statement 29   Human service professionals promote cooperation among related disciplines (e.g., psychology, counseling, social work, nursing, family and consumer sciences, medicine, education) to foster professional growth and interests within the various fields.

Statement 30   Human service professionals promote the continuing development of their profession. They encourage membership in professional associations, support research endeavors, foster educational advancement, advocate for appropriate legislative actions, and participate in other related professional activities.

Statement 31   Human service professionals continually seek out new and effective approaches to enhance their professional abilities.

The Human Service Professional's Responsibility to Employers

Statement 32   Human service professionals adhere to commitments made to their employers.

Statement 33   Human service professionals participate in efforts to establish and maintain employment conditions which are conducive to high quality client services. They assist in evaluating the effectiveness of the agency through reliable and valid assessment measures.

Statement 34   When a conflict arises between fulfilling the responsibility to the employer and the responsibility to the client, human service professionals advise both of the conflict and work conjointly with all involved to manage the conflict.

The Human Service Professional's Responsibility to Self

Statement 35   Human service professionals strive to personify those characteristics typically associated with the profession (e.g., accountability, respect for others, genuineness, empathy, pragmatism).

Statement 36   Human service professionals foster self-awareness and personal growth in themselves. They recognize that when professionals are aware of their own values, attitudes, cultural background, and personal needs, the process of helping others is less likely to be negatively impacted by those factors.

Statement 37   Human service professionals recognize a commitment to lifelong learning and continually upgrade knowledge and skills to serve the populations better.

SECTION II—STANDARDS FOR HUMAN SERVICE EDUCATORS

Human service educators are familiar with, informed by and accountable to the standards of professional conduct put forth by their institutions of higher learning; their professional disciplines, for example, American Association of University Professors (AAUP), American Counseling Association (ACA), Academy of Criminal Justice (ACJS), American Psychological Association (APA), American Sociological Association (ASA), National Association of Social Workers (NASW), National Board of Certified Counselors (NBCC), National Education Association (NEA), and the National Organization for Human Service Education (NOHSE).

Statement 38   Human service educators uphold the principle of liberal education and embrace the essence of academic freedom, abstaining from inflicting their own personal views/morals on students, and allowing students the freedom to express their views without penalty, censure or ridicule, and to engage in critical thinking.

Statement 39   Human service educators provide students with readily available and explicit program policies and criteria regarding program goals and objectives, recruitment, admission, course requirements, evaluations, retention and dismissal in accordance with due process procedures.

Statement 40   Human service educators demonstrate high standards of scholarship in content areas and of pedagogy by staying current with developments in the field of Human Services and in teaching effectiveness, for example learning styles and teaching styles.

Statement 41   Human service educators monitor students' field experiences to ensure the quality of the placement site, supervisory experience, and learning experience towards the goals of professional identity and skill development.

Statement 42   Human service educators participate actively in the selection of required readings and use them with care, based strictly on the merits of the material's content, and present relevant information accurately, objectively and fully.

Statement 43   Human service educators, at the onset of courses: inform students if sensitive/controversial issues or experiential/affective content or process are part of the course design; ensure that students are offered opportunities to discuss in structured ways their reactions to sensitive or controversial class content; ensure that the presentation of such material is justified on pedagogical grounds directly related to the course; and, differentiate between information based on scientific data, anecdotal data, and personal opinion.

Statement 44   Human service educators develop and demonstrate culturally sensitive knowledge, awareness, and teaching methodology.

Statement 45   Human service educators demonstrate full commitment to their appointed responsibilities, and are enthusiastic about and encouraging of students' learning.

Statement 46   Human service educators model the personal attributes, values and skills of the human service professional, including but not limited to, the willingness to seek and respond to feedback from students.

Statement 47   Human service educators establish and uphold appropriate guidelines concerning self-disclosure or student-disclosure of sensitive/personal information.

Statement 48   Human service educators establish an appropriate and timely process for providing clear and objective feedback to students about their performance on relevant and established course/program academic and personal competence requirements and their suitability for the field.

Statement 49   Human service educators are aware that in their relationships with students, power and status are unequal; therefore, human service educators are responsible to clearly define and maintain ethical and professional relationships with students, and avoid conduct that is demeaning, embarrassing or exploitative of students, and to treat students fairly, equally and without discrimination.

Statement 50   Human service educators recognize and acknowledge the contributions of students to their work, for example in case material, workshops, research, publications.

Statement 51   Human service educators demonstrate professional standards of conduct in managing personal or professional differences with colleagues, for example, not disclosing such differences and/or affirming a student's negative opinion of a faculty/program.

Statement 52   Human service educators ensure that students are familiar with, informed by, and accountable to the ethical standards and policies put forth by their program/department, the course syllabus/instructor, their advisor(s), and the Ethical Standards of Human Service Professionals.

Statement 53   Human service educators are aware of all relevant curriculum standards, including those of the Council for Standards in Human Services Education (CSHSE); the Community Support Skills Standards; and state/local standards, and take them into consideration in designing the curriculum.

Statement 54   Human service educators create a learning context in which students can achieve the knowledge, skills, values and attitudes of the academic program.

Source: National Organization for Human Services (1996). Retrieved September 10, 2006, from http://www.nationalhumanservices.org/ethics.html

The Holland Codes

APPENDIX **B**

The following offers descriptions of each of the six Holland Codes. You can informally determine your Holland Code by reading their descriptions and rank ordering your first three choices from the definitions of the six codes. For instance, I am a "SIA." Your first three choices, in rank order, is your code! An even more valid way would be to have your instructor have you take one of the established interest inventories, such as the **Self-Directed Search** (Holland, 1994) or the **Strong Interest Inventory** (CPP, 2009).

Realistic

Realistic persons like to work with equipment, machines, or tools, often prefer to work outdoors, and are good with manipulating concrete physical objects. These individuals prefer to avoid social situations, artistic endeavors, or intellectual tasks. They are often practical, robust, and have good physical skills. Realistic people tend to do well in work environments that promote the use of large motor skills, athletic and/or technical skills, and places where they do not have to take on leadership roles.

Some settings in which you might find realistic individuals include filling stations, farms, machine shops, construction sites, and power plants. Some typical jobs include forester, locksmith, animal trainer, farmer, machinist, geologist, mechanical engineer, cook, bricklayer, electrician, plumber, automobile or airplane mechanic, photographer, draftsperson, machine operator, and/or surveyor.

Investigative

Investigative persons like to think abstractly, problem solve, and investigate. These individuals feel comfortable with the pursuit of knowledge and with dealing with the manipulation of ideas and symbols. They prefer scientific methodology and feel comfortable with foreign languages, reading, arithmetic, and the arts. Investigative individuals prefer to avoid social situations and see themselves as introverted.

They tend to do well in work environments that promote independence, originality, and scholarly pursuits.

Some settings in which you might find investigative individuals include research laboratories, hospitals, universities, and government-sponsored research agencies. Some typical jobs include microbiologist, biologist, dentist, physician, chemist, scientist, physicist, research psychologist, geneticist, biochemist, civil engineer, assistant to scientist, dietitian, veterinarian, nurse practitioner, geologist, researcher, mathematician, computer programmer, and/or laboratory technician.

Artistic

Artistic individuals like to express themselves creatively, usually through artistic forms such as drama, art, music, and writing. They prefer unstructured activities in which they can use their imagination and creative side. They tend to prefer work environments that allow them to express their independence, sensitivity, and emotional side. They crave originality and flexibility at the workplace.

Some settings in which you might find artistic individuals include the theater, concert halls, libraries, art or music studios, dance studios, orchestras, photography studios, newspapers, and restaurants. Some typical jobs include comedian, actor, dancer, musician, conductor, designer, artist, writer, photographer, drama and art teacher, pastry chef, editor, sculptor, and/or music teacher.

Social

Social people are nurturers, helpers, caregivers and have high concern for others. They are introspective and insightful and prefer work environments in which they can use their intuitive and caregiving skills. They tend to be responsible citizens and usually have good communication skills. They prefer work settings where there is much social interaction and where they can use their social and helping skills.

Some settings in which you might find social people are government social service agencies, counseling offices, churches, schools, mental hospitals, reaction centers, personnel offices, and hospitals. Some typical jobs include counselor, psychologist, minister, speech therapist, social worker, psychiatric aid, social science teacher, chiropractor, nurse supervisor, human service worker, political scientist, nurse, sociologist, teacher, college professor, and/or educational administrator.

Enterprising

Enterprising individuals are self-confident, adventurous, bold, and sociable. They have good persuasive skills and prefer positions of leadership. They tend to dominate conversations and enjoy work environments in which they can satisfy their need for recognition, power, and expression. They tend to be good public speakers and appear emotionally stable.

Some settings in which you might find enterprising individuals include life insurance agencies, advertising agencies, political offices, real estate offices, new and used car lots, sales offices, and in management settings. Some typical jobs include life insurance agent, realtor, politician, broker, hotel clerk, sales manager, business executive, manager of personnel, car salesperson, and/or many jobs in which there is a need for management, supervision, or administration of programs.

Conventional

Individuals of the conventional orientation are stable, controlled, conservative, and sociable. They prefer working on concrete tasks and like to follow instructions. They like routine problem-solving and working with data. They would prefer a work environment that is orderly, neat, and in which their tasks are clear and spelled out. They value the business world and clerical tasks and tend to be good at computational skills.

Some settings in which you might find conventional people include banks, business offices, accounting firms, and medical records. Some typical jobs include data entry clerk, bookkeeper, accountant, stenographer, machine duplicator, receptionist, secretary, teller, banker, tax expert, credit manager, payroll clerk, file clerk, and/or a variety of other clerical positions.

Source: Reproduced by special permission of the Publisher, Psychological Assessment Resources, Inc., 16204 North Florida Avenue, Lutz, FL 33549, from *Making Vocational Choices*, Third Edition, Copyright 1973, 1985, 1992, 1997 by Psychological Assessment Resources, Inc. All rights reserved.

UNDERSTANDING YOUR HOLLAND CODE

After discovering which of the Holland codes most represents your personality type, you can find out which corresponding job environments best match you. For instance, a person with an investigative personality would want to find investigative jobs (e.g., scientist, mathematician). Brief descriptions of each of the personality types and some jobs that fit that type can be found with the descriptions of each Holland Code listed earlier. However, there are 30,000 jobs in the United States, and the ones listed represent only a small sample of these. Examine the descriptions and the sample jobs to see if they seem to fit the way you see yourself. Keep in mind that no description will perfectly fit any person.

Often it is important to find a job that not only matches your highest personality type but has qualities of your second and third orientation also. For instance, an individual who has a fairly high social and artistic orientation might be interested in jobs related to human services and teaching as they both have a social and artistic component to them.

Holland's research supported the notion that the six personality types could be viewed on a hexagon (see Figure B.1), with those codes that are next to one another being similar and those on opposite sides being different from one another. Probably, in discovering your personality codes, you have found that they are adjacent on the hexagon. This would make sense because the orientations adjacent to one another share more in common than do the types that are opposite. Similarly, most jobs do not exclusively follow one personality type but also offer some of the qualities of the orientation closest on the hexagon. If, however, you found that your highest personality types are not adjacent to one another (e.g., Conventional and Artistic), it is likely that you will have fewer job settings from which to choose. In some cases this will make your job search more difficult.

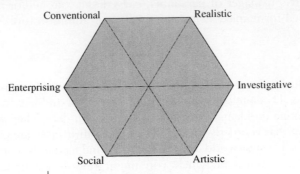

Figure B.1 | Holland Codes on Hexagon

Remember, there are approximately 30,000 jobs in this country, and, at this point, we are offering you only a small sample of the kinds of jobs that might fit your personality type. If you would like to examine other related jobs, there are a number of things you can do. First, you can go to a career counselor who, using a number of sophisticated instruments, can further the identification of your Holland personality type. Second, you can go online and visit the *Occupational Outlook Handbook* (*OOH*) (see http://www.bls.gov/oco/) or **O*NET Online** (see http://www.onetonline.org/), two government sources of occupational information. These important resources offer a listing of many jobs in the United States, and you can cross-reference the descriptions of the jobs and also see each job's Holland Code (go to "interests"). I think you will be surprised by the amount of information you will find.

Glossary

AACD *See* "American Association for Counseling and Development."

AAMFT *See* "American Association for Marriage and Family Therapy."

Ability Testing/Tests Any of a number of tests that measure an individual's cognitive capabilities. *See* "Achievement Testing" and "Aptitude Testing."

ACA *See* "American Counseling Association."

Academy of Certified Social Workers (ACSW) Established in 1960 by the "National Association of Social Workers," this association sets standards of practice in the field for master's-level social workers. Experienced social workers can hold a credential as an "ACSW." *See also* "QSCW" and "DSCW."

Acceptance Respecting people's ideals, thoughts, and emotions. One of the eight "Characteristics of the Effective Helper."

Accommodation The process of adapting new knowledge and experiences in such a way that one's understanding of the world is altered.

Accreditation The process of ensuring that programs meet minimal standards in addressing important competencies in a professional field. *See also* "Program Accreditation."

ACES *See* "Association for Counselor Education and Supervision."

Achievement Testing An "Ability Test" that measures what has been learned. Includes, *survey battery tests* that measure achievement based on what has been learned in schools; *diagnostic achievement tests* that are used to delve more deeply into areas of suspected learning problems; and *readiness tests* that are used to assess an individual's ability to move on to the next educational level.

ACSW *See* "Academy of Certified Social Workers."

Actualizing Tendency *See* "Self-actualizing Tendency."

ADA *See* "Americans with Disabilities Act."

Addams, Jane A social activist who established "Hull House" in Chicago in 1899 and who organized group discussions to help people with daily living skills. These groups are viewed as early group treatment.

Adjourning *See* "Stages of Group Development."

Adler, Alfred The developer of "Individual Psychology," sometimes called Adlerian therapy.

Adlerian Therapy *See* "Individual Psychology."

Administrative Supervision Administrative supervision is concerned with survivability of the agency and administrative supervisors focus on such things as managing costs, developing evaluation techniques, defining roles and functions of employees, encouraging or eliminating services, developing better ways of "Case Management," insisting on some forms of professional development (e.g., mandated reporting of abuse, affirmative action).

Administrator A human service worker who supervises community service programs.

Advanced Practice Registered Nurse *See* "Psychiatric-Mental Health Nurse."

Advice Giving The offering of recommendations or suggestions pertaining to a decision for a given situation. This type of response sometimes makes a client feel defensive. *See also* "Offering Alternatives" and "Information Giving."

Advocacy One aspect of social justice work in which the helper empowers the client to advocate for self and/or when the helper advocates for broader social issues which can benefit clients. *See also* "Advocacy Competencies."

Advocacy Competencies Competencies that describe advocacy in terms of three domains: the client, community, and

---

All capitalized words in quotation marks can be found alphabetically in the glossary.

public. Each of these domains is divided into two levels that include a focus on whether the helper is "acting on behalf" of the domain "or acting with" the domain. The competencies run from the microlevel (focus on client) to the macrolevel (focus on system).

Advocate A human service professional who champions and defends clients' causes and rights.

Affective/Impulsive The first stage of racism where a professional may respond impulsively and in a hostile fashion when discussing issues of diversity. Developmental theory formulated by "D'Andrea" and "Daniels." *See also* "Dualistic Rational," "Liberal," and "Principled Activist" stages.

Affirmation Expressing a positive attitude toward your client by reinforcing a client's existing way of being. *See also* "Encouragement."

Al Hajj Malik al-Shabaz The name adopted by "Malcolm X" following a pilgrimage to Mecca.

Almshouses Established by the "Poor Laws" of 1601, these were shelters for individuals who could not care for themselves.

Alternatives *See* "Offering Alternatives" and "Suggesting Alternatives."

American Association for Counseling and Development (AACD) Formerly "APGA," and currently "ACA."

American Association for Marriage and Family Therapy (AAMFT) A professional association for couple and family counselors.

American Counseling Association (ACA) The professional association for counselors.

American Personnel and Guidance Association (APGA) A professional association for counselors formed out of the "NVGA" and other associations and established in the 1950s. A forerunner of the "ACA."

American Psychiatric Association (APA) The professional association for psychiatrists.

American Psychiatric Nurses Association (APNA) The professional association for psychiatric nurses.

American Psychological Association (APA) The professional association for psychologists.

Americans with Disabilities Act **(ADA)** Enacted in 1992, ensures that qualified individuals with disabilities cannot be discriminated against in job application procedures, hiring, firing, advancement, compensation, fringe benefits, job training, and other terms, conditions, and privileges.

Anal Stage "Sigmund Freud's" second stage of psychosexual development, occurring between ages 1 and 3 years, whereby a child's emotional gratification is derived from bowel movements. *See also* "Oral Stage," "Genital Stage," "Latency Stage," "Phallic Stage," "Erogenous Zones," and "Psychosexual Stages of Development."

Analysis of Variance (ANOVA) A statistical measure that is used in quantitative research to examine differences or relationships between groups.

Analytical Psychology Developed by "Carl Jung," analytical therapists believe that early child-rearing develops a tendency to focus on one trait within each of two pairs of mental functions: sensation–intuition and thinking–feeling. They also believe we are born with an innate tendency to be extraverted or introverted. Our tendency to "become" these three traits (e.g., sensing, feeling, introverted) is called our psychological type. The complementary type (the psychological types you are not) resides in your personal unconscious and longs to be "heard." Analytical therapists also believe we all inherit an immeasurable number of primordial images called archetypes that are housed in the collective unconscious (mother archetype, father archetype, the shadow, God archetype). They provide the psyche with its tendency to perceive the world in certain ways and can sometimes interact with repressed material in the personal unconscious and cause complexes. *See also* "Psychodynamic Approaches."

ANOVA *See* "Analysis of Variance."

Antianxiety Agents One of five groups of "Psychotropic Medications." *See also* "Antidepressants," "Antipsychotics," "Mood-Stabilizing Drugs," and "Stimulants."

Antidepressants One of five groups of psychotropic medications. *See also* "Antianxiety Agents," "Antipsychotics," "Mood-Stabilizing Drugs," and "Stimulants."

Antideterministic The idea that we can change and go beyond factors that may have had an impact on our lives. Generally associated with the "Existential-Humanistic Approaches" to counseling. *See also* "Deterministic."

Antipsychotics One of five groups of psychotropic medications. *See also* "Antianxiety Agents," "Antidepressants," "Mood-Stabilizing Drugs," and "Stimulants."

APA *See* "American Psychiatric Association and the American Psychological Association."

APGA *See* "American Personnel and Guidance Association."

APNA *See* "American Psychiatric Nurses Association."

APRN *See* "Psychiatric-Mental Health Nurses."

Aptitude Testing Types of "Ability Tests" that measure what one is capable of learning. Includes *tests of intellectual and cognitive functioning* that encompass *intelligence tests* that are given one-to-one to measure general intellectual ability, *neuropsychological tests* to assess for suspected brain damage, *cognitive ability tests* given in groups to determine the potential of a student, *special aptitude tests* that focus on specific segments of ability, and *multiple aptitude tests* that measure a number of specific segments of ability as they relate to potential for success at jobs.

Aquinas, Thomas During the Middle Ages, Aquinas highlighted consciousness, self-examination, and inquiry as philosophies that dealt with the human condition.

Aristotle Has been termed the first psychologist because of his use of objectivity and reason in studying information.

Artifacts Symbols of a culture or group that can provide multiple meanings to assist in understanding the beliefs, values, and behaviors of that group. *See also* "Documents" and "Relics."

Assessment A broad array of evaluative procedures that yield information about a person. *See* "Informal Assessment," "Personality Testing," "Ability Testing," and the "Clinical Interview."

Assimilation The absorption of new information into an existing store of knowledge.

All capitalized words in quotation marks can be found alphabetically in the glossary.

Assistant to Specialist A human service professional who works closely with a highly trained professional as an aide and helper in servicing clients.

Association for Counselor Education and Supervision (ACES) Originally a division of "APGA" (now "ACA"), this organization was instrumental in originally setting standards for master's-level counseling programs.

Augustine During the Middle Ages, Augustine highlighted consciousness, self-examination, and inquiry as philosophies that dealt with the human condition.

Autonomy versus Shame and Doubt (Ages 1–3 Years) "Erik Erikson's" second stage of psychosocial development where the child begins to gain control over his or her body and explore the environment. Significant caretakers either promote or thwart autonomy during this stage. This stage's virtue is "will." *See also* "Virtue."

Bandura, Albert Behavioral researcher who was the originator of "Social Learning" theory, sometimes called "Modeling." Through his research, he showed that people have the capacity to repeat behaviors that we have observed—even at a much later time.

Beck, Aaron "Tim." Individual who developed "Cognitive Therapy."

Behavior Changer A human service professional who uses intervention strategies and counseling skills to facilitate client change.

Behavior Therapy Behaviorists believe that "Classical Conditioning," "Operant Conditioning," and "Social Learning" (or "Modeling") are all ways that a person can develop a specific personality style. By carefully analyzing how behaviors are conditioned, they suggest that helpers can develop behavioral techniques to eliminate undesirable behaviors. Some of the many techniques they use include positive reinforcement, extinction, systematic desensitization, relaxation exercises, assertiveness training, modeling, and the token economy. Well-known theorists and behavior therapists include "B. F. Skinner," "Ivan Pavlov," "John Watson," "Joseph Wolpe," and "Albert Bandura."

Belenky, Mary Field Formulated a theory of women's development of self called *Women's Way of Knowing.*

Berg, Insoo Kim One of the founders of "Solution-Focused Brief Therapy."

Binet, Alfred Developed the first individual intelligence test.

Bisexual A person who is attracted to men and to women.

Blank Slate *See* "Tabula Rasa."

Block Grants Federal funding to states that allows the state to decide which programs to fund.

Board-Certified Physician A certification that signifies a physician has met rigid requirements in one or more of a number of specialty areas.

Boundaries Barriers that mediate information flow into and out of a system. *See also* "Permeable Boundaries," "Rigid Boundaries," and "Semipermeable Boundaries."

Bracket In "Qualitative Research" the process researchers use to prevent their biases from affecting their conclusions and being able to stay open to differing opinions about the information received.

Brief Approaches to Counseling Any of a number of short-term approaches to helping that involves working on very focused problems and aims for practical change to relieve problems.

Broker A human service professional who helps clients find and use services.

Caregiver A human service professional who offers direct support, encouragement, and hope to clients.

Carkhuff, Robert Developed a 5 point scale to measure the ability to make an empathic response. *Level 3* responses are seen as accurately reflecting the client's affect and content. Responses below *Level 3* are seen as detracting, while responses above *Level 3* are seen as additive.

Carkhuff Scale *See* "Carkhuff, Robert."

Case Management The overall process involved in maintaining the optimal functioning of clients. Includes (1) treatment planning, (2) diagnosis, (3) monitoring medication, (4) case report writing, (5) managing client contact hours, (6) monitoring progress toward client goals, (7) making referrals, (8) follow-up, and (9) time management.

Case Report Writing A variety of different kinds of reports written about clients which may include, but are not

limited to, daily case notes, intake summaries, quarterly summaries, termination summaries, and reports that aid in educational and vocational planning. *See also* "SOAP Format." One aspect of the "Case Management" process.

Causal-Comparative Research A kind of quantitative research that examines intact groups instead of randomly assigning subjects to groups. Also called *Ex Post Facto* research.

Center for Credentialing and Education (CCE) The credentialing body that sets standards and develops a test for a human service professional to become a "Human Services—Board Certified Professional" (HS—BCP).

Certification Usually set by states or by national organizations, a credentialing that is more rigorous than registration but less rigorous than licensing. It often provides protection of a "title" (e.g., human service professional), but generally does not define scope of practice. *See also* "Registration," "Licensure," and "Credentialing."

Certified Family Therapist (CFT) A national certification sponsored by the "National Credentialing Academy" (NCA) open to those who have a master's in counseling or a related degree and a specialty in couples and family counseling.

Certified Rehabilitation Counselor (CRC) A credential that can be obtained by those who have obtained a master's degree in rehabilitation counseling.

Certified School Counselor A school counselor who is certified by his or her State Board of Education. Sometimes called "Licensed School Counselor." *See also* "Counselor."

Certified School Psychologist Generally, a certification that one gains after having successfully graduated from a state-approved school psychology program. Sometimes called "Licensed School Psychologist."

CFT *See* Certified Family Therapist.

Chaos *See* Integrative Approach.

Characteristics of the Effective Helper Eight characteristics important for helpers to embody if they are to be effective. They are "Acceptance," "Cognitive Complexity," "Competence," "Cross-Cultural Sensitivity,"

All capitalized words in quotation marks can be found alphabetically in the glossary.

"Empathy," "Genuineness," "Relationship Building," and "Wellness."

Charity Organization Society (COS) Arising in the United States in the 1800s, an organization of volunteers who tried to alleviate the conditions of poverty by entering the poorer districts of cities and helping the residents there.

Chickering, Arthur Formulated a theory of adult development of those who go through college.

Classical Conditioning Behavior change brought about by pairing a *conditioned stimulus* (such as the sound of a bell) with an *unconditioned stimulus* (such as the sight of food) until the conditioned stimulus alone evokes a response (such as salivation). Developed by "Ivan Pavlov," and expanded by "John Watson" and "Joseph Wolpe," among others.

Clinical Interview An assessment technique that allows the counselor to obtain an in-depth understanding of the client through an unstructured or structured interview process. See "Structured Interview," "Unstructured Interview," and "Semi-Structured Interview."

Clinical Psychologist See "Psychologist."

Closed Questions Questions that delimit the kinds of responses a client can make. See also "Questions."

Coalescence See "Integrative Approach."

Coding Process used in "Qualitative Research" to identify themes by breaking down large pieces of data into smaller parts that hold meaning with regard to the research question.

Cognitive-Behavioral Approaches A conceptual orientation that includes "Behavior Therapy," "Rational Emotive Behavior Therapy" ("REBT"), "Cognitive Therapy," "Reality Therapy," and other approaches to the helping relationship. To some degree, all of these approaches rely on learning theory and focus on the changing of behaviors and/or cognitions when assisting clients in the change process.

Cognitive-Behaviorists Theorists who believe in "Cognitive-Behavioral Approaches" to counseling.

Cognitive Complexity The ability to understand the world (and for human service professionals, to understand clients) in complex and multifaceted ways.

One of the eight "Characteristics of the Effective Helper."

Cognitive Structures Organized, mental ways of perceiving and responding to complex situations or stimulants. See also "Schemata."

Cognitive Therapy Developed by "Aaron (Tim) Beck," this approach suggests that individuals can be born with a predisposition toward certain emotional disorders that reveals itself under stressful conditions. It also proposes that genetics, biological factors, and experiences produce core beliefs that are responsible for automatic thoughts (fleeting thoughts about what we perceive and experience). Automatic thoughts result in a set of behaviors, feelings, and physiological responses. By understanding automatic thoughts and core beliefs, one can address and change them and prevent dysfunctional behaviors and distressful feelings. A number of cognitive and behavioral techniques are used to change automatic thoughts, core beliefs and their resulting dysfunctional behaviors and distressful feelings.

Collaboration Showing that you respect the client's opinion by eliciting feedback from the client about perceived progress, by hearing criticism about your skills, and by being willing to adjust the direction of the helping relationship.

Collective Perspective Clients who tend to focus more on the impact the community has on them in the helping relationship as opposed to a focus on self. See also "Individualistic Perspective."

College Counselor/Counseling A subspecialty of the counseling field. See "Counselor."

Commitment to Relativism The third stage of "William Perry's" theory of adult cognitive development, where a person maintains a relativistic outlook and commits to specific values and behaviors in his or her own life. See also "Dualism" and "Relativism."

Community Mental Health Centers Act Passed in 1963, this legislative act provided federal funds for the creation of comprehensive mental health centers across the country, which greatly changed the delivery of mental health services.

Community Planner A human service professional who designs, implements, and organizes new programs to service client needs.

Community Systems Communities, like any system, are affected by system dynamics as defined by "General Systems Theory." The effective human service professional knows how to affect change within a large system like this. Six steps for implementing change are accurately defining your problem, collaborating with community members, respecting community members, collaboratively developing strategies for change, implementing change strategies, and assessing the effectiveness of your strategies.

Compassion Fatigue/Vicarious Traumatization Syndrome The name given to the stress-related syndrome that affects mental health professionals as a result of working in a profession where one witnesses the saddest aspects of humanity.

Competence Being knowledgeable of the most recent professional research and trends and being able to apply it with clients. Having a thirst for knowledge. Knowing the limits of one's professional capabilities. One of the eight "Characteristics of the Effective Helper."

Complementary, Alternative, and Integrative Approaches Approaches that focus on nontraditional ways of healing to treat biological and mental health problems (e.g., massage, oils, rituals).

Concrete-Operational Stage "Jean Piaget's" third stage of cognitive development (ages 7–11 years) when a child starts to develop logical thinking. See also "Formal-operational Stage," "Pre-operational Stage," and "Sensorimotor Stage."

Conditions of Worth "Carl Rogers'" term for how conditions and opinions of significant others may lead to incongruity in individuals because peoples' need to be loved by significant others is so great that they act in a manner that others want them to act rather than be real or genuine.

Confidentiality The ethical guideline that stresses discretion and the knowledge of ethical, professional, and legal issues when retaining client information and knowing when confidentiality should be breached. See also "Privileged Communication."

Confrontation A counseling technique that emphasizes challenging others without being judgmental, argumentative, or aggressive. May include such

---

All capitalized words in quotation marks can be found alphabetically in the glossary.

responses as a high-level empathic response, suggesting alternatives, and pointing out discrepancies.

Congruence/Congruent *See* "Genuineness."

Conservation The notion that liquids and solids can be transformed in shape without changing their volume or mass.

Consultant A human service professional who seeks and offers knowledge and support to other professionals and meets with clients and community groups to discuss and solve problems.

Conventional Level "Lawrence Kohlberg's" second level of moral development (ages 9–18 years) when a person makes a moral decision based on peer approval or disapproval (Stage 3) or on established rules of what is right or wrong (Stage 4). *See also* "Preconventional Level" and "Postconventional Level."

Correlation Coefficient A statistics procedure where the relationships among two or more variables are examined. Correlations run, in hundredths, from 0 to minus 1 (negative correlation or inverse relationship) or from 0 to plus 1 (positive correlation or direct relationship). The closer to +1 or minus −1, the stronger the relationship.

Correlational Research The use of correlational coefficients to show the strength of the relationship between two or more sets of scores. *See also* "Simple Correlational Studies," "Predictive Correlational Studies," and "Quantitative Research."

Correlations *See* "Correlational Research."

COS *See* Charity Organization Society.

Council for Standards in Human Service Education (CSHSE) Founded in 1979, this organization focuses on education and training in the human service profession by setting national accreditation standards, helping to establish credentialing, and providing education-related materials.

Counseling Generally seen as the practice of working with a client that is short term and in the here and now and focused on surface issues, massaging personality, the conscious, moderate client revelations that can be mildly uncomfortable for the client. Contrast with "Psychotherapy."

Counseling Group Similar to a therapy group but with less self-disclosure and personality reconstruction expected; a meeting of individuals whose purpose is to effect behavior change and increase self-awareness.

Counseling Psychologist *See* "Psychologist."

Counseling Supervision An intensive, extended, and evaluative interpersonal relationship in which a senior member of a profession (1) enhances the professional skills of a junior person, (2) assures quality services to clients, and (3) provides a gatekeeping function for the profession.

Counselor An individual who has a master's degree in counseling. Includes subspecialities of school counselors, mental health counselors, college counselors, and rehabilitation counselors, among others.

Counterconditioning The process of applying new reinforcement contingencies in an effort to change behaviors.

Countertransference The process in which the helper's own issues interfere with effectively helping his or her clients. The unconscious transferring of thoughts, feelings, and attitudes onto the client.

Couple Counselor *See* "Couple and Family Counselor."

Couple and Family Counseling *See* "Couple and Family Counselors" and "Family Counseling."

Couple and Family Counselors Individuals who have a master's or doctoral degree in counseling or a related field and are specifically trained to conduct counseling with couples and families. *See also* "Family Counseling."

Covert Rules Unconscious or unspoken rules of behavior created by families that are partially responsible for the ways in which family members interact with one another. *See also* "Rules" and "Overt Rules."

CRC *See* "Certified Rehabilitation Counselor" ("CRC").

Credentialing Usually regulated by state or national legislation, a method of ensuring minimum competence in a field. Three types of credentialing are "Certification," "Licensure," and "Registration."

Crisis, Disasters, and Trauma Counseling A specialized area of training that

human service professionals will likely need to know about in the future.

Criterion-Referenced Test A test where the examinee's score is compared with the accomplishment of specific goals the examinee must attain. *See also* "Norm-Referenced Test."

Cross-Cultural Fairness In assessment, whether or not a test measures what it is supposed to measure in a consistent manner for all subgroups for which the test is given. One of the four qualities that make up "Test Worthiness."

Cross-Cultural Sensitivity Being sensitive to clients from nondominant groups and having the desire to learn about others in an effort to effectively counsel clients. One of the eight "Characteristics of the Effective Helper."

CSHSE *See* "Council for Standards in Human Service Education."

Cultural Anthropology *See* "Ethnographic Research."

Cultural Competence The gaining of the necessary attitudes, skills, and knowledge to be able to work with a wide variety of ethnically and culturally diverse clients. *See also* "Culturally Competent Helping."

Culturally Competent Helping The ability and readiness to understand the cultural identity of a client and to be cognizant of how the client's cultural heritage may impact the helping relationship. Also, understanding the unique issues of clients (individual identity), how culture impacts on them (their group identity), shared human experiences (the universal identity) and determining if a client relies more on an "Individualistic Perspective" (focus more on self) or a "Collective Perspective." *See also* "Cultural Competence."

Cultural Mosaic A society that has many diverse values and customs.

Culture The common values, habits, norms of behavior, symbols, artifacts, language, and customs that people may share.

D'Andrea, Michael with "Daniels," formulated a developmental theory that addressed "Stages of Racism of Helpers."

Daniels, Judy with "D'Andrea," formulated a developmental theory that addressed "Stages of Racism of Helpers."

All capitalized words in quotation marks can be found alphabetically in the glossary.

Data manager A human service professional who develops systems to gather facts and statistics as a means of evaluating programs.

DCSW *See* "Diplomate in Clinical Social Work."

de Shazer, Steve One of the founders of "Solution-Focused Brief Therapy."

Defense Mechanisms An unconscious mental process that allows a person to make compromises to avoid anxiety and to protect the ego. Some of the more common ones are *repression*, pushing out of awareness threatening or painful memories; *denial*, distorting reality to deny perceived threats to the person; *projection*, viewing others as having unacceptable qualities that the individual himself or herself actually has; *rationalization*, explaining away a bruised or hurt ego; and *regression*, reverting to behavior from an earlier stage of development that is a less demanding way of responding to anxiety (e.g., sucking one's thumb).

Deinstitutionalization A social change occurring in the late 1970s whereby patients who had been held against their will and were not in danger of hurting themselves or others were released from psychiatric hospitals. *See also* "Donaldson v. O'Connor."

Denial *See* "Defense Mechanisms."

Dependent Variable In true experimental research, a quantity that is measured following manipulation of the "Independent Variable"; an outcome measure.

Descriptive Statistics Used in the reporting of survey research and often includes measures of variability, measures of central tendency, percentages, and frequencies.

Deterministic The view that personality is determined early in life by such things as instincts, genetics, and early childhood development. Often associated with the psychodynamic approaches to counseling. *See also* "Antideterministic."

Developmental Model of Ethical Decision Making Models that attempt to understand the developmental level of the helper and assume that helpers who make decisions at higher levels of development come to conclusions in different and more complex ways than those who make decisions at lower levels of development. Based on such developmental researchers as "William Perry" and "Robert Kegan."

Developmental Stress Stress that is related to predicted developmental life stages in families (having your first child, puberty, etc.). *See also* "Situational Stress."

Developmental Tasks Expected milestones that all people go through as they age and are a natural, but sometimes painful, part of the life process (e.g., puberty, coupling, aging).

Diagnosis The process of classifying a client's behavior in order to treat the client more effectively. Often used in conjunction with "DSM-IV-TR"(soon to be "DSM-5"). One aspect of the "Case Management" process.

Diagnostic and Statistical Manual (DSM) Shortened term for any of the *DSM* manuals. *See also* "*DSM.*"

Diagnostic and Statistical Manual-IV (DSM-IV-TR) Developed by the "American Psychiatric Association," a manual that details the different types of mental illnesses and emotional problems. Axis I describes *Clinical Disorders and Other Conditions That May Be a Focus of Clinical Attention.* Axis II delineates *Personality Disorders and Mental Retardation.* Axis III explains *General Medical Conditions.* Axis IV describes *Psychosocial and Environmental Problems*, and Axis V offers a *Global Assessment of Functioning Scale. See also* "*Diagnostic and Statistical Manual-5.*"

Diagnostic and Statistical Manual-5 The newest diagnostic manual scheduled to be published in 2013. *See also* "*Diagnostic and Statistical Manual-IV-TR.*"

Diplomate in Clinical Social Work (DCSW) One of the most advanced national credentials an individual with a master's in social work can obtain. *See also* "ACSW" and "QCSW."

Discrepancies, Pointing Out A way of gently confronting a client by highlighting incongruence in the client's life between client's values and behaviors. *See also* "Confrontation."

Discrimination (as used in learning theory) In "Operant Conditioning," the ability of a person to respond selectively to one stimulus but not respond to a similar stimulus.

Discrimination (as used in understanding diversity issues) An active behavior that negatively affects individuals of ethnic, cultural, and racial groups.

Dix, Dorothea Fought for humane treatment of the mentally ill and helped to establish "modern" mental institutions.

Documentation The process of writing down the number of contact hours conducted with each client to ensure local, state, and federal funding regulations. One aspect of the "Case Management" process.

Documents Often used in "Ethnographic Research" and "Historical Research" documents are symbols of a culture or group that provide the researcher an understanding of the beliefs, values, and behaviors of the group. May include such things as diaries, personal letters, anecdotal record, official documents, communications, records, personnel files. *See also* "Artifacts" and "Relics."

Donaldson v. O'Connor The 1975 U.S. Supreme Court decision that stated that a person who is not dangerous to self or others could not be confined in a psychiatric hospital against his or her will. *See also* "Duty to Warn."

DSM Shortened term for *Diagnostic and Statistical Manual.* Used when referring to the current "*DSM*" being used.

DSM-IV-TR *See Diagnostic and Statistical Manual-IV-TR.*

DSM-5 *See Diagnostic and Statistical Manual-5.*

Dual Relationships The ethical guideline that stresses the importance of helpers avoiding dual relationships such as friendships and social relationships with clients when they can negatively impact upon the helping relationship.

Dualism The first stage in "William Perry's" theory of adult cognitive development, where a person views the world in terms of black or white, or right or wrong, and has little tolerance for ambiguity. *See also* "Relativism" and "Commitment to Relativism."

Dualistic Rational Stage The second stage of racism in which professionals learn to monitor their prejudices but still feel them. Developmental theory formulated by "D'Andrea" and "Daniels."

All capitalized words in quotation marks can be found alphabetically in the glossary.

See also "Affective/Impulsive," "Liberal," and "Principled Activist" stages.

Duty to Warn The ethical and sometimes legal obligation for a professional to take action if a client is in danger of harming himself or herself or someone else.

Dysfunctional Couples and Families The term used to describe families that have relational problems. Usually, such problems are the result of unfinished business that husbands and wives bring into the marriage that affects their marriage and, in turn, the family. In such families you often see blaming, boundaries that are too rigid or too permeable, and scapegoating. *See also* "Boundaries" and "Scapegoating."

EBSCO An electronic search engine that can assist when you are conducting research in education-related literature. *See also* "ERIC" and "PsychINFO."

Education for All Handicapped Children Act Enacted in 1975, a federal law that guarantees an education in the least restrictive environment to individuals with a disability who are between the ages of 3 and 21 years. This act mandates the states to fund the services. *See also* "Public Law 94-142" (PL 94-142).

Educational Resources Information Center (ERIC) An electronic search engine that can assist when you are conducting research in education-related literature. *See also* "EBSCO" and "PsychINFO."

Eclecticism *See* "Integrative Approach to Counseling."

Ego According to Freudian theory, the conscious portion of the psyche that is the mediator between the person and reality, especially in the functioning of the person's perception of and adaptation to reality. Ruled by the "Reality Principle." *See also* "Id," "Superego," and "Structures of Personality."

Ego Integrity versus Despair (Later Life) "Erik Erikson's" last stage of "Psychosocial Development" where the older person examines whether or not he or she has successfully mastered the preceding developmental tasks. Such mastery will lead to a sense of integrity, whereas lack of mastery will lead to despair. This stage's virtue is "wisdom." *See also* "Virtue."

Ellis, Albert Founder of "Rational Emotive Behavior Therapy" ("REBT").

EMDR *See* "Eye Movement Desensitization Therapy."

Empathic Response, Higher Level Gently pointing out to the client, through empathy, hidden parts of self. *See also* "Confrontation."

Empathy Originally derived from the German word *Einfühlung*, empathy has become a core counseling skill. Popularized by "Carl Rogers" and listed as one of his three core conditions of helping along with "Genuineness" ("Congruence") and "Unconditional Positive Regard," it is today viewed as the ability to understand another person's feelings and situation in the world. High-level empathic responses are seen as helping a client see hidden parts of himself or herself. One of the eight "Characteristics of the Effective Helper."

Encounter Group A group in which expressions of feelings are encouraged and which leads to new self-awareness.

Encouragement Expressing a positive attitude toward your client by reinforcing his or her ability to perform a task. *See also* "Affirmations."

ERIC *See* "Educational Resources Information Center."

Erikson, Erik Developed a humanistically based, psychosocial and developmental theory that stressed the influences of social forces. Founder of the "Psychosocial Development" model (*see* specific stages).

Erogenous Zones The psychoanalytic term used to describe places on the body from which sexual satisfaction is derived as a result of the individual's psychosexual development. *See also* "Psychosexual Stages of Development."

Esalen One of the first places to offer a variety of different types of in-depth group experiences and other humanistically oriented growth experiences.

Ethical Decision-Making Models Any of a number of models that assist a helper when faced with difficult and complex ethical decisions. *See* "Problem-solving," "Moral," and "Developmental Models."

Ethical Guidelines *See* "Ethical Standards."

Ethical Standards Codes developed by professional associations to aid the

professional in making sound ethical decisions.

Ethical Standards of Human Service Professionals Ethical guidelines adopted by "NOHS" in 1996 that reflect the unique perspective of the human service professional. *See* Appendix A.

Ethnicity When a group of people share long-term patterns of behavior that include specific cultural and social patterns such as a similar language, values, religion, foods, and artistic expressions.

Ethnocentric The potentially harmful assumption that one's view of the world is the same as his or her client's.

Ethnographic Interviews A common method used in ethnographic research which includes asking open-ended questions to ascertain information about how the interviewees construct meaning and make sense of their world.

Ethnographic Research Involves the description and understanding of human cultures through immersion within the cultures. Sometimes called *cultural anthropology*. *See* "Qualitative Research."

Evaluations Ways of determining if a program offered has been effective and what can be done to improve it (e.g., a workshop, conference, class). *See* "Formative Evaluation" and "Summative Evaluation."

Evaluator A human service professional who assesses client programs and ensures that agencies are accountable for services provided.

Ex Post Facto Research *See* "Causal-Comparative Research."

Existential-Humanistic *See* "Existential-Humanistic Approaches" and "Existential Therapy."

Existential-Humanistic Approaches A conceptual orientation that includes "Existential Therapy," "Person-Centered Counseling," "Gestalt Therapy," and other approaches to the helping relationship. Based loosely on some of the early existential philosophers and humanistic theorists, all of these approaches focus on struggles of living, how individuals construct meaning, the subjective reality of the client ("Phenomenological Approach"), and the ability of clients to change, fulfill their potential, and move toward "Self-Actualization." They all tend to deemphasize the role of the unconscious

---

All capitalized words in quotation marks can be found alphabetically in the glossary.

and focus on consciousness and/or awareness. They are more optimistic than many other approaches and all are "Antideterministic."

Existential Therapy An "Existential-Humanistic Approach" to counseling that suggests we are born into a world that has no inherent meaning, that we all struggle with the basic questions about life, and that we alone can create meaning and purpose. They believe we all have the ability to live authentically and experience fully, but sometimes avoid doing so because we are fearful of looking at our existence, including our ultimate demise, which is death or non-being. They suggest that anxiety and struggles are natural part of living and are messages about how we live and relate to others. They also believe we can choose to live meaningfully and experience a limited sense of freedom. Two well-known theorists are "Viktor Frankl" and "Rollo May." An "Anti-deterministic" approach."

Extinction In "Operant Conditioning," a principle that a behavior will cease if it is not reinforced.

Eye Contact One means of communicating nonverbally. *See also* "Nonverbal Behavior."

Eye Movement Desensitization Therapy (EMDR) An approach which has clients focus on rapid eye movements, or some other rhythmic stimulation (e.g., tapping), while imagining a traumatic or troubling event.

Family Counseling Using any of a number of advanced training techniques to help families change. May include such approaches as strategic family therapy, family therapy from a communication perspective, structural family therapy, multigenerational family therapy, experiential family therapy, psychodynamic family therapy, cognitive-behavioral family therapy, and narrative family therapy. Most human service professionals are trained to do family guidance and would refer to family therapists if family counseling is needed. *See also* "Family Guidance."

Family Counselor *See* "Couple and Family Counselor."

Family Educational Rights and Privacy Act (FERPA) This 1974 federal act grants parents the right to access their children's educational records.

Family Guidance Activities that may include knowing how to recognize when to refer clients to couple and family counselors, suggesting workshops to attend, offering reading materials regarding how families interact, and giving basic advice on family matters. *See also* "Family Counseling."

Family Therapy *See* "Family Counseling."

Federal Emergency Management Agency (FEMA) The federal agency charged with addressing crises and disasters in the United States. FEMA has developed some key principles for crisis counseling.

FEMA *See* "Federal Emergency Management Agency."

Feminist Therapy *See* "Gender-Aware Therapy."

FERPA *See* "*Family Educational Rights and Privacy Act.*"

Follow-Up The process of ensuring that clients are managing well after the helping relationships have ended. One aspect of the "Case Management" process.

Formal-Operational Stage "Jean Piaget's" fourth stage of cognitive development (ages 11–16 years), when a child can think abstractly, consider more than one aspect of a problem at one time, and understand more complex meanings. *See also* "Concrete-Operational Stage," "Preoperational Stage," and "Sensorimotor Stage."

Formative Evaluation The assessment of a program during its implementation to gain feedback about its effectiveness and to allow for change in the program as needed. Also called "Process Evaluation."

Forming *See* "Stages of Group Development."

Fowler, James Formulated a theory of faith development.

Frankl, Viktor An "Existential-Humanistic" theorist who developed one approach to "Existential Therapy."

Freedom of Information Act Enacted in 1974, this federal law allows individuals to have access to any records maintained by a federal agency that contain personal information about the individual.

Frequencies One way of reporting results in "Descriptive Statistics."

Freud, Sigmund Founder of "Psychoanalysis," the first comprehensive approach to psychotherapy. Freud developed his theory in the late 1800s after dabbling with hypnosis. He realized that many of his patients' symptoms had psychological, not physical origins. His psychosexual model of development offered one perspective on how personality is formed.

Friendly Visitors Volunteers who worked with the poor and deprived for "Charity Organization Societies." Frequently stressed moral judgment and religious values while helping these individuals.

"GAF" Scale *See* "Global Assessment of Functioning Scale."

Galt, John Minson, II Tried to employ more humane methods of treating the mentally ill in the public mental hospitals of the 1800s.

Galton, Sir Francis One of the first experimental psychologists.

Gay Usually, referring to men who have a same-sex attraction. Sometimes used to refer to lesbians. *See also* "Lesbian" and "Queer."

Gender-Aware Therapy Inclusive of *feminist therapy* and *men's issues therapy*, these approaches assume that that gender is central to the helping relationship, view problems within a societal context, encourage helpers to actively address gender injustices, encourage the development of a collaborative and equal relationship, acknowledge how language is passed down through culture and affects one's sex-role identity, and respect the client's right to choose the gender roles appropriate for himself or herself regardless of political correctness.

General Systems Theory The postulation that any living system (individual, family, community, institution, and so on) has a regulatory mechanisms that includes "Boundaries" and which develop a unique "Homeostasis" while it interacts with other systems. *See also* "Hierarchy."

Generalist The term used to describe the interdisciplinary knowledge and work of the human service professional.

Generalization In "Operant Conditioning," the tendency for stimuli that are similar to a conditioned stimulus to take

---

All capitalized words in quotation marks can be found alphabetically in the glossary.

on the power of the conditioned stimulus.

Generativity versus Stagnation (Middle/Late Adulthood) "Erik Erikson's" seventh stage of "Psychosocial Development" where the healthy adult becomes concerned about the meaningfulness of his or her life through such activities as work, volunteering, parenting, and community activities. This stage's "virtue" is "caring." *See also* "Virtue."

Genital Stage "Sigmund Freud's" fifth and final stage of psychosexual development, occurring at puberty and continuing through the lifespan, where sexual energy is focused on social activities and love relationships and where unresolved issues of earlier stages emerge. *See also* "Oral Stage," "Anal Stage," "Latency Stage," "Phallic Stage," "Erogenous Zones," and "Psychosexual Stages of Development."

Genuineness The quality of expressing one's true feelings. Being congruent or "in sync" with one's feelings, thoughts, and behaviors. Popularized by "Carl Rogers" and listed as one of his three core conditions of helping along with empathy and unconditional positive regard. One of the eight "Characteristics of the Effective Helper." Sometimes called "Congruence."

Gestalt Therapy Founded by "Fritz Perls," Gestalt therapy suggests we are born with the capacity to embrace an infinite number of personality dimensions. With the mind, body, and soul operating in unison, the individual is in a constant state of need identification and need fulfillment. However, parental dictates, social mores, and peer norms prevent a person from attaining a need and results in resistances or blockages to the experiencing of the person's needs. Needs therefore get pushed out of awareness. Because experience=awareness=reality, Gestalt therapists believe that allowing oneself to experience self enables one to understand resistances and blockages and to break free from them, live a saner life, and become whole. An "Antideterministic" approach. *See also* "Existential-Humanistic Approaches."

Gilligan, Carol Questioned some of the work of "Lawrence Kohlberg" and stated that the moral development of girls and women was different than that of boys and men in that women value connectedness and interdependence and view the relationship as primary when making moral decisions whereas men valued autonomy and independence.

Glasser, William Founder of "Reality Therapy."

GLBT An acronym that stands for gay, lesbian, bisexual, and transgender. *See also* "Gay," "Lesbian," "Bisexual," and "Transgendered."

Global Assessment of Functioning Scale ("GAF" Scale) The "fifth" axis of *DSM-IV-TR*, this scale helps clinicians assess the level of functioning of a client by rating the client from 1 to 100.

Gould, Roger Formulated a theory of adult psychological development.

Great Society The term given to the numerous social programs generated by President Lyndon Johnson.

Griggs v. Duke Power Company A Supreme Court decision asserting that tests used for hiring and advancement at work must show that they can predict job performance for all groups.

Grounded Theory A research process in which a broad research question is examined in a multitude of ways that eventually leads to the emergence of a theory. Process elements include preparing, data collection, note taking, coding, and writing. *See* "Qualitative Research."

Group Dynamics The ways in which groups interact.

Group Leadership Styles Various techniques adopted by group leaders that are based on the personality of the leader and on the stage of group development.

Group Membership Behavior Behaviors taken on by group members that are a function of the personality of the member and the stage of group development. Behaviors often mimic those in one's "real" life.

Groups Whenever individuals function together in a systematic manner, they are considered a group. All groups are affected by systems theory and can be understood by examining the dynamic interaction of its members and how that interaction results in specific communication patterns, power dynamics, hierarchies, and the system's unique homeostasis. Groups that assist in personal growth include "Self-Help Groups," "Psychoeducational Groups," and "Counseling and Therapy Groups."

Guidance Groups *See* "Psychoeducational Groups."

Hall, G. Stanley Founder of the "American Psychological Association."

Head Start Program A federally funded program, started in the 1970s, that provides an intellectually stimulating and nurturing environment to disadvantaged preschool children.

Health Insurance Portability and Accountability Act (**HIPAA**) Ensures the privacy of client records and limits sharing of such information.

Health Maintenance Organization Act Passed in 1973, this act focused on the expansion of health maintenance organizations and related programs (e.g., preferred provider organizations [PPO]; employee assistance programs [EAP]).

Heinz Dilemma, The A "Moral Dilemma" given to adolescent boys that helped "Lawrence Kohlberg" formulate his theory of moral development.

Heterosexism The conscious discrimination, denigration, or stigmatizing of a person for nonheterosexual behaviors. Preferred over the word "Homophobia."

Heuristic The process of gathering information that can be used in an investigation. Something that is researchable.

Hierarchy In systems, how the system defines who tends to be the rule makers and who tends to be in charge.

HIPAA *See* "*Health Insurance Portability and Accountability Act.*"

Hippocrates Greek philosopher who was one of the first individuals in recorded history to reflect on the human condition.

Historical Research A type of "Qualitative Research" which relies on the systematic collection of information through a literature review to describe and analyze conditions and events from the past in an effort to answer a research question.

Holland Code Six codes used to describe one's personality type that can be matched to specific jobs. The codes include: *realistic types*, who are individuals who are practical and have good physical skills; *investigative types*, who are introverted individuals interested in problem solving; *artistic types*, who are individuals who can skillfully express

---

All capitalized words in quotation marks can be found alphabetically in the glossary.

their imaginations; *social types* who are verbally skilled individuals who enjoy social situations and care for others; *enterprising types* who are persuasive people who like to lead, and *conventional types*, who are individuals who think in concrete terms and prefer clerical tasks.

Homeostasis The tendency for a system to maintain its unique equilibrium. A systems' homeostasis is not "bad" or "good." It simply is.

Homophobia The implication that there is a disorder within a person who makes that person discriminate, denigrate, or stigmatize another due to his or her sexual orientation. The word "Heterosexism" is, today, preferred by many.

HS—BCP *See* "Human Services Board Certified Practitioner."

Hull House A "Settlement House" established by "Jane Addams" in Chicago in 1899.

Human Service Professionals Persons who have earned an associate's or bachelor's degree, and less commonly a graduate degree, in human services or a closely related field and who work in a wide variety of human service agencies within the social services.

Human Services—Board Certified Practitioner (HS—BCP) This credential, developed by the "Center for Credentialing and Education" ("CCE"), can be obtained by human service professionals if they have adequate education, training, and have passed the credentialing exam.

Humanistic Approach Developed by "Carl Rogers," "Abraham Maslow," and others, this approach to counseling tends to be nondirective, facilitative, and present-centered in comparison with the more directive and past-focus approach of psychoanalysis and the more goal-oriented approach of "Cognitive-Behaviorists."

Hypothesis An assumption or a proposition that is derived from prior research and allows us to examine phenomena. *See also* "Research Question."

IAMFC *See* International Association of Marriage and Family Counselors.

Id According to Freudian theory ("Psychoanalysis"), the unconscious portion of the psyche that is the source of instinctual drives and needs. *See also*

"Ego," "Superego," "Pleasure Principle," and "Structures of Personality."

IDEA *See* "*Individuals with Disabilities Education Act.*"

Identified Patient In a family, the individual who is blamed for a behavior problem when actually the family "owns" the problem.

Identity versus Role Confusion (Adolescence) "Erik Erikson's" fifth stage of psychosocial development, in which adolescents begin to identify the temperament, values, interests, and abilities they hold. Self-understanding can lead to a strong sense of identity, whereas lack of self-understanding can lead to role confusion. This stage's "virtue" is "fidelity." *See also* "Virtue."

IEP *See* "Individual Education Plan."

Imperial Stage Stage 2 of "Robert Kegan's" constructive model of development, where a person can begin to control impulses and where needs, interests, and wishes become primary. *See also* "Incorporative Stage," "Impulsive Stage," "Interpersonal Stage," "Institutional Stage," and "Interindividual Stage."

Impulsive Stage Stage 1 of "Robert Kegan's" constructive model of development, where a person has limited control over his or her actions and acts spontaneously to have needs met. *See also* "Incorporative Stage," "Imperial Stage," "Interpersonal Stage," "Institutional Stage," and "Interindividual Stage."

Incongruity As pertains to conditions of worth, the state of being inconsistent within oneself; that is, ignoring one's true beliefs and values and adopting significant others' beliefs and values in order to gain acceptance.

Incorporative Stage Stage 0 of "Robert Kegan's" constructive model of development, where a person is self-absorbed and has no sense of being separate from the outside world. *See also* "Imperial Stage," "Impulsive Stage," "Interpersonal Stage," "Institutional Stage," and "Interindividual Stage."

Independent Variable In "True Experimental Research," the variable that is being manipulated to examine its effect on some outcome measure. *See also* "Dependent Variable."

Individual Education Plan A plan, developed by a school team, that

determines what kinds of services a child with a learning disability will receive.

Individual Perspective Clients who tend to focus on self for answers to problems as opposed to outside groups, such as the family or culture from which they come. *See also* "Collective Perspective."

Individual Psychology Developed by "Alfred Adler," individual psychology suggests that memories of early childhood experiences result in our character or personality. Believing that as children we all experience feelings of inferiority, Adler suggested that if we learn how to respond to such feelings in healthy ways, we will move toward wholeness, completion, and perfection. Feelings of inferiority, can, however, develop negative private logic, which results in compensatory behaviors that are maladaptive and/or neurotic. Although a "Psychodynamic Approach," individual psychology is seen as less "Deterministic," and more optimistic in that a person can change through education and therapy.

Individualistic Perspective Clients who tend to focus more on self in the helping relationship as opposed to a more collective or community perspective. *See also* "Collective Perspective."

***Individuals with Disabilities Education Act* (IDEA)** A federal law that ensures the rights of individuals with disabilities to receive educational services within the least restrictive environment (update of "*Public Law 94-142*").

Indivisible Self One model that views wellness as the conglomeration of five factors: creative self, coping self, social self, essential self, and physical self as well as the individual's context.

Inductive Analysis Used in qualitative data collection to determine the patterns and categories that emerge from data.

Industrial Revolution Beginning after the Civil War, this economic and social revolution resulted in individuals being drawn to urban settings and set the stage for the need for vocational guidance and is an early marker of the beginning of the counseling profession.

Industry versus Inferiority (Ages 6–12 Years) "Erik Erikson's" fourth stage of psychosocial development where the child begins to examine what he or she does well. High self-worth or feelings of inferiority can be formed in this stage.

All capitalized words in quotation marks can be found alphabetically in the glossary.

This stage's "virtue" is "competence." *See also* "Virtue."

Informal Assessment Procedures Any of a number of assessment instruments that are generally less valid and reliable but easily developed by the examiner. Some of the more common informal procedures include *rating scales, observation, classification systems* (e.g., feeling word checklists), *records and personal documents, environmental assessment* (checklist of problems in the client's environment), and *performance-based assessment* (basing a person's ability on performance rather than an "Ability Test").

Information Flow The manner in which information flows into and out of systems. Affected by "Boundaries," "Hierarchies," and system "Rules."

Information Giving The communication of factual knowledge. *See also* "Offering Alternatives" and "Advice Giving."

Informed Consent Notifying clients of and getting clients' agreement on some of the basic issues related to the helping relationship before the interview. Usually conducted during the first stage of counseling (Rapport and Trust Building).

Initiative versus Guilt (Ages 3–5 Years) "Erik Erikson's" third stage of development where the child explores the environment and gains an increased sense of independence. Caretakers either encourage or thwart exploration. This stage's "virtue" is "purpose." *See also* "Virtue."

Instincts As postulated by "Sigmund Freud," drives (e.g., sex and aggression) that are regulated as a function of parenting received in early childhood. *See also* "Psychoanalysis."

Institutional Racism When an agency or organization purposely, or out of ignorance, supports policies or behaviors that are racist.

Institutional Review Board This board is required by any institution that receives federal funds, with its purpose being to assure the ethical nature of research being conducted.

Institutional Stage Stage 4 of "Robert Kegan's" constructive model of development, where a person has separated his or her values from others' and has a

strong sense of personal autonomy and self-reliance. *See also* "Incorporative Stage," "Imperial Stage," "Impulsive Stage," "Interpersonal Stage," and "Interindividual Stage."

Integrative Approach to Counseling Formerly called "Eclecticism," an integrative approach implies that the helper has drawn his or her approach to helping from a number of different theoretical orientations. The development of an integrative approach can be seen as moving from *chaos*, in which the helper is new to the field and has no firm theory from which he or she works; to *coalescence*, where there is movement toward the adherence of one theoretical approach; to *multiplicity*, where helpers have thoroughly learned one theory and are beginning to gain knowledge and use of other theories; to *metatheory*, where the professional begins to wonder about underlying commonalties and themes among theories and begins to integrate these major themes into his or her own, unique approach.

Interindividual Stage Stage 5 of "Robert Kegan's" constructive model of development, where a person maintains a separate sense of self while accepting feedback from others in order to grow and change. *See also* "Incorporative Stage," "Imperial Sage," "Impulsive Stage," "Interpersonal Stage," and "Institutional Stage."

International Association of Marriage and Family Counselors A professional association for couple and family counselors. A division of the "American Counseling Association."

Interpersonal Stage Stage 3 in "Robert Kegan's" constructive model of development, where a person cannot separate his or her own sense of being from family, friends, or community groups. *See also* "Incorporative Stage," "Imperial Stage," "Impulsive Stage," "Institutional Stage," and "Interindividual Stage."

Intimacy versus Isolation (Early Adulthood/Adulthood) "Erik Erikson's" sixth stage of psychosocial development where, if the young adult has achieved a sense of self, he or she is ready to develop intimate relationships. Lack of self-understanding leads to isolation. This stage's "virtue" is "love." *See also* "Virtue."

Introjection Unconsciously adopting significant others' beliefs and values. "swallowing whole" others' points of view.

Joining A term that "Salvadore Minuchin" used to describe the manner in which individuals build relationships with clients. *See also* "Relationship Building."

Journal of Human Services The peer-reviewed journal of the "National Organization of Human Services."

Jung, Carl Founder of the Jungian analytical approach. *See* "Analytical Therapy."

Jungian Therapy *See* "Analytical Therapy."

Kegan, Robert An adult developmental theorist who believes that individuals can pass through as many as six stages in life: incorporative, impulsive, imperial, interpersonal, institutional, and interindividual. *See* definitions for each stage. *See also* "Subject/Object Theory."

Kitchener, Karen Examined the role of moral principles in the making of ethical decisions. Believed ethical decision making should revolve around the following principles: autonomy, nonmaleficence, beneficence, justice, fidelity, and veracity.

Kohlberg, Lawrence Examined moral development by examining how children and young adults responded to "Moral Dilemmas."

Kuhn, T. S Developed the concept of the "Paradigm Shift."

Latency Stage Sigmund Freud's fourth stage of psychosexual development, occurring between age 5 years and the onset of puberty, where the child replaces sexual feelings with socialization. *See also* "Oral Stage," "Anal stage," "Genital Stage," "Phallic Stage," "Erogenous Zones," and "Psychosexual Stages of Development."

LCSW *See* "Licensed Clinical Social Worker."

Learning Theorists Any theorist who believes that "Learning Theory" is the basis for personality development.

Learning Theory Theories that propose behaviors and/or cognitions are reinforced and become the basis for the development of personality. *See also* "Operant Conditioning," "Classical

All capitalized words in quotation marks can be found alphabetically in the glossary.

Conditioning," "Modeling (Social Learning)," and "Cognitive Theories."

Least Restrictive Environment Related to "PL 94-142" and the "IDEA" it ensures the right of a child with a disability to be given an education within the public schools in the least restrictive manner; that is, "mainstreamed" as much as possible.

Lesbian Women who have a same-sex attraction. *See also* "Queer."

Levinson, Daniel and Judy Formulated theories of male and female adult development over the lifespan.

Lewin, Kurt Developed the "National Training Laboratory" ("NTL") to examine group dynamics or the ways in which groups tend to interact.

Liberal Stage The third stage of racism where professionals can understand different viewpoints when working with clients from nondominant cultures. Developmental theory formulated by "D'Andrea" and "Daniels." *See also* "Affective/Impulsive," "Dualistic Rational," and "Principled Activist" stages.

Licensed Clinical Social Worker (LCSW) An individual who has earned a master's degree in social work ("MSW") and has met specific state requirements to obtain licensure.

Licensed Marriage and Family Therapist (LMFT) An individual who has obtained a master's degree in couples and family counseling may be able to obtain a license in this area if the individual has met specific state requirements.

Licensed Physician An individual who has earned a medical degree and has met specific state requirements to obtain licensure as a physician.

Licensed Professional Counselor (LPC) An individual who has earned a master's degree in counseling and has met specific state requirements to obtain licensure.

Licensed Psychologist An individual who has earned a doctoral degree in clinical or counseling psychology and has met specific state requirements to obtain licensure.

Licensed School Counselor *See* "Certified School Counselor."

Licensed School Psychologist *See* "Certified School Psychologist."

Licensure This most rigorous form of credentialing is generally set by the state

and requires a minimum educational level, usually a state or national exam, and additional documentation of expertise such as evidence of posteducation supervision. Often protects the title and the scope of practice of the professional. *See also* "Certification," "Registration," and "Credentialing."

Life-Span Development Theories Models of understanding the development of the person that stress that individuals continue to grow throughout their lives. *See also* "Erik Erikson," "Stages of Psychosocial Development," "Robert Kegan," and "Subject/Object Theory."

Link, The The newsletter of the "National Organization of Human Services."

Listening Skills A counseling technique that stresses being able to hear the client and enable the establishment of a trusting, open relationship.

LMFT *See* "Licensed Marriage and Family Therapist."

Loevinger, Jane Formulated a theory of ego development and examined how individuals develop interpersonally, cognitively, and morally over the lifespan.

Logical Analysis The process used in qualitative research to understand the information collected. It involves reviewing the data, synthesizing results, and drawing conclusions and generalizations.

LPC *See* "Licensed Professional Counselor."

MAC *See* "Master Addiction Counselor."

Malcolm X A well-known African-American leader who embodied many of the characteristics of self-actualized individuals. *See* "Al Hajj Malik al-Shabaz."

Managed Health Care Includes HMOs, PPOs, and EAPs, which are designed to help contain health care costs.

Maslow, Abraham One of the founders of the field of the "Existential-Humanistic Approaches" to counseling and education. *See also* "Maslow's Hierarchy of Needs."

Maslow's Hierarchy of Needs In "Abraham Maslow's" hierarchical theory, the postulation that lower-order needs must be fulfilled before

higher-order needs; the order of needs fulfillment is (1) physiological, (2) safety, (3) love and belonging, (4) self-esteem, and (5) "self-actualization."

Master Addiction Counselor A national certification in substance abuse counseling sponsored by the "National Board for Certified Counselors" ("NBCC").

May, Rollo A leader in the "Existential-Humanistic Approach" to counseling and a person who developed one approach to "Existential Therapy."

McKinney Act Enacted in 1987, this act provides funding for services to assist the poor and homeless, including job training, literacy programs, child care, and transportation, as well as subsidized counseling.

McPheeters, Harold Received a grant for the funding of some of the first mental health programs at community colleges and thus is considered by some to be the founder of the human services field.

Mead, Margaret Made "Ethnographic Research" popular through her studies of aboriginal youth in Samoa.

Mean A statistical property referring to the average of all test scores of the group. *See also* "Measures of Central Tendency," "Median," and "Mode."

Measures of Central Tendency Those statistical concepts that provide information about the middle range of scores. *See also* "Mean," "Median," "Mode."

Measures of Variability Those statistical concepts that provide information on how much scores vary. *See also* "Standard Deviation" and "Range."

Median A statistical property referring to the middle test score, or the point where 50% of examinees score above and 50% score below. *See also* "Measures of Central Tendency," "Mean," and "Mode."

Mehrabian, Albert A researcher in the early 1970s who demonstrated that words accounted for 7% of what was being communicated, while voice intonation accounted for 38% and body language for about 55%.

Meichenbaum, Donald A "Cognitive Therapist" who believes that it is not only the behavior of the individual that

---

All capitalized words in quotation marks can be found alphabetically in the glossary.

becomes reinforced, but the ways in which the individual thinks.

Melting Pot The misnomer that various values and customs of different cultures become integrated and subsumed into the larger culture. *See* "Cultural Mosaic."

Men's Issues Therapy *See* "Gender-Aware Therapy."

Mental Health Counselor/Counseling A subspecialty in the counseling profession. *See* "Counselor."

Mental Health Study Act Passed in 1955, this act was a broadly based effort to study the diagnosis and treatment of mental illness.

Mesmer, Franz A contemporary of "Freud" who influenced him to practice hypnosis. The name from which the word *mesmerized* was derived.

Metatheory *See* "Integrative Approach."

Microaggressions Conscious or unconscious discrimination that includes brief, subtle, and common putdowns or indignities directed toward individuals from diverse cultures.

Microcounseling Skills Training A relatively quick way of training helpers in which the learning of specific basic helping skills is focused upon one at a time.

Milgram, Stanley Conducted controversial deceptive research that was one factor that eventually led to restraints on the ways research could be conducted. *See also* "Institutional Review Board."

Minority Any group of people who are being singled out because of their cultural or physical characteristics and who are being systematically oppressed by those individuals who are in a position of power. *See also* "Nondominant Group."

Minuchin, Salvadore Developed structural family therapy and highlighted the importance of understanding situational crises and developmental milestones when working with families. *See also* "Family Counseling."

Miracle Question A "Solution-Focused Brief Therapy" technique that involves asking the client how the future would look if the client's problem(s) were miraculously solved.

Mixed Methods Combining quantitative and qualitative methods of research in one's research design. *See also* "Quantitative Research" and "Qualitative Research."

Mobilizer A human service professional who organizes client and community support to provide needed services.

Mode A statistical property referring to the most frequent test score of the group. *See also* "Measures of Central Tendency," "Mean," and "Median."

Modeling The acquisition of behavior patterns through the viewing of models in social situations. As a counseling skill, the purposeful or subtle ways that the helper can demonstrate new behaviors for the client. Sometimes called "Social Learning." Developed by "Albert Bandura."

Moral Dilemmas Problems of a moral nature that have no clear-cut answers. Given to children by "Lawrence Kohlberg" that gave direction for his moral development theory. *See also* the "Heinz Dilemma."

Moral Models of Ethical Decision Making Ethical decision-making models that stress moral principles in ethical decision making, such as *principles* that can guide the helper or *virtues* the helper should consider. *See* also "Kitchener," "Principle Ethics Model," and "Virtue Ethics Model."

Motivational Interviewing A helping approach which assumes that motivation is the key to change and offers four basic principles to motivate clients: showing empathy, pointing out discrepancies, rolling with resistance, and supporting self-efficacy.

MSW Master's in Social Work.

Multiple Relationships *See* "Dual Relationships."

Narrative Therapy A "Postmodern Approach" that suggests reality is a social construction and that each person's reality is maintained through his or her narrative or language discourse. Values held by those in power are often disseminated through language and become the norms against which individuals compare themselves. Therefore, problems individuals have, including mental disorders, are seen as a function of how people compare themselves to what they have been told are the "norms" of society. Thus, individuals sometimes end up believing their lives are filled with problems that are demonstrated by the *problem-saturated stories* or *narratives* they generate. By being humble, asking respectful questions, listening to exceptions to the problem-saturated stories, and listening to more subtle positive stories, narrative therapists help clients create new, *preferred stories*. *See also* "Postmodernism" and "Social Constructionism."

NASW *See* "National Association of Social Workers."

National Association of Social Workers (NASW) The professional association for social workers.

National Board for Certified Counselors An organization that sponsors certification of counselors as "National Certified Counselors" ("NCCs") and in other specialty areas.

National Certified Counselor (NCC) Certification as a counselor that requires a master's degree and additional training and supervision.

National Credentialing Academy (NCA) The organization offers credentialing as a "Certified Family Therapist" ("CFT").

National Defense Education Act (NDEA) Passed in 1958 as a direct response to the Soviet Union's launching of *Sputnik*, the act provided funding for the expansion of counseling programs in schools in order to identify gifted students.

National Institute of Mental Health (NIMH) Created by the U.S. Congress in the late 1940s, this agency was the federal government's first real effort in confronting mental health issues and resulted in systematic research and training in the mental health field.

National Mental Health Study Act Passed in 1955, this act funded a broadly based effort to study the diagnosis and treatment of mental illness that resulted in the passage of the *"Community Mental Health Centers Act"* of 1963.

National Organization for Human Services (NOHS) Founded in 1975 as the National Organization for Human Service Education, this professional association provides a link between human service educators, practitioners, and organizations; supports the credentialing

All capitalized words in quotation marks can be found alphabetically in the glossary.

of human service professionals; provides educative materials, ethical guidelines, and workshops for human service professionals; supports creative approaches toward meeting clients' needs; and promotes the professional identity of human service professionals. The association has six regions, a journal called the *"Journal of Human Services"* (formerly, "Human Service Education"), a newsletter called *"The Link,"* a national conference, and much more.

National Organization for Human Service Education *See* "National Organization for Human Services."

National Training Laboratory (NTL) Founded in the 1940s by Kurt Lewin and other prominent theorists, this institution examines group dynamics and trains individuals to understand the special interactions that occur in groups.

National Vocational Guidance Association (NVGA) Founded in 1913 as a professional association for vocational guidance counselors, it is considered to be the forerunner of the "American Counseling Association" ("ACA").

NBCC *See* National Board for Certified Counselors.

NCA *See* National Credentialing Academy.

NCC *See* National Certified Counselor.

NDEA *See National Defense Education Act.*

Needs Assessment The process of determining and addressing needs or "gaps" between current conditions and desired conditions and are often used to improve an existing structure, such as an organization or some aspects of a community.

Negative Reinforcement In "Operant Conditioning," any stimulus that, when removed following a response, increases the likelihood of that response.

Neo-Freudian Approaches Although still emphasizing early child-rearing, the conscious, and the unconscious, these approaches tend to focus more on psychosocial factors, relationships in the building of self, and play down the influence of instincts. They also tend to be less deterministic than the classic psychodynamic approaches. Some include "Erik Erikson's" psychosocial theory, object relation theories, relational theories, and intersubjectivity theories.

NIMH *See* "National Institute of Mental Health."

NOHS *See* "National Organization for Human Services."

NOHSE *See* "National Organization for Human Service Education."

Nondirective, Humanistic Approach Involves trusting the client's ability to develop the strategies for change in the helping process. This view is in opposition to directive counseling.

Nondominant Group A term used instead of the word *minority* due to negative conations sometimes associated with that word. *See* "Minority."

Nonstandardized Assessment Procedures that are not necessarily given under the same conditions and in the same manner at each administration. *See also* "Standardized Assessment."

Nonverbal Behavior Communication that is not verbal, such as through one's posture, tone of voice, eye contact, personal space, and touch.

Norming *See* "Stages of Group Development."

Norm-Referenced Test Assessment instruments in which examinees' scores can be compared to those of their peer or norm group. *See also* "Criterion-Referenced Test."

NTL *See* "National Training Laboratory."

NVGA *See* "National Vocational Guidance Association."

Observation In qualitative research, this is an examination of a situation that uses descriptive information gathering. In assessment, it is an informal assessment procedure in which a professional, significant other, or client observes a targeted behavior.

Occupational Outlook Handbook (OOH) Published by the federal government, a sourcebook on occupations that includes future outlook, nature of the work, type of training needed, and expected wages and employment conditions.

Offering Alternatives A response that suggests to the client that there may be a number of ways to tackle the problem and suggests a variety of alternatives from which the client can choose. *See also* "Information Giving" and "Advice Giving."

O*NET Online Developed by the United States Department of Labor, this online resource offers comprehensive information on close to 1,000 occupations, including information on worker characteristics, worker requirements, experience requirements, occupational requirements, workforce characteristics, and occupation-specific information.

OOH *See* "Occupational Outlook Handbook."

Open Questions Questions that allow for a wide variety of responses. *See also* "Questions."

Operant Conditioning The shaping of behavior, which is brought about through the use of positive reinforcement and/or negative reinforcement. Developed by "B. F. Skinner."

Operationalize To take an abstract construct (e.g., empathy) and develop a means to define, measure, and quantify it.

Oral Histories In "Qualitative Research," an interview with an individual who has participated in the event or observed the event in question.

Oral Stage "Sigmund Freud's" first stage of psychosexual development, occurring between birth and age 1, in which a child's emotional gratification is derived from intake of food, by sucking, and later by biting. *See also* "Anal Stage," "Genital Stage," "Latency Stage," "Phallic Stage," "Erogenous Zones," and "Psychosexual Stages of Development."

Organizational Systems Organizational systems, such as agencies, follow the basic tenets of "General Systems Theory." Thus, issues related to "Boundaries," "Rules," "Hierarchy," and "Homeostasis" all play a role in the system dynamics. Human service professionals need to know how to work effectively within such systems.

Outcome Evaluation *See* "Summative Evaluation."

Outreach Worker A human service professional who may go out into the community to work with clients.

Overt Rules Clearly defined rules made by families that affect how members of the family interact with one another. *See also* "Covert Rules."

Paradigm Shift The concept that knowledge builds on itself, that new discoveries are based on past

All capitalized words in quotation marks can be found alphabetically in the glossary.

knowledge, and that when current knowledge no longer explains the way things work, a new view of understanding the world is in order. Popularized by T. S. "Kuhn."

Parsons, Frank Founder of vocational guidance and an important figure in the subsequent development of the counseling profession.

Participant Observers Research in which information is gathered by a researcher who joins or lives with a group, interacts with its members, and takes notes about their interactions.

Pause Time The amount of silence between statements made during an interview; may be adjusted to meet the expectations of people from different cultures.

Pavlov, Ivan Behavioral researcher who was the originator of "Classical Conditioning" through his research which showed that a hungry dog that salivated when shown food would learn to salivate to a tone if that tone were repeatedly paired or associated with the food.

Percentages One way of reporting results in "Descriptive Statistics."

Performing *See* "Stages of Group Development."

Perls, Fritz An "Existential-Humanistic" theorist who developed Gestalt therapy.

Permeable Boundaries When boundaries in a system allow information to come in and be "digested" or analyzed, and then that information is allowed to adjust the system in a healthy manner. *See also* "Rigid Boundaries" and "Semipermeable Boundaries."

Perry, William An adult development theorist who emphasized the learning process and cognitive development of college students. *See also* "Dualism," "Relativism," and "Commitment to Relativism."

Person-Centered Counseling Developed by "Carl Rogers" and part of the "Existential-Humanistic Approach" to counseling, this approach suggests we all have an actualizing tendency to reach our full potential. This tendency, however, can be thwarted by an individual's desire to be regarded by significant others, who, will sometimes place conditions of worth on the individual. Such

conditions result in an incongruent self. Person-centered helpers suggest that the way to facilitate change is by the helper exhibiting empathy, unconditional positive regard, and congruence (genuineness). An "Antideterministic" approach. *See also* "Existential-Humanistic Approaches."

Personal Space One means of communicating nonverbally. *See also* "Nonverbal Behavior."

Personality Assessment Tests that assess the affective realm. Personality assessment includes *objective personality tests*, which measure aspects of personality through some kind of forced choice method (e.g., true/false questions); *projective testing*, which assesses personality by having individuals respond to unstructured stimuli and then making interpretations about their responses (e.g., "inkblots"); and *interest inventories*, which assess an individual's likes and dislikes related to the world of work. Interest inventories are used exclusively for career counseling.

Phallic Stage "Sigmund Freud's" third stage of psychosexual development, occurring between ages 3 and 5 years, when the child becomes aware of his or her and the opposite sex's genitals and receives pleasure from self-stimulation. *See also* "Oral Stage," "Anal Stage," "Latency Stage," "Genital Stage," "Erogenous Zones," and "Psychosexual Stages of Development."

Piaget, Jean A cognitive developmental theorist who examined child development. *See also*, the "Sensorimotor," "Preoperational," "Concrete-Operational," and "Formal-Operational" stages of development.

PL 94–142 *See* "Public Law 94–142."

Plato An early Greek philosopher who considered problems of the human condition to have physical, moral, and spiritual origins.

Pleasure Principle The principle by which the "Id" functions.

Poor Laws Established by the English government in 1601, this was one of the first attempts at legislating aid for the poor. In many ways, the American system of social welfare was modeled after the Poor Laws.

Positive Psychology A number of approaches, such as "Well-Being

Therapy," which assume that humans are capable of good and bad but it is important to focus mostly on the positive aspects of self.

Positive Regard A trait humanists consider necessary for creating a nurturing environment. *See also* "Acceptance."

Positive Reinforcement In "Operant Conditioning," any stimulus that, when presented following a response, increases the likelihood of that response.

Postconventional Level "Lawrence Kohlberg's" third level of moral development (age 14 years and older) when a person makes a moral decision based on acceptance of a social contract that is related to democratically recognized universal truths (Stage 5), or individual conscience based on universal principles and moral values that are not necessarily held by others (Stage 6). *See also* "Conventional Level" and "Preconventional level."

Postmodern Approaches A conceptual orientation that includes "Narrative Therapy," "Solution-Focused Brief Therapy," "Gender-Aware Therapy," and other approaches to the helping relationship. Based on the philosophies of postmodernism and social constructionism, postmodern approaches question many assumptions about what is "truth" and believe that language usage propagates beliefs that people end up viewing as truth. These approaches question many of the assumptions of other therapies, such as the belief that certain "diagnoses" or "intrinsic" problems exist. Instead, they believe clients develop problems due to the rules and language developed by those who are in powerful position (e.g., the aristocracy, the wealthy, those in positions of power). The purpose of these approaches is to help clients see how they have become a prisoner to the language and rules used in society and to help them use new language and find new solutions to their problems. *See also* "Postmodernism" and "Social Constructionism."

Postmodernism Postmodernism questions many of the basic assumptions taken for granted as a result empiricism and the scientific method and suggests there is no one way to understand the world, no foundational set of rules to make sense of who we are, and no one way of understanding a person. These

---

All capitalized words in quotation marks can be found alphabetically in the glossary.

individuals question "truth" and question many of the basic tenets of popular therapies that suggest certain structures cause mental health problems (e.g., "Id," "Ego," "Superego," "Self-Actualization" tendency, and core beliefs).

Postmodernists In this context, individuals like "Michael White" and David Epston who believe in "Postmodernism" and have developed "Postmodern Approaches" to counseling.

Posture One means of communicating nonverbally. *See also* "Nonverbal Behavior."

Power Differentials Differing degrees of control, authority, or influence over others which can be real or perceived and are a function of such things as race, class, gender, occupation. socioeconomic status, or a host of other factors.

Practicality The usefulness of a test, considering such factors as cost, length, ease of administration, and ease of interpretation. One of the four qualities that make up "Test Worthiness."

Preconventional Level "Lawrence Kohlberg's" first level of moral development (ages 2–9) when a person makes a moral decision based on perceived power others hold and the desire to avoid punishment (Stage 1), or the egocentric desire to satisfy one's own need to gain personal rewards (Stage 2). *See also* "Conventional Level," and "Postconventional Level."

Predictive Correlational Studies When statistical relationships are used to predict scores on one variable to scores on one or more other variables. *See also* "Simple Correlational Studies."

Prejudice Judging a person or a group based on preconceived notions about the group.

Preoperational Stage "Jean Piaget's" second stage of cognitive development (ages 2–7 years) when a child develops language ability and can maintain mental images. A child in this stage responds intuitively rather than act in a manner that might seem to be logically correct. *See also* "Concrete-operational Stage," "Formal-operational stage," and "Sensorimotor stage."

Primary Prevention Concentrating on the prevention of emotional problems and promoting a wellness outlook.

See also "Secondary Prevention" and "Tertiary prevention."

Primary Sources Using original records, as opposed to secondary sources, in collecting data for research. Particularly important in "Historical Research."

Principle Ethics Model Any of a number of models that suggest ethical decision making should revolve around moral principles. *See* "Kitchener" and *see* "Moral Models of Ethical Decision Making."

Principled Activist The fourth stage of racism where the professional can understand and accept that all people hold varying values and beliefs. In this stage, the helper is ready to embrace social justice actions. Developmental theory formulated by "D'Andrea" and "Daniels." *See also* "Affective/Impulsive," "Dualistic Rational," and "Liberal" stages.

Privileged Communication As determined by the state, the legal right of a professional (lawyer, priest, physician, or licensed therapist) to not reveal information about a client.

Probability Level The statistical level set to determine significance between groups and whether or not the results could be found by chance alone. For instance, much research will set its probability at the .05 level ($p < 0.5$), which means that the likelihood that the results happened by chance is less than 5 out of 100.

Problem-Solving Models Models that provide the helper with a step-by-step, practical, approach to ethical decision making that are useful for the beginning clinician.

Process Evaluation *See* "Formative Evaluation."

Professional Disclosure Statement A written statement, given to the client, describing such issues as the limits of confidentiality, the length of the interview, the helper's credentials, the limits of the relationship, the helper's theoretical orientation, legal concerns, fees for service, and agency rules that might affect the client. Usually given in the first stage of counseling (Rapport and Trust Building Stage).

Program Accreditation As set by the "Council for Standards in Human Service Education" ("CSHSE"), program

accreditation acknowledges that human service programs have met minimal standards in the training of human service professionals.

Program Evaluation Assessing a program to determine if it has achieved its goals and objectives and has worth and value.

Projection *See* "Defense Mechanisms."

"Psy.D." *See* "Psychologist."

Psychiatric-Mental Health Nurse A nurse who has received specialized training as a mental health professional. The advanced psychiatric-mental health nurse is called an Advanced Practice Registered Nurse (APRN).

Psychiatrist A physician who generally has completed a residency in psychiatry— that is, has completed extensive training in some kind of mental health setting.

PsycINFO An electronic search engine used to review psychology-related literature. *See also* "ERIC" and "EBSCO."

Psychoanalysis Developed by "Freud," the belief that instincts (e.g., hunger, thirst, survival, aggression, and sex) are strong motivators of behavior and satisfying them is mostly an unconscious process. "Defense Mechanisms" (e.g., rationalizing, repression) are developed to manage instincts. Early child-rearing practices, as applied through the oral, anal, and phallic psychosexual stages in the first six years of life, are responsible for how defenses are developed and result in normal or abnormal personality development. Effects of early childhood practices are observed in adolescence and adulthood in what are called the latency and genital psychosexual stages. A Deterministic approach. *See also* "Psychodynamic Approaches."

Psychodynamic Approaches A conceptual orientation that includes "Psychoanalysis," "Analytical Therapy" ("Jungian Therapy"), "Individual Therapy" ("Adlerian Therapy"), and other approaches to the helping relationship. To some degree, all suggest an unconscious and a conscious effect of the functioning of the person in some deeply personal and dynamic ways, all look at early child-rearing practices as important in the development of personality, and all believe that the past and the dynamic interaction of the past with

---

All capitalized words in quotation marks can be found alphabetically in the glossary.

conscious and unconscious factors are important in the therapeutic process.

Psychoeducational Groups Groups that are focused on educating participants to prevent future problems. Formerly called guidance groups, but changed due to the negative connotation of the word *guidance.*

Psychologist Generally, a person who holds a doctoral degree in counseling psychology, clinical psychology, or a "Psy.D."; has completed an internship at a mental health facility; and has passed specific state requirements to obtain licensure as a "Psychologist."

Psychosexual Stages of Development As posited by "Sigmund Freud," stages of development that affect the emerging personality as a function of developing erogenous zones. *See also* "Oral Stage," "Anal Stage," "Phallic Stage," "Latency Stage," "Genital Stage," Erogenous Zones," and "Psychoanalysis."

Psychosocial Development The notion, posited by "Erik Erikson," that social forces impact the development of our psyche and that different psychosocial forces affect us at varying periods in our lives.

Psychosocial Forces The notion that social forces affect the development of our psyche (e.g., parenting, peer relationships, work relationships).

Psychotherapist Although generally not licensed by states, on a practical level, a person who has an advanced degree in psychology, social work, or counseling and who works in a mental health setting or in private practice, providing individual, marital, or group counseling.

Psychotherapy Generally seen as the practice of working long-term with a client in the "there and then" and focusing on life stories, deep-seated issues, personality reconstruction, the unconscious, deep client revelations, which can be painful for the client. Contrast with "Counseling."

Psychotropic Medications Medications that affect psychological functioning, which are often classified into five groups: "Antianxiety Agents," "Antidepressants," "Antipsychotics," "Mood-Stabilizing Drugs," and "Stimulants."

Public Law 94–142 (PL 94–142) The *"Education for All Handicapped Children Act"* which ensures the right to an

education within the least restrictive environment for individuals between the ages of 3 and 21 who have a disability. *See also "Individuals with Disabilities Education Act* (IDEA)."

Punishment In "Operant Conditioning," applying an aversive stimulus following a behavior in an effort to decrease a specific behavior. This method of changing behavior is not particularly effective as it can lead to undesirable side effects (e.g., counteraggression).

QCSW *See* "Qualified Clinical Social Worker."

Qualified Clinical Social Worker (QCSW) A credential that implies more experience than the ACSW but less than the QCSW. *See also* "ACSW" and "DCSW."

Qualitative Research Research in which there are multiple ways of viewing knowledge and that one can make sense of the world by immersing oneself in the research situation in an attempt to provide possible explanations for the problem being examined. *See* "Grounded Theory," "Ethnographic Research," and "Historical Research."

Quantitative Research Research that assumes that there is an objective reality within which research questions can be formulated and scientific methods used to measure the probability that certain behaviors, values, or beliefs either cause or are related to other behaviors, values, or beliefs. *See* "True Experimental Research," "Causal-Comparative (Ex Post Facto) Research," "Correlational Research," and "Survey Research."

Queer Traditionally seen as a derogatory word to describe gays and lesbians, in recent years this word has been embraced by the "GLBT" community as a means of regaining power and not buying into existing ways of seeing the world.

Questions A counseling skill used to uncover patterns, gather information quickly, induce self-exploration, challenge the client to change, or move a client along quickly to preferred goals. *See* "Closed Questions," "Open Questions," "Solution-Focused Questions," "Tentative Questions," and "'Why' Questions."

Race Traditionally, a division of people who share common genetic and biological characteristics. With gene pools

having been mixed for a variety of reasons over the centuries, and with recent genetic research showing that genetic differences between any two people is extremely small, the concept of races has been challenged in recent years.

Racism The belief that one race is superior to another.

Random Assignment Assigning subjects to various treatment groups in a randomized fashion. *See also* "True Experimental Research."

Range A statistical property referring to the spread of test scores from highest to lowest for the group. *See also* "Measures of Variability" and "Standard Deviation."

Rational Emotive Behavior Therapy Developed by "Albert Ellis," REBT suggests we are born with the potential for rational or irrational thinking, and it is the belief about an event that is responsible for one's reaction to the event. Thus, an *Activating* event (A) precedes the *Beliefs* about the event, and it is the beliefs that result in the Consequences or the feelings and behaviors that follow (A → B → C). Irrational beliefs (iB) result in negative feelings and behaviors and rational beliefs (rB) result in appropriate and reasonable feelings and behaviors. Ellis offers three core irrational beliefs that many people buy into. Helpers assist clients in *Disputing* irrational beliefs by changing their thoughts and by having them practice new behaviors. *See also* "Cognitive-Behavioral Approaches."

Rationalization *See* "Defense Mechanisms."

Reality Principle The principle by which the "Ego" is ruled.

Reality Therapy Developed by "William Glasser," reality therapy suggests we are born with five needs: survival, love and belonging, power, freedom, and fun—which can be satisfied only in the present. Reality therapists believe we have a quality world that contains pictures in our mind of the people, things, and beliefs most important to meeting our needs. We make choices based on these pictures, although we can only choose actions and thoughts; feelings and our physiology result from those choices. Language we use reflects the kinds of choices we have made. At any point in one's life, one can evaluate one's

---

All capitalized words in quotation marks can be found alphabetically in the glossary.

behaviors, thoughts, feelings, and physiology, and make new choices by acting and thinking differently and using more positive language. Although a "Cognitive-Behavioral Approach," it also has "Existential-Humanistic."

Reductionistic The idea, proposed by early learning theorists, that the development of personality can be reduced to behavioral contingencies, such as "Positive Reinforcement" and "Negative Reinforcement."

Referral The process and reason for having your client see another helper or professional. Involves discussing the referral with the client, obtaining permission for the referral, monitoring the client's progress with the referral, and ensuring "Confidentiality." One aspect of the "Case Management" process.

Registration The least vigorous type of credentialing. See also "Certification," "Licensure," and "Credentialing."

Regression See "Defense Mechanisms."

Rehabilitation Act Enacted in 1973, this law ensured access to vocational rehabilitation for adults, based on three conditions: a severe physical or mental disability, a disability that interferes with obtaining or maintaining a job, and employment that is feasible.

Rehabilitation Counselor/Counseling A subspecialty in the counseling field. See "Counselor."

Relationship Building The idea that it is critical to find some mechanism that allows one to build effective relationships with clients. Relationships are formed in many different ways, depending on the personality of the helper. One of the eight "Characteristics of the Effective Helper." Closely related to what some have called the "Working Alliance."

Relativism The second stage in "William Perry's" theory of adult cognitive development, where a person thinks abstractly, allows for differing opinions, is empathic, is sensitive to context, and understands there are many ways to view the world. See also "Dualism" and "Commitment to Relativism."

Reliability The consistency of test scores; a measure of the accuracy of a test. Some of the more common types of reliability are *internal consistency*, *split-half reliability*, *parallel forms reliability*, and *test–retest reliability*. One of the

four qualities that make up "Test Worthiness."

Relics Often used in "Historical Research," any of a variety of objects that can provide evidence about the past event in question. See also "Documents" and "Artifacts."

Religion Organized or unified set of practices and beliefs that have moral underpinnings and define a group's way of understanding the world. See also "Spirituality."

Repression See "Defense Mechanisms."

Research Question Based on prior research and theory, a question that is developed to examine a particular problem. See also "Hypothesis."

RESPECTFUL Model Developed by "D'Andrea," and "Daniels" an acronym that speaks to the ingredients needed by the culturally competent mental health professional. Includes understanding religion, economic class, sexual identity, psychological development, ethnicity, chronological disposition, trauma, family history, unique physical traits, and language.

Review of the Literature A thorough examination of major research done in a particular area, found from books, journal articles, and computerized abstracts.

Richmond, Mary Developed one of the first social work training programs.

Rigid Boundaries When "Boundaries" are so inflexible that they do not allow much information into families or out of families. Often see in families where abuse has taken place and in which there are secrets. See also "Permeable Boundaries" and "Semipermeable Boundaries."

Rogers, Carl One of the founders of the field of humanistic counseling and education as well as the person who developed "Person-Centered Counseling." Proponent of the importance of "Empathy," "Congruence" ("Genuineness"), and "Unconditional Positive Regard" in the helping relationship. Also was one of the first to develop group counseling techniques which became the forerunner of the "*Encounter Group*" movement. See also "Humanistic Approach."

Rule Makers See "Hierarchy."

Rules See "Covert Rules" and "Overt Rules."

Rush, Benjamin Known for his progressive and humanistic treatment of the mentally ill in the first "modern" mental institutions.

Satir, Virginia A social worker who was instrumental in popularizing a systemic approach to counseling. Developed the communication approach to family counseling. See also "Couple and Family Counseling."

Scapegoat An individual, within a system, who is unconsciously given the blame for problems in the system.

Schedules of Reinforcement In "Operant Conditioning," the numerous ways in which a stimulus can be arranged to reinforce behavior, based on elapsed time and frequency of responses.

Schemata Organized, mental ways of perceiving and responding to complex situations or stimulants. See also "Cognitive Structures."

School Counselor A subspecialty within the counseling field. See "Counselor."

School Psychologist An individual who holds a master's degree in school psychology and has expertise in conducting testing and assessment and in assisting in the development and implementation of behavior plans for children.

SDS See "Self-Directed Search."

Secondary Prevention Focuses on the control of nonsevere mental health problems. See also "Primary Prevention" and "Tertiary prevention."

Secondary Sources Documents or verbal information obtained from sources that did not actually experience the event; used by researchers in collecting data for historical studies.

Self-Actualization The process of becoming real, true to self, and reaching one's potential. The highest need on "Maslow's Hierarchy of Needs."

Self-Actualized Person "Abraham Maslow's" term for a person who has reached "Self-Actualization." This person tends to be in touch with himself or herself, can hear feedback from others, is nondogmatic, accepting, empathic, genuine, and introspective. See "Maslow's Hierarchy of Needs."

Self-Actualizing Tendency The tendency for individuals to move toward becoming whole or to move toward

---

All capitalized words in quotation marks can be found alphabetically in the glossary.

genuineness and realness in the expression of who they are.

Self-Directed Search (SDS) A type of interest inventory that uses the "Holland Code."

Self-Disclosure When the helper reveals to the client personal information about himself or herself purposefully or unwittingly. Often intentionally used by helpers to provide a model to the client of effective ways of coping.

Self-Help Groups Sometimes called support groups, their purpose is to educate, affirm, and enhance the existing strengths of the group members.

Selye, Hans Stated that stress is a healthy response to a changing situation, but can become unhealthy if not properly dealt with by the individual.

Semipermeable Boundaries As pertains to "General Systems Theory," a framework that allows information to enter the system and be processed and incorporated. "Boundaries" that are too rigid prevent information from coming into or leaving the system. Boundaries that are too permeable do not allow the system to maintain its identity. *See also* "Rigid Boundaries" and "Permeable Boundaries."

Semi-Structured Interview A cross between an "Unstructured" and "Structured Interview."

Sensorimotor Stage Jean Piaget's first stage of cognitive development (from birth to 2 years) when the child responds only to physical and sensory experiences. *See also* "Concrete-Operational Stage," "Formal-Operational Stage," and "Preoperational Stage."

Settlement Houses Houses where individuals would go to live within a poor community to help those in need. *See* "Settlement Movement," "Jane Addams," and "Hull House."

Settlement Movement Arising in the United States in the 1800s, the attempt by social activists, while living with the poor, to change communities through community action and political activities. *See* "Settlement Houses," "Jane Addams," and "Hull House."

Sexism Discrimination, denigration, or stigmatizing of another due to his or her gender.

Sexual Prejudice Negative attitudes targeted toward homosexual, bisexual,

heterosexual, or transgendered individuals.

Shamans Individuals who have special status because of their healing and sometimes mystical powers.

Silence A skill used by the human service professional to help a client reflect on what he or she has been saying; it allows the helper to process the session and formulate his or her next response.

Simple Correlational Studies A type of correlational research that explores the relationship between two variables. *See also* "Predictive Correlational Studies."

Situational Stress In families, unexpected stress that affects the family (e.g., a job loss, natural disaster). *See also* "Developmental Stress."

Skill Standards Twelve competencies, and skills associated with them, identified in a national project as being important to the work of the human service professional. The competencies are participant empowerment; communication; assessment; community and service networking; facilitation of services; community and living skills and supports; education, training, and self-development; advocacy, vocational, educational, and career support; crisis intervention; organizational participation; and documentation.

Skinner, B. F. Behavioral researcher who was the originator of "Operant Conditioning." Through his research, he showed that animals would learn specific behaviors if the behavior just emitted was reinforced. His and other learning theories are sometimes used to explain the development of personality. *See also* "Behavior Therapy" and "Cognitive-Behavioral Approaches."

SOAP Format A popular type of case report that stands for Subjective, Objective, Assessment, and Plan.

Social Casework Having its roots in charity organization societies, the process by which the needs of a client are examined and a treatment plan is designed to facilitate client growth.

Social Class The grouping of people according to such things as wealth, ancestry, position, and the ranking and subsequent perception of an individual's worth to society based on this grouping.

Social Construction A construct developed by people in positions of power and believed by many people in society. Not necessarily "truth." *See also* "Social Constructionism."

Social Constructionism This philosophy has to do with how values are transmitted through language by the social milieu (e.g., family, culture, and society) and suggests that the person is constantly changing with the ebb and flow of the influences of significant others, culture, and society. Social constructionists generally agree that those in positions of power control the type of language that is used in cultures and society and thus individuals who are not in power (e.g., nondominant groups such as minorities and women) are at a disadvantage and may be oppressed by the power structure that prevails. Part of the basis of the "Postmodern Approaches" to counseling.

Social Constructionists Those who believe in "Social Constructionism."

Social Justice Impacting the broader system (e.g., agencies, cities, country) to affect positive change for clients. *See also* "Advocacy."

Social Learning *See* "Modeling."

Social Worker Although this person can hold a bachelor's or master's degree, in recent years the term has applied mostly to those who hold a master's degree in social work. These individuals often work with human service professionals.

Solution-Focused Brief Therapy (SFBT) Developed by "Steve de Shazer," "Insoo Kim Berg," and others, this postmodern approach suggests that problems are the result of language passed down by families, culture, and society, and dialogues between people. Pathology, for all practical purposes, is not inherently found within the person (inside the person). They suggest there is no reason to spend time looking "inside" the person or spending a lot of time looking at the past. They build collaborative relationships and have clients establish preferred goals, so they can move from a problem focus to a solution focus in as few as six sessions. One particular technique that has received widespread recognition is the "Miracle Question." *See also* "Postmodernism" and "Social Constructionism."

All capitalized words in quotation marks can be found alphabetically in the glossary.

Solution-Focused Questions Questions used to help clients quickly reach their goals. They include preferred goals questions, evaluative questions, coping questions, and solution-focused questions. Often used in brief treatment modalities. *See also* "Questions."

Southern Regional Education Board (SREB) Relative to human services, this board developed 13 roles and functions necessary for a qualified human service professional.

Spirituality Seen as residing in a person, not a group, spirituality defines the person's understanding of self, self in relationship to others, and self in relationship to a self-defined higher power or lack thereof. *See also* "Religion."

Spontaneous Recovery In "Operant Conditioning," after treatment for behavior change, the recurrence of former, unwanted behaviors.

SREB *See* Southern Regional Education Board.

Stages of Group Development The typical stages that a group progresses through in the group process, including the pregroup stage ("Forming"), initial stage ("Forming"), transition stage ("Storming" then "Norming"), work stage ("Performing"), and closure stage ("Adjourning").

Stages of the Helping Relationship A series of predictable stages that clients pass through in the helping relationship. They include rapport and trust building, problem identification, deepening understanding and goal-setting, work, and closure.

Stages of Psychosocial Development As developed by "Erik Erikson," eight stages of life-span development that affect the formation of the personality and is characterized by a specific virtue or strength (see specific stages). *See also* "Virtue."

Stages of Racism A developmental theory by "Daniels" and "D'Andrea" that suggests helpers will pass through stages of racism that include affect/impulsive, dualistic rational, liberal, and principled activist stages (see each stage).

Standard Deviation A statistical property referring to the amount, on average, that test scores vary from the mean. *See also* "Measures of Variability" and "Range."

Standard of Care As suggested by "Gilligan," the concept that relative to moral decisions, as compared to men, women tend to be more concerned about the effect their choices have on others, whereas men are more concerned about a sense of justice being maintained.

Standardized Assessment An assessment instrument that is administered in the same way every time it is given; the test results may be compared with those of a norm group. An example is the Scholastic Aptitude Test (SAT). *See also* "Nonstandardized Assessment."

Stereotypes Rigidly held beliefs about a group of people based on the false assumption that most or all members of the group have certain behaviors or beliefs that tend to be unique to that group.

Stimulants One of five groups of psychotropic medications. *See also* "Antianxiety Agents," "Antidepressants," "Antipsychotics," "Mood-Stabilizing Drugs," and "Stimulants."

Stoltenberg, Carl Formulated a theory of development as it relates to how mental health professionals learn while under supervision.

Storming *See* "Stages of Group Development."

Strength *See* "Virtue."

Stress The normal physiological and psychological response to changing situations. In moderation, it is a healthy response; however, too much stress can cause psychological and physical problems.

Strong Interest Inventory An interest inventory that examines one's likes and dislikes as well as one's personality orientation toward the world of work. The test uses the "Holland Codes," and is used in career counseling.

Structured Interview A type of clinical interview which allows the examinee to respond to a set of preestablished items verbally or in writing. *See also* "Unstructured Interview" and "Semi-Structured Interview."

Structures of Personality Collectively, the id, ego, and superego. *See also* "Id," "Ego," "Superego," and "Psychoanalysis."

Subject/Object Theory The basis for "Robert Kegan's" constructive model of development which suggests that individuals pass through specific developmental stages in constructing their unique way of making meaning of the world.

Suggesting Alternatives A means of gently confronting a client by offering new ways of viewing the world. *See also* "Confrontation."

Summative Evaluation The assessment of a program after it is completed. Also called "Summative Evaluation."

Superego According to Freudian theory ("Psychoanalysis"), the partly conscious portion of the psyche that internalizes parental and societal rules that reward or punish the individual through a system of moral attitudes, conscience, and a sense of guilt. *See also* "Id," "Ego," "Psychoanalysis," and "Structures of Personality."

Supervisee The individual whose work is being overseen by another in a supervisory relationship.

Supervision *See* "Administrative Supervision" and "Counseling Supervision."

Supervisor The individual who oversees the practice of a supervisee during supervision. A good supervisor is empathic, flexible, genuine, open, and has a strong alliance with the supervisee.

Survey Research Research where specific information is gathered from a target population using a questionnaire. *See* "Quantitative Research."

Tabula Rasa Latin phrase meaning "smoothed or erased tablet"; refers to the mind in its blank or empty state before receiving outside impressions.

Tarasoff Case The landmark case that set a precedent for the responsibility that mental health professionals have regarding confidentiality and acting to prevent a client from harming self or others.

Teacher/Educator A human service professional who tutors, mentors, and models new behavior for clients.

Tentative Questions Questions that are akin to an empathic response and are more facilitative when trying to build a relationship with a client and for client self-exploration. *See also* "Questions."

Tertiary Prevention Concentrates on the control of serious mental health problems. *See also* "Primary Prevention" and "Secondary Prevention."

All capitalized words in quotation marks can be found alphabetically in the glossary.

Test Worthiness Four qualities that, together, make up the worthiness of an assessment instrument. They are "Validity," "Reliability," "Practicality," and "Cultural Fairness."

Theory A comprehensive system of doing counseling that enables the helper to understand his or her clients, apply techniques, predict change, and evaluate results.

Therapy Group A meeting of individuals whose purpose is to effect behavior change and increase self-awareness; similar to a counseling group but with more self-disclosure and personality reconstruction expected.

Time Management The planning of activities involved in the "Case Management" process.

Tone of Voice One means of communicating nonverbally. *See also* Nonverbal Behavior.

Touch One means of communicating nonverbally. *See also* "Nonverbal Behavior."

Transference The redirection of both negative and positive feelings and desires, especially those unconsciously retained from childhood, toward a helper.

Transgendered A person who does not identify with his or her birth sex and lives in congruence with the sex to which he or she identifies.

Treatment Planning The accurate assessment of client needs that results in the formation of client goals. Is conducted through such means as a clinical interview, testing, and informal assessment techniques. One aspect of the "Case Management" process.

Triangulating In "Qualitative Research," this means to collect data in multiple ways thereby increasing the validity or trustworthiness of the information being obtained.

True Experimental Research Research in which one randomly assigns subjects to particular groups and manipulates the independent variable(s), to measure the effect of the variable(s) on the outcome. *See also* "Dependent Variable,"

"Independent Variable," and "Random Assignment."

Trust versus Mistrust (Ages Birth–1 Year) "Erik Erikson's" first stage of psychosocial development where the infant develops a sense of trust or mistrust based on the type of caretaking received. This stage's "virtue" is "hope." *See also* "Virtue."

t-test A statistical measure that is used in "Quantitative Research" to examine differences between groups.

Unconditional Positive Regard Accepting a person without strings attached. One of "Carl Rogers'" core conditions of helping along with empathy and congruence. *See also* "Acceptance."

Unconscious Proposed by early psychodynamic theorists, the idea that there is a hidden part of all individuals which motivates behavior in complex ways. The goal of many counseling approaches today is to make parts of the unconscious conscious.

Unfinished Business Unresolved problems and experiences brought from an earlier life stage that affect interpersonal relationships.

Unstructured Interview An interview which does not have a preestablished list of items or questions and client responses to helper inquiries establish the direction for follow-up questioning. *See also* "Semi-structured Interview" and "Structured Interview."

Vaillant, George. E Formulated a theory of adult development that was unique in that it spoke to how adults overcome major psychiatric illnesses.

Validity (in "Assessment") The ability of a test to measure what it is supposed to measure. Some of the more popular types of validity are *content validity, concurrent validity, predictive validity,* and *construct validity.* One of the four qualities that make up "Test Worthiness."

Validity (in "Quantitative Research") The ability to control extraneous variables when conducting research.

Variable Any quality or characteristic that can be measured. *See also* "Dependent Variable" and "Independent Variable."

View of Human Nature Describes how a person comes to understand the reasons people are motivated to do the things they do and can include such things as the impact of early-childhood, instincts, genetics, social forces, and a variety of other beliefs about personality development.

Virtue Relative to the "Stages of Psychosocial Development" of "Erik Erikson," a virtue (or "strength") is the specific age-related developmental task that individuals must master.

Virtue Ethics Model Any of a number of models that suggests ethical decision making should be based on the helper's character. For instance, some suggest that helpers should be prudent and tentative in their decision making, maintain integrity, be respectful, and be benevolent. *See* "Moral Models of Ethical Decision Making."

Watson, John One of the first to apply the concepts of classical conditioning to the clinical setting.

Well-Being Therapy *See* "Positive Psychology."

Wellness Ensuring individuals attend to their personal issues and examine all aspects of their lives. One of the eight "Characteristics of the Effective Helper." *See also* "Indivisible Self."

White, Michael One of the persons who developed "Narrative Therapy."

"Why" Questions A type of question sometimes used in the helping relationship. "Why" questions, however, are generally not recommended because they tend to make clients feel defensive.

Wolpe, Joseph One of the first to apply the concepts of "Classical Conditioning" to the clinical setting.

Working Alliance *See* "Relationship Building."

Wundt, William One of the first experimental psychologists.

All capitalized words in quotation marks can be found alphabetically in the glossary.

References

Aasheim, L. L. (2010). Guidance/ psychoeducational groups. In D. Capuzzi, D. R. Gross, & M. D. Stauffer (Eds.), *Introduction to group work* (5th ed., pp. 282–307). Denver, CO: Love Publishing.

Adam, B. D. (2007). Homophobia and heterosexism. In R. George (Ed.), *Blackwell encyclopedia of sociology.* Retrieved from http://www. blackwellreference.com.proxy.lib. odu.edu/subscriber/uid=2165/ tocnode?query=heterosexism& widen=1&result_number=1 &from=search&fuzzy_0&type= std&id=g9781405124331_chunk_ g978140512433114_ss1-43&slop=1

Adams, R. E., Figley, C. R., & Boscarino, J. A. (2008). The Compassion Fatigue Scale: Its sue with social workers following urban disaster. *Research in Social Work Practice, 18*(3), 238–250. doi: 10.1177/1049731507310190

Addams, J. (1910). *Twenty years at Hull House.* New York: Macmillan.

Agazarian, Y. M. (2008). Introduction to a theory of living human systems and systems-centered practice. In G. M. Saiger, S. Rubenfeld, & M. D. Dluhy (Eds.), *Windows into today's group therapy* (pp. 23–31). New York: Routledge.

Altekruse, M. K., & Wittmer, J. (1991). Accreditation in counselor education. In F. O. Bradley (Ed.), *Credentialing in counseling* (pp. 81–85).

Alexandria, VA: Association for Counselor Education and Supervision.

American Association of Marriage and Family Therapists. (2002–2011). *Press and media information.* Retrieved from http://www.aamft. org/iMIS15/AAMFT/Press/ Press_Information/Content/ Press_Info/Press_Page.aspx? hkey=747f43c1-d238-4c85-a4a2- cbe0acab6876

American Counseling Association. (2005). *Code of ethics.* Retrieved from http://www.counseling.org/ Resources/CodeOfEthics/TP/Home/ CT2.aspx

American Counseling Association. (2011a). *About us.* Retrieved from http://www.counseling.org/ AboutUs/Default.aspx?

American Counseling Association. (2011b). *Home page.* Retrieved from http://www.counseling.org/

American Nurses Credentialing Center. (2011). *Home page.* Retrieved from http://www.nursecredentialing.org/

American Psychiatric Association. (2000). *Diagnostic and statistical manual of mental disorders* (4th ed., text revision). Washington, DC: Author.

American Psychiatric Association. (2010). *DSM-5: The future of psychiatric diagnosis.* Retrieved May 28, 2010, from http://www. dsm5.org/Pages/Default.aspx

American Psychiatric Association. (2011). *About APA.* Retrieved from http://www.psych.org/ FunctionalMenu/AboutAPA.aspx

American Psychiatric Nurses Association. (n.d.a). *Home page.* Retrieved from http://www.apna.org/

American Psychiatric Nurses Association. (n.d.b). *Mission.* Retrieved from http://www.apna. org/i4a/pages/index.cfm? pageid=3334

American Psychological Association. (1954). *Technical recommendations for psychological tests and diagnostic techniques.* Washington, DC: Author.

American Psychological Association. (2003). *Careers for the 21st century* [Brochure]. Washington, DC: Author.

American Psychological Association. (2007). *Guidelines for psycho- logical practice with girls and women.* Washington, DC: Author.

American Psychological Association. (2011a). *About us.* Retrieved from http://www.apa.org/about/index. aspx

American Psychological Association. (2011b). *Effects of poverty, hunger, and homelessness on children and youth.* Retrieved from http://www. apa.org/pi/families/poverty.aspx

Anastasi, A. (1992). What counselors should know about the use and interpretation of psychological tests. *Journal of Counseling and Development, 70,* 610–615.

Anastasi, A., & Urbina, S. (1997). *Psychological testing* (7th ed.). Englewood Cliffs, NJ: Prentice-Hall.

Anderson, T., Lunnen, K. M., & Ogles, B. M. (2010). Putting models and techniques in context. In B. L. Duncan, S. D. Miller, B. E. Wampold, & M. A. Hubble (Eds.), *The heart and soul of change* (2nd ed., pp. 143–166). Washington, DC: American Psychological Association.

Andrews, J. (2001). Group work's place in social work: A historical analysis. *Journal of Sociology & Social Welfare, 28*(4), 45–65.

Appignanesi, R., & Zarate, O. (2004). *Introducing Freud.* Royton, UK: Icon Books.

Armstrong, J. (2010). How effective are minimally trained/experienced volunteer mental health counsellors? Evaluation of CORE outcome data. *Counselling & Psychotherapy Research, 10*(1), 22–31. doi: 10.1080/14733140903163284

Arredondo, P. (1999). Multicultural counseling competencies as tools to address oppression and racism. *Journal of Counseling and Development, 77*(1), 102–108.

Arthur, M. L. (2007). Race. In G. Ritzer (Ed.), *Blackwell encyclopedia of sociology.* Retrieved from http://www.blackwellreference.com/subscriber/tocnode?id=g978140 5124331_chunk_g978140512 433124_ss1-1

Association for Assessment in Counseling. (2003). *Responsible users of standardized tests.* Retrieved from http://aac.ncat.edu/Resources/documents/RUST2003%20v11%20Final.pdf

Association for Counselor Education and Supervision. (1990). Standards for counseling supervisors. *Journal of Counseling and Development, 69,* 30–36.

Association for Specialists in Group Work. (2000). *Professional standards for the training of group workers.* Retrieved from http://www.asgw.org/PDF/training_standards.pdf

Atkinson, D. R. (2004a). Addressing the mental health needs of ethnic minorities. In D. R. Atkinson (Ed.), *Counseling American minorities* (pp. 57–80). New York: McGraw-Hill.

Atkinson, D. R. (2004b). Defining populations and terms. In D. R. Atkinson (Ed.), *Counseling American minorities* (6th ed., pp. 3–26). Boston, MA: McGraw-Hill.

Atkinson, D. R. (2004c). Within-group differences among ethnic minorities. In D. R. Atkinson (Ed.), *Counseling American minorities* (6th ed., pp. 27–56). New York: McGraw-Hill.

Bacon, F. (1997). *Francis Bacon essays.* Hertfordshire, England: Wordsworth. (Original work published 1597)

Baldwin, S. A., Wampold, B. E., & Imel, Z. E. (2007). *Journal of Consulting and Clinical Psychology, 75*(6), 842–852. doi:10.1037/0022-006X.75.6.842

Bandura, A. T. (1977). *Social learning theory.* Englewood Cliffs, NJ: Prentice Hall.

Bandura, A. T., Ross, D., & Ross, S. A. (1963). Imitation of film-mediated aggressive models. *Journal of Abnormal and Social Psychology, 67,* 3–11. doi:10.1037/h0048687

Barker, P. (2007). *Basic family therapy* (5th ed.). Ames, IA: Blackwell Science Ltd.

Bartram, D. (2001). *American Psychological Association (APA) test user qualifications task force.* Retrieved from http://www.intestcom.org/APA_Test_Use_Task_Force.htm

Baruth, L. G., & Huber, C. H. (1984). *An introduction to marital theory and therapy.* Prospect Heights, IL: Waveland Press.

Barz, M. L. (2001). Assessing suicide hotline volunteers' empathy and motivations. *Dissertation Abstracts International: Section B: The Sciences & Engineering, 62*(3-B), 1563. (US: University Microfilms International No.AAI3009882)

Beck, J. (1995). *Cognitive therapy: Basics and beyond.* New York: Guilford Press.

Beck, J. (2005). *Cognitive therapy for challenging problems.* New York: Guilford Press.

Bedi, R. P. (2006). Concept mapping the client's perspective on counseling alliance formation. *Journal of Counseling Psychology, 53*(1), 26–35.

Benjamin, A. (2001). *The helping interview, with case illustrations.* Boston, MA: Houghton Mifflin.

Berger, J. M., Levant, R., McMillan, K. K., Kelleher, W., & Sellers, A. (2005). Impact of gender role conflict, traditional masculinity ideology, alexithymia, and age on men's attitudes toward psychological help seeking. *Psychology of Men & Masculinity, 6*(1), 73–78. doi:10.1037/1524-9220.6.1.73

Bernard, J. M., & Goodyear, R. K. (2009). *Fundamentals of clinical supervision* (4th ed.). Upper Saddle River, NJ: Pearson.

Best, J. W., & Kahn, J. V. (2006). *Research in education* (10th ed.). Boston, MA: Allyn & Bacon.

Beutler, L. E., Malik, M., Alimohamed, S., Harwood, T. M., Talebi, H., Noble, S., et al. (2004). Therapist variables. In M. J. Lambert (Ed.), *Bergin and Garfield's handbook of psychotherapy and behavior change* (5th ed., pp. 227–306). New York: Wiley.

Bike, D., Norcross, J., & Schatz, D. (2009). Process and outcomes of psychotherapists' personal therapy: Replications and extensions 20 years later. *Psychotherapy: Theory, Research, Practice, Training, 46,* 19–31. doi:10.1037/a0015139

Binet, A., & Simon, T. (1916). *The intelligence of the feeble-minded.* Baltimore, MD: Williams & Wilkins Company.

Bloom, J. (1996). *Credentialing professional counselors for the 21st century.* Retrieved from ERIC database (ED399498).

Bloomgarden, A., & Mennuti, R. B. (2009). Therapist self-disclosure: Beyond the taboo. In A. Bloomgarden & R. B. Mennuti (Eds.), *Psychotherapist revealed: Therapists speak about self-disclosure in psychotherapy* (pp. 3–16). New York: Taylor and Francis Group.

Bodenhorn, N., & Lawson, G. (2003). Genetic counseling: Implications for community counselors. *Journal of Counseling & Development, 81*(4), 497–501.

Bohart, A. C., Elliot, R., Greenberg, L. S., & Watson, J. C. (2002). Empathy. In J. C. Norcross (Ed.), *Psycho-therapy relationships that work: Therapist contributions and responsiveness to patients* (pp. 89–108). New York: Oxford University Press.

Borders, L. D., & Brown, L. L. (2005). *The new handbook of counseling supervision.* Mahwah, NJ: Erlbaum.

Bowen, M. (1976). Theory in the practice of psychotherapy. In P. J. Guerin (Ed.), *Family therapy: Theory and practice* (pp. 42–90). New York: Gardner Press.

Bowen, M. (1978). *Family therapy in clinical practice*. New York: Jason Aronson.

Brabender, V., & Fallon, A. (2009). *Group development in practice: Guidance for clinicians and researchers on stages and dynamics of change*. Washington, DC: American Psychological Association.

Brammer, L. M., & MacDonald, G. (2003). *The helping relationship: Process and skills* (8th ed.). Boston, MA: Allyn & Bacon.

Bright, J., & Earl, J. (2009). *Amazing resumes: What employers want to see—And how to say it* (2nd ed.). Indianapolis, IN: JIST works.

Brinson, J., & Denby, R. (2008). Cultural competency course work, personal counseling or both: What influences students' ability to work effectively with culturally diverse clients. *Journal of Human Services, 28,* 44–68.

Brooks-Gunn, J. (2004). Intervention and policy as change agents for young children. In P. L. Chase-Lansdale, K. Kiernan, & R. J. Friedman (Eds.), *Human development across lives and generations: The potential for change* (pp. 293–342). New York: Cambridge University Press.

Brooks-Harris, J. E. (2008). *Integrative multitheoretical psychotherapy*. Boston, MA: Houghton Mifflin.

Brown, C. G., Weber, S., & Ali, S. (2008). Women's body talk: A feminist narrative approach. *Journal of Systemic Therapies, 27*(2), 92–104.

Brown, L. C., & Bryan, T. C. (2007). Feminist therapy with people who self-inflict violence. *Journal of Clinical Psychology, 63*(11), 1121–1133. doi:10.1002/jclp.20419

Brown, N. (1998). *Psychoeducational group counseling*. Bristol, PA: Taylor & Francis.

Buckley, M. R. (2010). Grounded theory methodology. In C. J. Sheperis, J. C. Young, & M. H. Daniels (Eds.), *Counseling research: Quantitative, qualitative, and mixed methods* (pp. 115–150). Upper Saddle River, NJ: Pearson.

Buckley, T. R., & Franklin Jackson, C. F. (2005). Diagnosis in racial-cultural practice. In R. T. Carter (Ed.), *Handbook of racial-cultural psychology and counseling: Theory and research* (Vol. 2, pp. 286–296). Hoboken, NJ: John Wiley.

Budman, S. H., & Gurman, A. S. (1988). *Theory and practice of brief therapy*. New York: Guilford Press.

Bureau of Justice Statistics. (2010). *Prison inmates at midyear 2009—Statistical tables*. Retrieved from http://bjs.ojp.usdoj.gov/index.cfm?ty=pbdetail&iid=2200

Burger, W. (2011). *Human services in contemporary America* (8th ed.). Belmont, CA: Brooks/Cole.

Burlingame, G., & Krogel, J. (2005). Relative efficacy of individual versus group psychotherapy. *International Journal of Group Psychotherapy, 55*(4), 607–611. doi:10.1521/ijgp.2005.55.4.607

Burlingame, G. M., MacKenzie, K. R., & Strauss, B. (2004). Small group treatment: Evidence for effectiveness and mechanism of change. In M. J. Lambert (Ed.), *Bergin and Garfield's handbook of psychotherapy and behavior change* (5th ed., pp. 647–696). New York: Wiley.

Buscaglia, L. (1972). *Love*. Thorofare, NJ: Slack.

Cameron, S., & Turtle-Song, I. (2002). Learning to write case notes using the SOAP format. *Journal of Counseling and Development, 80,* 286–292.

Capuzzi, D., & Gross, D. R. (2010). Group work: An introduction. In D. Capuzzi, D. R. Gross, & M. D. Stauffer (Eds.), *Introduction to group work* (5th ed., pp. 3–38). Denver, CO: Love Publishing.

Carey, B. (2011, May 21). Need therapy? A good man is hard to find. *New York Times*. Retrieved from http://www.nytimes.com/2011/05/22/health/22therapists.html?_r=1&emc=eta1

Carkhuff, R. (1969). *Helping and human relations* (Vol. 2). New York: Holt, Rinehart & Winston.

Carkhuff, R. (2009). *The art of helping in the twenty-first century* (9th ed.). Amherst, MA: Human Resource Development Press.

Carlson, J., & Sperry, L. (Eds.). (2000). *Brief therapy with individuals and couples*. Phoenix, AZ: Zeig, Tucker, and Theisen.

Center for Credentialing and Education. (2011). *Human Services—Board Certified Practitioner exam candidate handbook*. Retrieved from http://www.cce-global.org/Downloads/HS-BCPHandbook.pdf

Center for Credentialing and Education. (n.d.). *Human Services—Board Certified Practitioner*. Retrieved from http://www.cce-global.org/HSBCP

Centers for Disease Control and Prevention. (2002). *Key statistics from the national survey of family health*. Retrieved from http://www.cdc.gov/nchs/nsfg/abc_list_s.htm

Centers for Disease Control and Prevention. (2007). *Advancing HIV prevention: New strategies for a changing epidemic*. Retrieved from http://www.cdc.gov/hiv/topics/prev_prog/AHP/default.htm

Centers for Disease Control and Prevention. (2010). *HIV and AIDS in the United States*. Retrieved from http://www.cdc.gov/hiv/resources/factsheets/us.htm

Centers for Disease Control and Prevention. (2011a). *National marriage and divorce rate trends*. Retrieved from http://www.cdc.gov/nchs/nvss/marriage_divorce_tables.htm

Centers for Disease Control and Prevention. (2011b). *National survey of family growth*. Retrieved from http://www.cdc.gov/nchs/nsfg/abc_list_s.htm

Chambers, C. A. (1963). *Seedtime of reform: American social service and social action 1918–1933*. St. Paul: North Central Publishing Company.

Chang, C. Y., Hays, D. G., & Milliken, T. F. (2009). Addressing social justice issues in supervision: A call for client and professional advocacy. *The Clinical Supervisor, 28,* 20–35. doi:10.1080/07325220902855144

Chaplin, J. P. (1975). *Dictionary of psychology* (2nd ed.). New York: Dell.

Chinman, M. J., Bailey, P., Frey, J., & Rowe, M. (2001). Developing the case management relationship with seriously mentally ill homeless individuals. In F. Flach (Ed.), *Directions in rehabilitation counseling, 2001* (Vol. 22, pp. 107–119). New York: Hathcrleigh Co., Ltd.

Chopra, D. (2009). *Reinventing the body, resurrecting the soul*. New York: Random House.

Cipriani, R. (2007). Religion. In R. George (Ed.), *Blackwell encyclopedia of sociology*. Retrieved from http://www.blackwellreference.com/subscriber/tocnode?id=g9781405124331_chunk_g978140512433124_ss1-48

Clark, L. A., & Watson, D. (2008). Temperament: An organizing paradigm for trait psychology. In O. P. John, R. W. Robins, & L. A. Pervin (Eds.), *Handbook of personality: Theory and research* (3rd ed., pp. 265–287). New York: The Guilford Press.

Clawson, T., Henderson, D. A., Schweiger, W. K., & Collins, D. R. (2008). *Counselor preparation: Programs, faculty, trends* (12th ed.). New York: Brunner-Routledge.

Close, G. (2001). Community development. In T. McClam & M. Woodside (Eds.), *Human service challenges in the 21st century* (pp. 243–252). Birmingham, AL: Ebsco Media.

Clubok, M. (1984). Four-year human services programs: How they differ from social work. *Journal of the National Organization of Human Service Educators, 6*, 1–6.

Clubok, M. (1987). Human services: An "aspiring" profession in search of a professional identity. In R. Kornick (Ed.), *Curriculum development in human services education* [Monograph Series, Issue No. 5]. Council for Standards in Human Service Education.

Clubok, M. (1997). Baccalaureate-level human services and social work: Similarities and differences. *Human Service Education, 17*(1), 7–18.

Clubok, M. (2001). The aging of America. In T. McClam & M. Woodside (Eds.), *Human service challenges in the 21st century* (pp. 339–346). Birmingham, AL: Ebsco Media.

Cobia, C. D., Carney, J. S., Buckhalt, J. A., Middleton, R. A., Shannon, D. M., Trippany, R., et al. (2005). The doctoral *portfolio*: Centerpiece of a comprehensive system of evaluation. *Counselor Education and Supervision, 44*(4), 242–254.

Cogan, D. B. (1989). A theoretical perspective on the supervision of field work students. In C. Tower (Ed.), *Field work in human service education* (pp. 40–52). Knoxville, TN: Council for Standards in Human Service Education.

Cogan, D. B., & O'Connell, G. R. (1982). Models of supervision: A five-year review of the literature. *Journal of the National Organization of Human Service Educators, 4*, 12–17.

Connors, J., & Caple, R. (2005). A review of group systems theory. *Journal for Specialists in Group Work, 30*(2), 93–110. doi: 10.1080/01933920590925940

Constantine, M. C., & Sue, D. W. (2005). *Strategies for building multicultural competence in mental health and educational settings*. Hoboken, NJ: John Wiley.

Constantine, M. G., Smith, L., Redington, R. M., & Owens, D. (2008). Racial microaggressions against Black counseling and counseling psychology faculty: A central challenge in the multicultural counseling movement. *Journal of Counseling and Development, 86*(3), 348–355.

Cooper, J. O., Heron, T. E., & Heward, W. L. (2007). *Applied behavior analysis* (2nd ed.). Columbus, Ohio: Merrill.

Corey, G. (2008). *Theory and practice of group counseling* (7th ed.). Belmont, CA: Brooks/Cole.

Corey, G. (2009). *Theory and practice of counseling and psychotherapy* (8th ed.). Belmont, CA: Brooks/Cole.

Corey, G., Corey, M. S., & Callanan, P. (2011). *Issues and ethics in the helping professions* (8th ed.). Belmont, CA: Brooks/Cole.

Corey, G., Haynes, R., Moulton, P., & Muratori, M. (2010). *Clinical supervision in the helping professions: A practical guide* (2nd ed.). Alexandria, VA: American Counseling Association.

Corey, M. S., Corey, G., & Corey, C. (2010). *Groups: Process and practice* (8th ed.). Belmont, CA: Brooks/Cole.

Cottone, R. R. (2001). A social constructivism model of ethical decision making in counseling. *Journal of Counseling and Development, 79*(1), 39–45.

Cottone, R. R., & Claus, R. E. (2000). Ethical decision-making models: A review of the literature. *Journal of Counseling and Development, 78*, 275–283.

Cottone, R. R., & Tarvydas, V. M. (2007). *Counseling ethics and decision-making* (3rd ed.). Upper Saddle River, NH: Merrill.

Council for Standards in Human Service Education. (2010). *Overview of the CSHSE national standards*. Retrieved from http://www.cshse.org/standards.html

Council for Standards of Human Service Education. (2011a). *About CSHSE: The CSHSE history*. Retrieved from http://www.cshse.org/accreditation.html

Council for Standards of Human Service Education. (2011b). *Accredited programs*. Retrieved from http://www.cshse.org/accreditation.html

Council for Standards of Human Service Education. (n.d.). *Overview of the CSHSE national standards*. Retrieved from http://www.cshse.org/standards.html

CPP. (2009). *Strong Interest Inventory*. Retrieved from https://www.cpp.com/products/strong/index.aspx

Crandell, T. L., Crandell, C. H., & Vander Zanden, J. M. (2008). *Human development* (9th ed.). New York: McGraw-Hill.

Cummings, N. A. (1990). The credentialing of professional psychologists and its implications for the other mental health disciplines. *Journal of Counseling and Development, 68*, 490.

D'Andrea, M. (1996, November 19). *Multicultural counseling*. Presentation at Old Dominion University, Norfolk, VA.

D'Andrea, M., & Daniels, J. (1991). Exploring the different levels of multicultural counseling training in counselor education. *Journal of Counseling and Development, 70*(1), 78–85.

D'Andrea, M., & Daniels, J. (1992, September). *The structure of racism: A developmental framework*. Paper presented at the Association for Counselor Education and Supervision National Conference, San Antonio, TX.

D'Andrea, M., & Daniels, J. (2005, July). A socially responsible approach to counseling, mental health care. *Counseling Today, 48*(1), 36–38.

D'Andrea, M., & Heckman, E. F. (Eds.). (2008). Multicultural counseling [Special issue]. *Journal of Counseling and Development, 86*(3).

de Shazer, S. (1988). *Clues: Investigating solutions in brief therapy*. New York: Norton.

Deal, H. D. (2003). The relationship between critical thinking and interpersonal skills: Guidelines for clinical supervision. *The Clinical Supervisor, 22*(2), 3–19. doi: 10.1300/J001v22n02_02

Diambra, J. F. (2000). Human services: A bona fide profession in the 21st century. *Human Service Education, 20,* 3–9.

Diambra, J. F. (2001). Human services: The past as prelude. In T. McClam & M. Woodside (Eds.), *Human service challenges in the 21st century* (pp. xvii–xxii). Birmingham, AL: Ebsco Media.

Diambra, J. F., McClam, T., Woodside, M., & Kronick, R. F. (2006). Student growth and development in a human service major. *Journal of Human Services, 26,* 49–57.

Dieser, R. (2005). Understanding how Jane Addams and Hull-House programs bridged cross-cultural differences: Leisure programs and contact theory. *Journal of Human Services, 25,* 53–63.

DiGiovanni, M. (Ed.). (2009). *Council for standards in human service education legacy: Past, present, and future* [Monograph]. Chicago, IL: Council for Standards in Human Service Education.

Dolgoff, R., Loewenberg, F. M., & Harrington, D. (2009). *Ethical decisions for social work practice* (8th ed.). Belmont, CA: Brooks/Cole.

Donaldson v. O'Connor, 422 U.S. 563 (U.S. Supreme Ct., 1975).

Dykeman, W. (1997). Poverty: What are we to make of its gnawing existence in our midst? *Human Service Education, 17*(1), 3–5.

Editorial Page Editor. (2005, July 30). Debunking the concept of race. *New York Times,* p. A28.

Egan, G. (1975). *The skilled helper.* Monterrey, CA: Brooks/Cole.

Egan, G. (2010). *The skilled helper: A problem management and opportunity-development approach to helping* (9th ed.). Belmont, CA: Brooks/Cole.

Ellis, A., & Harper, F. A. (1997). *A guide to rational living* (3rd ed.). North Hollywood, CA: Wilshire.

Ellis, A., & MacLaren, C. (2005). *Rational emotive behavior therapy: A therapist's guide* (2nd ed.). Atascadero, CA: Impact Publishers.

Ellwood, R. S. (1993). *Introducing religion from inside and outside* (3rd ed.). North Hollywood, CA: Wilshire.

Emerson, R. W. (1880). *Works of Ralph Waldo Emerson: Letters and social aims* (Vol. IV). Boston, MA: Houghton, Osgood, and Company.

Encyclopedia of Black America. (1981). New York: McGraw-Hill.

Eriksen, K., & Kress, V. (2005). *Beyond the DSM story: Ethical quandaries, challenges, and best practices.* Thousand Oaks, CA: Sage.

Eriksen, K., & Kress, V. (2006). The DSM and the professional counseling identity: Bridging the gap. *Journal of Mental Health Counseling, 28,* 202–217.

Eriksen, K., & Kress, V. (2008). Gender and diagnosis: Struggles and suggestions for counselors. *Journal of Counseling and Development, 86,* 152–162.

Erikson, E. H. (1968). *Identity: Youth and crisis.* New York: Norton.

Erikson, E. H. (1998). *The life cycle completed.* New York: Norton.

Evans, A. C., Delphin, M., Simmons, R., Omar, G., & Tebes, J. (2005). Developing a framework for culturally competent systems care. In R. T. Carter (Ed.), *Handbook of racial-cultural psychology and counseling: Theory and research* (Vol. 2, pp. 492–513). Hoboken, NJ: John Wiley.

Evans, D. R., Hearn, M. T., Uhlemann, M. R., & Ivey, A. E. (2011). *Essential interviewing: A programmed approach to effective communication* (8th ed.). Pacific Grove, CA: Brooks/Cole.

Evenson, T. L., & Holloway, L. L. (2003). Promoting professionalism in human service education. *Human Service Education, 23*(1), 15–24.

Exploring Religious America. (2002, April 26). *A poll conducted for religion and ethics newsweekly and U.S. News & World Report.* Retrieved from http://www.pbs.org/wnet/religionandethics/week534/specialreport.html

Farber, B. A. (2006). *Self-disclosure in psychotherapy.* New York: The Guilford Press.

Federal Emergency Management Agency. (n.d.). *Crisis counseling assistance and training program.* Retrieved from http://www.fema.gov/pdf/media/factsheets/2009/dad_crisis_counseling.pdf

Federal Register. (1977). *Regulation Implementing Education for All Handicapped Children Act of 1975* (PL.94-142), 42(163), 42474–42518.

Ferch, S. R. (2000). Meanings of touch and forgiveness: A hermeneutic phenomenological inquiry. *Counseling and Values, 44*(3), 155–173.

Flavell, J. H. (1963). *The developmental psychology of Jean Piaget.* New York: Van Nostrand.

Foster, S., & Gurman, A. S. (1985). Family therapies. In S. J. Lynn & J. P. Garske (Eds.), *Contemporary psychotherapies: Models and methods* (pp. 377–418). Columbus, OH: Merrill.

Foster-Fishman, P. G., & Behrens, T. R. (2007). Systems change reborn: Rethinking our theories, methods, and efforts in human services reform and community-based change. *American Journal Community Psychology, 39,* 191–196.

Fowler, J. W. (1995). *Stages of faith: The psychology of human development and the quest for meaning.* New York: Harper & Row. (Original work published 1981)

Freedman, J., & Combs, G. (1996). *Narrative therapy: The social construction of preferred realities.* New York: W. W. Norton and Company.

Freud, S. (2003). *An outline of psychoanalysis* (Rev. ed., J. H. Ragg-Kirby, Trans.). New York: Penguin Group. (Original work published in 1940)

Fullerton, S. (1990a). A historical perspective of the baccalaureate level human service professional. *Human Service Education, 20*(1), 53–62.

Fullerton, S. (1990b). Development of baccalaureate-level professional education in human services. In S. Fullerton & D. Osher (Eds.), *History of the human services movement* [Monograph Series, Issue No. 7] (pp. 57–70). Council for Standards in Human Service Education.

Gabbard, G. O. (1995). Are all psychotherapies equally effective? *The Menninger Letter, 3*(1), 1–2.

Gall, M. D., Gall, J. P., & Borg, W. R. (2010). *Applying educational research: How to read, do, and use research to solve problems* (6th ed.). Boston, MA: Pearson.

Gallup. (2010). *Gay and lesbian rights.* Retrieved from http://www.gallup.

com/poll/1651/Gay-Lesbian-Rights. aspx

Garfield, S. L. (1998). *The practice of brief psychotherapy* (2nd ed.). New York: Wiley.

Garske, G. G. (2009). Psychiatric disability: A biopsychosocial challenge. In I. Marini & M. A. Stebnicki (Eds.), *The professional counselor's desk reference* (pp. 647–654). New York: Springer.

Gater, L. (2011). Prison mental health treatment: Trying to keep up with the outside world. *Corrections Forum, 20*, 16–52.

Gay, L. R., Mills, G. E., & Airasian, P. W. (2009). *Educational research: Competencies for analysis and applications* (9th ed.). Upper Saddle River, NJ: Pearson.

Gazda, G. M. (1989). *Group counseling: A developmental approach* (4th ed.). Boston, MA: Allyn & Bacon.

Gelso, C. J., & Carter, J. A. (1994). Components of the psychotherapy relationship: Their interaction and unfolding during treatment. *Journal of Counseling Psychology, 41*(3), 296–306. doi:10.1037/0022-0167.41.3.29

Gelso, C. J., Kelley, F. A., Fuertes, J. N., Marmarosh, C., Holmes, S. E., Costa, C., et al. (2005). Measuring the real relationship in psychotherapy: Initial validation of the therapist form. *Journal of Counseling Psychology, 52*(4), 640–649. doi:10.1037/0022-0167.52.4.640

Gerrig, R., & Zimbardo, P. G. (2010). *Psychology and life* (19th ed.). Upper Saddle River, NJ: Pearson.

Gert, B. (2005). *Morality* (Rev. ed.). New York: Oxford University Press.

Gilligan, C. (1982). *In a different voice: Psychological theory and women's development.* Cambridge, MA: Harvard University Press.

Gilligan, C. (2008). *Kyra.* New York: Random House.

Gingerich, W. J., & Eisengart, S. (2000). Solution-focused brief therapy: A review of outcome research. *Family Process, 39*(4), 477–498. doi:10.1111/j.1545-5300.2000.39408.x

Gladding, S. (2008). *Groups: A counseling specialty* (5th ed.). New York: Merrill.

Gladding, S. (2009). *Counseling: A comprehensive profession* (6th ed.). Upper Saddle River, NJ: Merrill.

Gladding, S., & Newsome, D. W. (2010). *Clinical mental health counseling in community and agency settings* (3rd ed.). Upper Saddle River, NJ: Merrill.

Glasser, W., & Glasser, C. (2007). *Eights lessons for a happier marriage.* New York: HarperCollins.

Gleissner, J. D. (2010). *How bad is the crisis in America's prisons?* Retrieved from http://www.corrections.com/articles/26861-how-bad-is-the-crisis-in-america-s-prisons-

Gompertz, K. (1960). The relation of empathy to effective communication. *Journalism Quarterly, 37,* 535–546.

Good, G. E., & Brooks, G. R. (2005). *The new handbook of psychotherapy and counseling with men: A comprehensive guide to settings, problems, and treatment approaches.* New York: Wiley.

Good, G. E., Gilbert, L. A., & Scher, M. (1990). Gender aware therapy: A synthesis of feminist therapy and knowledge about gender. *Journal of Counseling and Development, 68,* 376–380.

Goodman, J., Schlossberg, N. K., & Anderson, M. L. (2006). *Counseling adults in transition: Linking practice with theory* (3rd ed.). New York: Springer Publishing Company.

Gray, L. A. (2005). Introduction to international perspectives of human services. In L. A. Gray (Ed.), *Human services: International perspectives* [Monograph Series]. Council for Standards in Human Serviced Education.

Gray, L. A. (Ed.). (2005, October). *Human services: International perspectives* [Monograph]. Chicago, IL: Council for Standards in Human Service Education.

Greer, M. (2005, June). Keeping them hooked in. *APA Monitor, 36*(6), 60.

Griggs v. Duke Power Company, 401 U.S. 424(1971).

Grob, G. N. (1996). Creation of the National Institute of Mental Health. *Public Health Reports, 111*(4), 378–381.

Guerrero, L. K., & Floyd, K. (2006). *Nonverbal communication in close relationships.* Mahwah,

New Jersey: Lawrence Erlbaum Associates.

Hackney, H., & Cormier, L. S. (2009). *The professional counselor: A process guide to helping* (6th ed.). Upper Saddle River, NJ: Pearson.

Haley, J. (1973). *Uncommon therapy.* New York: Norton.

Haley, J. (1976). *Problem-solving therapy.* San Francisco: Jossey-Bass.

Haley, J. (2009). *Jay Haley: The family therapist.* Retrieved from http://www.jay-haley-on-therapy.com/html/family_therapy.html

Halstead, R. W. (2007). *Assessment of client core issues.* Alexandria, VA: American Counseling Association.

Hansen, J. C., Rossberg, R. H., & Cramer, S. H. (1994). *Counseling: Theory and process* (5th ed.). Boston, MA: Allyn & Bacon.

Haynes, S., & Sweitzer, H. F. (2005). An evolving journal for an evolving organization. *Human Service Education, 25,* 5–7.

Haynes, S. H. (2011). The effects of victim-related contextual factors on the criminal justice system. *Crime & Delinquency, 52*(2), 298–328. doi:10.1177/0011128710372190

Health Maintenance Organization Act of 1973, 42 U.S.C. A§ 300e.

Heppner, P. P., Wampold, B. E., & Kivlighan, D. M. (2008). *Research design in counseling* (3rd ed.). Belmont, CA: Wadsworth.

Herek, G. M. (2000). The psychology of sexual prejudice. *Current Directions in Psychological Science, 9*(1), 19–22. doi:10.1111/1467-8721.00051

Herr, E. L., Cramer, S. H., & Niles, S. G. (2004). *Career guidance and counseling through the life span: Systematic approaches* (6th ed.). Boston, MA: Pearson/Allyn & Bacon.

Hershenson, D. B., Power, P. W., & Waldo, M. (2003). *Community counseling: Contemporary theory and practice.* Long Grove, IL: Waveland Press.

Hicks-Coolick, A., & Millsap, T. (2001). Meeting the needs of incarcerated parents and their children: Challenges in the 21st century. In T. McClam & M. Woodside (Eds.), *Human service challenges in the 21st century* (pp. 19–28). Birmingham, AL: Ebsco Media.

Higgs, J. A. (1992). Dealing with resistance: Strategies for effective group. *Journal for Specialists in Group Work, 17*(2), 67–73.

Hill, C. E. (2009). *Helping skills: Facilitating exploration, insight, and action* (3rd ed.). Washington, DC: APA.

Hill, C. E., & Knox, S. (2002). Self-disclosure. In J. C. Norcross (Ed.), *Psychotherapy relationships that work: Therapist contributions and responsiveness to patients* (pp. 255–266). New York: Oxford University Press.

Hinkle, J. S., & O'Brien, S. (2010). The Human Services—Board Certified Practitioner: An overview of a new national credential. *Journal of Human Services, 30*, 23–28.

Holland, J. L. (1994). *The self-directed search* (Rev. ed.). Odessa, FL: Psychological Assessment Resources.

Horwitz, A. V. (2002). *The social control of mental illness*. Clinton Corners, NY: Percheron Press.

Hosie, T. (1991). Historical antecedents and current status of counselor licensure. In F. O. Bradley (Ed.), *Credentialing in counseling* (pp. 23–52). Alexandria, VA: Association for Counselor Education and Supervision.

Houser, R. (2009). *Counseling and educational research: Evaluation and application* (2nd ed.). Thousand Oaks, CA: Sage.

Human Services— Board Certified Practitioner. (2011, February 1). *Press releases*. Retrieved from http://www.cce-global.org/HSBCP/PressReleases

Humphreys, K. (2004). *Circles of recovery: Self-help organizations for addictions*. New York: Cambridge University Press.

Iannone, A. P. (2001). *Dictionary of world philosophy*. New York: Routledge.

Ivey, A., & Gluckstein, N. (1974). *Basic attending skills: An introduction to microcounseling and helping*. North Amherst, MA: Microtraining Associates.

Ivey, A. E., Ivey, M., & Zalaquett, C. P. (2010). *Intentional interviewing and counseling: Facilitating client development in a multicultural society* (7th ed.). Belmont, CA: Brooks/Cole.

Jacobs, E. E., Masson, R. L., & Harvill, R. L. (2009). *Group counseling: Strategies and skills* (6th ed.). Belmont, CA: Brooks/Cole.

Jayakar, P. (1996). *J. Krishnamurti: A biography*. New York: Penguin Books. (Original work published 1986)

Jenkins, R. (2007). Ethnicity. In R. George (Ed.), *Blackwell encyclopedia of sociology* [Electronic version]. Retrieved from www.blackwellreference.com/subscriber/tocnode?id=g9781405124331_chunk_g978140512433111_ss1-68

Jennings, L. (2007). Prejudice. In R. George (Ed.), *Blackwell encyclopedia of sociology*. Retrieved from http://www.blackwellreference.com.proxy.lib.odu.edu/subscriber/uid=2165/tocnode?id=g9781405124331_chunk_g978140512433122_ss1-97

Johnson, J. (2009). Whether states should create prescription power for psychologists. *Law and Psychology Review, 33*, 167–178.

Jones, L. K. (1994). Frank parsons' contribution to career counseling. *Journal of Career Development, 20*(4), 287–294.

Jongsma, A. E., Jr., & Peterson, L. M. (2003). *The complete adult psychotherapy treatment planner* (3rd ed.). New York: Wiley.

Kadushin, D., & Harkness, A. (2002). *Supervision in social work* (4th ed.). New York: Columbia University Press.

Kahn, M. (2001). *Between therapist and client: The new relationship* (Rev. ed.). New York: W. H. Freeman/Owl.

Kaplan, D. (2006, March 1). *Counseling Today online: Ethics update*. Retrieved from http://www.counseling.org/Publications/CounselingTodayArticles.aspx?AGuid=e6b5t6f3-9fca-4519-8b44-b22355ae4db7

Kaplan, M., & Cuciti, P. L. (Eds.). (1986). *The Great Society and its legacy: Twenty years of U.S. social policy*. Durham, NC: Duke University Press.

Kees, N. L. (2005). Women's voices, women's lives: An introduction to the special issue on women and counseling. *Journal of Counseling and Development, 83*, 259–261.

Kegan, R. (1982). *The evolving self*. Cambridge, MA: Harvard University Press.

Kegan, R. (1994). *In over our heads*. Cambridge, MA: Harvard University Press.

Kincaid, S. (2004a). Introduction and council survey. In S. Kincaid (Ed.), *Technology in human services: Using technology to improve quality of life* [Monograph] (pp. 1–5). Council for Standards in Human Service Education.

Kincaid, S. (Ed.). (2004b). *Technology in human services: Using technology to improve quality of life* [Monograph]. Council for Standards in Human Service Education.

Kincaid, S. O., & Andresen, S. A. (2010). Higher education accountability and the CSHSE accreditation process. *Journal of Human Services, 30*, 8–17.

King, P. M. (1978). William Perry's theory of intellectual and ethical development. In L. Knefelkamp, C. Widick, & C. L. Parker (Eds.), *Applying new developmental findings* (pp. 34–51). San Francisco, CA: Jossey-Bass.

Kinkaid, S. O., & Andresen, S. A. (2010). Higher education accountability and the CSHSE accreditation process. *Journal of Human Services, 30*, 8–17.

Kitchener, K. S. (1984). Intuition, critical evaluation and ethical principles: The foundation for ethical decisions in counseling psychology. *The Counseling Psychologist, 12*(3), 43–45. doi:10.1177/0011000084123005

Klaw, E., & Humphreys, K. (2004). The role of peer led mutual help groups in promoting health and well-being. In L. DeLucia-Waack, D. A. Gerrity, C. R. Kalodner, & M. T. Riva (Eds.), *Handbook of group counseling and psychotherapy* (pp. 630–640). Thousand Oaks, CA: Sage Publications.

Klein, M. H., Kolden, G. G., Michels, J. L., & Chisholm-Stockard, S. (2001). Congruence or genuineness. *Psychotherapy, 38*(4), 396–400. doi:10.1037/0033-3204.38.4.396

Kleist, D., & Bitter, J. R. (2009). In J. Bitter (Ed.), *Theory and practice of family therapy and counseling* (pp. 43–65). Belmont, CA: Brooks/Cole.

Kohlberg, L. (1963). The development of children's orientations towards a moral order: I. Sequence in the developmental of moral thought. *Vita Humana, 6*, 11–33.

Kohlberg, L. (1981). *The philosophy of moral development: Moral stages and the idea of justice.* San Francisco, CA: Harper and Row.

Kohlberg, L. (1984). *The psychology of moral development: The nature and validity of moral stages.* San Francisco: Harper & Row.

Kosmin, B. A., & Keysar, A. (2008). *American religious identification survey.* Hartford, CO: Trinity College.

Kress, V. E. W., Eriksen, K. P., Rayle, A. D., & Ford, S. J. W. (2005). The DSM-IV-TR and culture: Considerations for counselors. *Journal of Counseling and Development, 83,* 97–104.

Kubler-Ross, E., & Kessler, D. (2005). *On grief and grieving.* New York: Scribner.

Kuhn, T. S. (1962). *The structure of scientific revolutions.* Chicago: University of Chicago Press.

Kuriansky, J. (2008). A clinical toolbox for cross-cultural counseling and training. In U. P. Gielen, J. G. Draguns, & J. M. Fish (Eds.), *Principles of multicultural counseling and therapy.* New York: Routledge.

Kursmark, L. M. (2011). *Best resumes for college students and new grads: Jump-start your career* (3rd ed.). Indianapolis, IN: JIST Works.

Lamar, J. (1992). The problem with you people. *Esquire, 117,* 90–91, 94.

Lambert, M. J. (Ed.). (2004). *Bergin and Garfield's handbook of psychotherapy and behavior change* (5th ed.). New York: Wiley.

Lanci, J. R. (1997). *A new temple for Corinth: Rhetorical and archaeological approaches to Pauline imagery* (5th ed.). New York: Peter Lang Publishing.

Lanci, J. R. (1999). *Texts, rocks, and talk: Reclaiming biblical Christianity* (5th ed.). Collegeville, MN: Michael Glazier/Liturgical Press.

Law, I. (2007). Discrimination. In R. George (Ed.), *Blackwell encyclopedia of sociology.* Retrieved from http://www.blackwellreference.com/subscriber/tocnode?id=g9781405124331_chunk_g981405124333110_ss2-27

Lawson, G. (2007). Counselor wellness and impairment: A national survey. *Journal of Humanistic Counseling, Education and Development, 46(1),* 20–34.

Layne, C. M., & Hohenshil, T. H. (2005). High-tech counseling revisited. *Journal of Counseling and Development, 83,* 222–227.

Leary, M. R. (2007). *Introduction to behavioral research methods* (5th ed.). Boston, MA: Allyn & Bacon.

Lees, J. (2011). Counselling and psychotherapy in dialogue with complementary and alternative medicine. *British Journal of Guidance and Counseling, 39,* 117–130.

Levinson, D. (1978). *The seasons of a man's life.* New York: Knopf.

Lieberman, M. A., & Keith, H. (2002). Self-help groups and substance abuse: An examination of Alcoholics Anonymous. In D. W. Brook & H. Spitz (Eds.), *The group therapy of substance abuse* (pp. 203–221). New York: Haworth Press.

Linda, S., Miller, G., & Johnson, P. (2000). *Counseling and spirituality: The use of emptiness and the importance of timing.* Paper presented at the Annual Conference of the American Counseling Association Washington, DC. Retrieved from ERIC database (ED442021).

Lindner, E. (Ed.). (2009). *Yearbook of American and Canadian churches.* Nashville, TN: Abingdon Press.

Linstrum, K. S. (2005). The effects of training on ethical decision making skills as a function of moral development and context in master-level counseling students. *Dissertation Abstracts International Section A: Humanities & Social Sciences 65(9-A), 2005,* 3289. (US: University Microfilms International)

Lipps, T. (1960). Empathy, inner imitation, and sense feelings. In M. M. Rader (Ed.), *A modern book of esthetics: An anthology* (3rd ed., pp. 374–381). New York: Holt, Rinehart, and Winston. (Original work published 1903)

List of psychotherapies. (2011). *Wikipedia, The free encyclopedia.* Retrieved from http://en.wikipedia.org/wiki/List_of_psychotherapies

Livneh, H., & Antonak, R. F. (2005). Psychosocial adaptation to chronic illness and disability: A primer for counselors. *Journal of Counseling and Development, 83,* 12–20.

Lovell, C. (1999). Empathic-cognitive development in students of

counseling. *Journal of Adult Development, 6(4),* 195–203. doi: 10.1023/A:1021432310030

Lum, C. (2009). *Federal information resources for professional counselors.* Alexandria, VA: American Counseling Association.

Lum, D. (2004). *Social work practice and people of color: A process-stage approach* (5th ed.). Pacific Grove, CA: Brooks/Cole.

MacDonald, A. J. (2003). Research in solution-focused brief therapy. In B. O'Connell & S. Palmer (Eds.), *Handbook of solution-focused therapy* (pp. 12–24). Thousand Oaks, CA: Sage.

Macht, J. (1990). A historical perspective. In S. Fullerton & D. Osher (Eds.), *History of the human services movement* [Monograph Series, Issue No. 7] (pp. 9–22). Council for Standards in Human Service Education.

Macionis, J. J. (2009). *Sociology* (13th ed.). Upper Saddle River, NJ: Prentice Hall.

Madsen, K., & Leech, P. (2007). *The ethics of labeling in mental health.* Jefferson, NC: MacFarland & Company.

Madson, M. B., Loignon, A. C., & Lane, C. (2009). Training in motivational interviewing: A systematic review. *Journal of Substance Abuse Treatment, 36,* 101–109.

Malcolm, X., & Haley, A. (2001). *The autobiography of Malcolm X.* New York: Ballantine.

MANTA. (2011). *8,304 mental health services companies in the U.S.* Retrieved from http://www.manta.com/mb_35_D003F7SK_000/mental_health_services

Maramba, G. G., & Nagayama Hall, G. C. (2002). Meta-analysis of ethnic match as a predictor of dropout, utilization, and level of functioning. *Cultural Diversity and Ethnic Minority Psychology, 8,* 290–297.

Marchand, M. M. (2010). Application of Paulo Freire's *Pedagogy of the Oppressed* to human services education. *Journal of Human Services, 30,* 43–53.

Marmarosh, C. L., Markin, R. D., Gelso, C. J., Majors, R., Mallery, C., & Choi, J. (2009). The real relationship in psychotherapy: Relationships to adult attachments, working alliance, transference, and therapy outcome. *Journal of Counseling Psychology, 56*(3), 337–350. doi:10.1037/a0015169

Maroda, K. J. (2009). Less is more: An argument for the judicious use of self-disclosure. In A. Bloomgarden & R. B. Mennuti (Eds.), *Psychotherapist revealed: Therapists speak about self-disclosure in psychotherapy* (pp. 17–29). New York: Taylor and Francis Group.

Maslow, A. H. (1954). *Motivation and personality.* New York: Harper & Row.

Maslow, A. H. (1968). *Toward a psychology of being* (2nd ed.). Princeton, NJ: Van Nostrand.

Maslow, A. H. (1970). *Motivation and personality* (Rev. ed.). New York: Harper & Row.

Matsumoto, D. (2006). Culture and nonverbal behavior. In V. Manusov & M. L. Patterson (Eds.), *The SAGE handbook of nonverbal communication* (pp. 219–236). Thousand Oaks, CA: Sage Publishing.

McAuliffe, G. (Ed.). (2008a). *Culturally alert counseling: A comprehensive introduction.* Los Angeles, CA: Sage Publications.

McAuliffe, G. (2008b). What is culturally alert counseling? In G. McAuliffe (Ed.), *Culturally alert counseling: A comprehensive introduction* (pp. 2–44). Los Angeles, CA: Sage Publications.

McAuliffe, G., & Eriksen, K. (Eds.). (2010). *Handbook of counselor preparation: Constructivist, Developmental, and Experiential approaches.* Thousand Oaks/ Alexandria, CA/VA: Sage/ Association for Counselor Education and Supervision.

McAuliffe, G., Goméz, E., & Grothaus, T. (2008). Race. In G. McAuliffe (Ed.), *Culturally alert counseling: A comprehensive introduction* (pp. 105–145). Los Angeles, CA: Sage Publications.

McCarthy, J., & Holliday, E. L. (2004). Help-seeking and counseling within a traditional male gender role: An examination from a multicultural perspective. *Journal of Counseling and Development, 82,* 25–30.

McClam, T. (1997a). Baccalaureate-level human services and social work: Similarities and differences. *Human Service Education, 17*(1), 29–36.

McClam, T. (1997b). Human service education: Back to the future.

Human Service Education, 17(1), 29–35.

McClam, T., & Woodside, M. R. (1989). A conversation with Dr. Harold McPheeters. *Human Service Education, 9*(1), 1–9.

McClam, T., Woodside, M. R., & Cole-Zakrzewski, K. (2005). A survey of human service educators: A longitudinal study. *Human Service Education, 25*(1), 65–73.

McDaniels, C., & Watts, G. A. (1994). Frank Parsons: Light, information, inspiration, cooperation [Special issue]. *Journal of Career Development, 20*(4).

McMillan, J. H., & Schumacher, S. (2010). *Research in education: Evidence-based inquiry* (7th ed.). Boston: Allyn & Bacon.

McMillen, D. P. (2001). The future of human services: Models of service delivery. In T. McClam & M. Woodside (Eds.), *Human service challenges in the 21st century* (pp. 229–242). Birmingham, AL: Ebsco Media.

McPheeters, H. (1990). Developing the human services generalist concept. In S. Fullerton & D. Osher (Eds.), *History of the human services movement* [Monograph Series, Issue No. 7] (pp. 31–40). Council for Standards in Human Service Education.

Mead, M. (1961). *Coming of age in Samoa: A psychological study of primitive youth for western civilization.* New York: Morrow.

Meara, N. M., Schmidt, L. D., & Day, J. D. (1996). Principles and virtues: A foundation for ethical decisions, policies, and character. *The Counseling Psychologist, 24*(9), 4–77 doi:10.1177/0011000096241002

Mehrabian, A. (1971). *Silent messages.* Belmont, CA: Wadsworth.

Meichenbaum, D. (1977). *Cognitive behavior modification: An integrative approach.* New York: Basic Books.

Mejia, X. (2005). Gender matters: Working with adult male survivors of trauma. *Journal of Counseling and Development, 83,* 29–40.

Milgram, S. (1965). Some conditions of obedience and disobedience to authority. *Human Relations, 18,* 56–76.

Milgram, S. (1974). *Obedience to authority.* New York: Harper & Row.

Milliken, T. F. (2004). The impact of cognitive development on White school counselor interns' perspectives and perceived competencies for addressing the needs of African American students (Doctoral dissertation, College of William and Mary, 2003). *Dissertation Abstracts International, 65*(02A), 420.

Milliken, T. F., & Neukrug, E. (2009). Perceptions of ethical behaviors of human service professionals. *Human Service Education, 29*(1), 35–48.

Milliken, T. F., & Neukrug, E. S. (2010). An introduction to the special section on professional standards in human services. *Journal of Human Services, 30,* 5–7.

Minuchin, S. (1974). *Families and family therapy.* Cambridge, MA: Harvard University Press.

Minuchin, S. (1981). *Family therapy techniques.* Cambridge, MA: Harvard University Press.

Morrow, S. (2004). Finding the "yes" within ourselves: Counseling lesbian and bisexual women. In D. R. Atkinson & G. Hackett (Eds.), *Counseling diverse populations* (3rd ed., pp. 366–387). Boston, MA: McGraw-Hill.

Murdin, L. (2000). *How much is enough? Endings in psychotherapy and counseling.* New York: Routledge.

Mussen, P. H., Conger, J. J., & Kagan, J. (1969). *Child development and personality.* New York: Harper & Row.

Mwaba, K., & Pedersen, P. (1990). Relative importance of intercultural, interpersonal, and psychopathological attributions in judging critical incidents by multicultural counselors. *Journal of Multicultural Counseling and Development, 18,* 106–117.

Myers, J. E., & Harper, M. C. (2004). Evidence-based effective practice with older adults. *Journal of Counseling and Development, 82,* 207–218.

Myers, J. E., & Sweeney, T. J. (2008). Wellness counseling: The evidence base and practice. *Journal of Counseling and Development, 86*(4), 482–493.

Napier, A., & Whitaker, C. (1978). *The family crucible.* New York: Harper & Row.

Napier, R. W., & Gershenfeld, M. K. (2004). *Groups: Theory and experience* (7th ed.). New York: Houghton Mifflin Company.

National Alliance of Direct Support Professionals. (2008). *Making a world of difference in people's lives: Community support skill standards (CSSS).* Retrieved from http://www.nadsp.org/orglibrary/csss.asp

National Association of Social Workers. (2011a). *About NASW.* Retrieved from http://www.naswdc.org/nasw/default.asp

National Association of Social Workers. (2011b). *NASW credentialing center.* Retrieved from http://www.socialworkers.org/credentials/default.asp

National Board for Certified Counselors. (2011). *Understanding NBCC's national certifications.* Retrieved from http://www.nbcc.org/OurCertifications

National Coalition for the Homeless. (2009). *How many people experience homelessness?* Retrieved from http://www.nationalhomeless.org/factsheets/How_Many.html

National Human Genome Research Project. (2010). *From blueprint to you.* Retrieved from http://www.genome.gov/Pages/Education/Modules/BluePrintToYou/BlueprintCoverto2.pdf

National Institute of Mental Health. (2008). *The numbers count: Mental disorders in America.* Retrieved from http://wwwapps.nimh.nih.gov/health/publications/the-numbers-count-mental-disorders-in-america.shtml http://www.nimh.nih.gov/health/publications/the-numbers-count-mentaldisorders-in-america/index.shtml

National Institute of Mental Health. (2010). *Mental health medications: Complete index.* Retrieved from http://www.nimh.nih.gov/health/publica tions/mental-health-medications/complete-index.shtml#pub1

National Law Center on Homelessness & Poverty. (2010). *Homelessness and poverty in America.* Retrieved from http://www.nlchp.org/hapia.cfm

National Organization of Human Services. (1996). *Ethical standards of human service professionals.* Retrieved from http://www.nationalhumanservices.org/index.php?option=com_content&view=article&id=43&Itemid=90

National Organization of Human Services. (2009a). *About: Regions.* Retrieved from http://www.nationalhumanservices.org/index.php?option=com_content&view=article&id=81&Itemid=87

National Organization of Human Services. (2009b). *Home.* Retrieved from http://www.nationalhumanservices.org/

National Organization of Human Services. (2009c). *What is human services?* Retrieved from http://www.nationalhumanservices.org/index.php?option=com_content&view= article&id=88&Itemid=89

National Training Laboratory. (2008). *About NTL.* Retrieved from http://www.ntl.org/inner.asp?id=177&category=2

Naugle, A. E., & Maher, S. (2003). Modeling and behavioral rehearsal. In W. O'Donohue, U. J. Fisher, & S. C. Hayes (Eds.), *Cognitive behavior therapy: Applying empirically supported techniques in your practice* (pp. 238–246). Hoboken, NJ: John Wiley & Sons.

Neukrug, E. (1980). The effects of supervisory style and type of praise upon counselor trainees' level of empathy and perception of supervisor (Doctoral dissertation, University of Cincinnati, 1980). *Dissertation Abstracts International, 41*(04A), 1496.

Neukrug, E. (1987). The brief training of paraprofessional counselors in empathic responding. *New Hampshire Journal for Counseling and Development, 15*(1), 15–19.

Neukrug, E. (1998). Support and challenge: Use of metaphor as a higher-level empathic response. In H. Rosenthal (Ed.), *Favorite counseling and therapy techniques* (pp. 139–141). Bristol, PA: Accelerated Development.

Neukrug, E. (2001). Medical breakthroughs: Genetic research and genetic counseling, psychotropic medications, and the mind-body connection. In T. McClam & M. Woodside (Eds.), *Human service challenges in the 21st century* (pp. 115–132). Birmingham, AL: Ebsco Media.

Neukrug, E. (2002). *Skills and techniques for human service professionals: Counseling environment, helping skills,* *treatment issues.* Pacific Grove, CA: Brooks/Cole.

Neukrug, E. (2011). *Counseling theory and practice.* Belmont, CA: Brooks/Cole.

Neukrug, E. (2012). *The world of the counselor* (4th ed.). Belmont, CA: Brooks/Cole.

Neukrug, E., & Fawcett, R. (2010). *Essentials of testing and assessment: A practical guide for counselors, social workers, and psychologists* (2nd ed.). Pacific Grove, CA: Brooks/Cole.

Neukrug, E., Lovell, C., & Parker, R. (1996). Employing ethical codes and decision-making models: A developmental process. *Counseling and Values, 40,* 98–106.

Neukrug, E., & Milliken, T. (2008). Activities to enhance the cultural competence of human services students. *Human Service Education, 28,* 17–28.

Neukrug, E., Milliken, T., & Shoemaker, J. (2001). Counselor seeking behaviors of NOHSE practitioners, educators, and trainees. *Human Service Education, 21,* 45–48.

Neukrug, E., & Schwitzer, A. M. (2006). *Skills and tools for today's counselors and psychotherapists: From natural helping to professional counseling.* Pacific Grove, CA: Brooks/Cole.

Newport, F. (2009, December 24). *Gallup: This Christmas, 78% of Americans identify as Christian.* Retrieved from http://www.gallup.com/poll/124793/This-Christmas-78-Americans-Identify-Christian.aspx

Nichols, M. P., & Schwartz, R. C. (2008). *Family therapy: Concepts and methods* (8th ed.). Boston, MA: Allyn & Bacon.

Nichols, M. P., & Schwartz, R. C. (2009). *The essentials of family therapy* (4th ed.). Boston, MA: Allyn & Bacon.

Niles, S. (Ed.). (2009). Special section: Advocacy competencies. *Journal of Counseling and Development, 87*(3).

Norcross, J. C. (2010). The therapeutic relationship. In B. L. Duncan, S. D. Miller, B. E. Wampold, & M. A. Hubble (Eds.), *The heart and soul of change* (2nd ed., pp. 113–142). Washington, DC: American Psychological Association.

Norcross, J. C., Bike, D. H., & Evans, K. L. (2009). The therapist's therapist: A replication and extension 20 years later. *Psychotherapy: Theory, Research, Practice, & Training, 46,* 32–41. doi:10.1037/a0015140

Norcross, J. C., Bike, D. H., Evans, K. L., & Schatz, D. M. (2008). Psycho-therapists who abstain from personal therapy: Do they practice what they preach? *Journal of Clinical Psychology, 64*(12), 1368–1376. doi:10.1002/jclp.20523

Nye, R. D. (1992). *The legacy of B. F. Skinner: Concepts and perspectives, controversies and misunderstandings.* Pacific Grove, CA: Brooks/Cole.

Nye, R. D. (2000). *Three psychologies: Perspectives from Freud, Skinner, and Rogers* (6th ed.). Belmont, CA: Brooks/Cole.

O'Donohu, W., Fisher, U. J., & Hayes, S. C. (Eds.). (2003). *Cognitive behavior therapy: Applying empirically supported techniques in your practice.* Hoboken, NJ: John Wiley & Sons.

O'Leary, E. (2006). The need for integration. In E. O'Leary & M. Murphy (Eds.), *New approaches to integration in psychotherapy* (pp. 3–12). New York: Routledge.

O'Leary, E., & Murphy, M. (2006). *New approaches to integration in psychotherapy.* New York: Routledge.

Orlinsky, D. E., Ronnestad, M. H., & Willutzki, U. (2004). Fifty years of psychotherapy process outcome research: Continuity and change. In M. J. Lambert (Ed.), *Bergin and Garfield's handbook of psycho-therapy and behavior change* (5th ed., pp. 307–389). New York: Wiley.

Osher, D. (1990). More than needs and service: The antecedent and concurrent social conditions that influenced the human services movement. In S. Fullerton & D. Osher (Eds.), *History of the human services movement* [Monograph Series, Issue No. 7] (pp. 23–30). Council for Standards in Human Service Education.

Parsons, F. (1989). *Choosing a vocation.* Garrett Park, MD: Garrett Park. (Original work published 1909)

Pease, A., & Pease, B. (2006). *The definitive book of body language.* New York: Bantam Books.

Pence, G. E. (2008). *Medical ethics: Accounts of ground breaking cases* (6th ed.). New York: McGraw-Hill.

Pepinsky, H. B. (2001). Counseling psychology: History. In W. E. Crawford & C. B. Nemeroff (Eds.), *The Corsini encyclopedia of psychology and behavioral science* (Vol. 1, pp. 375–379). New York: Wiley.

Perry, W. G. (1970). *Forms of intellectual and ethical development in the college years: A scheme.* New York: Holt, Rinehart, & Winston.

Phillips, S. J. (2007). A comprehensive look at the legislative issues affecting advanced nursing practice. *Nurse Practitioner, 32*(1), 14–17. doi: 10.1097/00006205-200701000-00006

Pieterse, A. L., Evans, S. A., Risner-Butner, A., Collins, N. M., & Mason, L. B. (2009). Multicultural competence and social justice training in counseling psychology and counselor education: A review and analysis of a sample of multicultural course syllabi. *The Counseling Psychologist, 37,* 93–115. doi: 10.1177/0011000008319986

Piot, P., Bartos, M., Larson, H., Zewdie, D., & Mane, P. (2008). Coming to terms with complexity: A cal to action for HIV prevention. *The Lancet, 372*(9641), 845–859. doi: 10.1016/S0140-6736(08)60888-0

Planalp, S., & Knie, K. (2002). How to do emotions with words: Emotionality in conversations. In S. R. Fussell (Ed.), *The verbal communication of emotions: Interdisciplinary perspectives* (pp. 55–77). Mahwah, NJ: Erlbaum.

Polcin, D. L. (2006). Reexamining confrontation and motivational interviewing. *Addictive Disorders and Their Treatment, 54*(4), 201–209.

Ponton, R., & Duba, J. (2009). The "ACA Code of Ethics": Articulating counseling's professional covenant. *Journal of Counseling & Development, 87*(1), 117–121.

Pope, M. (2008). Culturally appropriate counseling considerations for lesbian and gay clients. In P. B. Pedersen, J. G. Draguns, W. J. Lonner, & J. E. Trimble (Eds.), *Counseling across cultures* (6th ed., pp. 201–222). Thousand Oaks, CA: Sage.

Pope, M., & Sveinsdottir, M. (2005). Frank, we hardly knew ye: The very personal side of Frank Parsons. *Journal of Counseling and Development, 83,* 105–115.

Pottick, K. J. (1988). Jane Addams revisited: Practice theory and social economics. *Social Work with Groups, 11,* 11–26. doi: 10.1300/J009v11n04_04

Pressly, P. K., & Heesacker, M. (2001). The physical environment and counseling: A review of theory and research. *Journal of Counseling and Development, 79,* 148–160.

Preston, J. D., O'Neal, J. H., & Talaga, M. C. (2010). *Handbook of clinical psychopharmacology for therapists* (6th ed.). Oakland, CA: New Harbinger Publications.

Prieto, L. R., & Scheel, K. R. (2002). Using case documentation to strengthen counselor trainees' case conceptualization skills. *Journal of Counseling and Development, 81,* 11–21.

Pritts, T. A., Wang, Q., Sun, X., Moon, M. R., Fischer, D. R., Fischer, J. E., et al. (2000). Induction of the stress response in vivo decreases nuclear factor-kappa B activity in jejunal mucosa of endotoxemic mice. *Archives of Surgery, 135*(7), 860–866.

Puma, M., Bell, S., Cook, R., Heid, C., Shapiro, G., Broene, P., et al. (2010). *Head Start impact study. Final report.* Retrieved from ERIC database (ED507845).

Remley, T. P., & Herlihy, B. (2010). *Ethical, legal, and professional issues in counseling* (3rd ed.). Upper Saddle River, NJ: Prentice Hall.

Rice, F. P. (2001). *Human development: A life-span approach* (4th ed.). Upper Saddle River, NJ: Prentice Hall.

Ridley, C. R., Liddle, M. C., Hill, C. L., & Li, L. C. (2001). Ethical decision making in multicultural counseling. In J. G. Ponterotto, J. M. Casas, L. A. Suzuki, & C. M. Alexander (Eds.), *Handbook of multicultural counseling* (2nd ed., pp. 165–188). Thousand Oaks, CA: Sage.

Riva, M. T., Wachtel, M., & Lasky, G. B. (2004). Effective leadership in group counseling and psychotherapy: Research and practice. In J. L. DeLucia-Waack, D. A. Gerrity, C. R. Kalodner, & M. T. Riva (Eds.), *Handbook of group counseling and psychotherapy* (pp. 37–48). Thousand Oaks, CA: Sage Publications.

Roach, L. F., & Young, M. E. (2007). Do counselor education programs promote wellness in their students?

Counselor Education and Supervision, 47(1), 29–45.

Roberts, M. C., Brown, K. J., Johnson, R. J., & Reinke, J. (2005). Positive psychology for children: Development, prevention, and promotion. In C. R. Snyder & S. J. Lopez (Eds.), *Handbook of positive psychology* (pp. 663–675). New York: Oxford University Press.

Rockinson-Szapkiw, A. J., & Silvey, R. J. (2010). Using a wiki for collaboration and learning in helping profession education: A pilot study. *Journal of Human Services, 30,* 71–80.

Rogers, C. R. (1942). *Counseling and psychotherapy.* Boston, MA: Houghton Mifflin.

Rogers, C. R. (1951). *Client-centered therapy.* Boston, MA: Houghton Mifflin.

Rogers, C. R. (1957). The necessary and sufficient conditions of therapeutic personality change. *Journal of Consulting Psychology, 21,* 95–103. doi:10.1037/h0045357

Rogers, C. R. (1959). A theory of therapy, personality and interpersonal relationships as developed in the client-centered framework. In S. Koch (Ed.), *Psychology: A study of science, vol. 3. Formulations of the person and the social context* (pp. 184–256). New York: McGraw-Hill.

Rogers, C. R. (1961). Ellen West and loneliness. In H. Kirschenbaum & V. L. Henderson (Eds.), *The Carl Rogers reader* (pp. 157–167). Boston, MA: Houghton Mifflin.

Rogers, C. R. (1970). *Carl Rogers on encounter groups.* New York: Harper & Row.

Rogers, C. R. (1980). *A way of being.* Boston, MA: Houghton Mifflin.

Rogers, C. R. (1986). Reflection of feelings. *Person-Centered Review, 1*(4), 375–377.

Rothwell, N. (2005). How brief is solution focused brief therapy? A comparative study. *Clinical Psychology and Psychotherapy, 12,* 402–405. doi:10.1002/cpp.458

Routh, D. K. (2000). Clinical psychology: History of the field. In A. E. Kazdin (Ed.), *Encyclopedia of psychology* (Vol. 2, pp. 113–118). New York: Oxford University Press.

Royse, D., Thyer, B. A., & Padgett, D. K. (2006). *Program evaluation: An introduction* (5th ed.). Belmont, CA: Brooks/Cole.

Russell-Miller, M. (2001). Social service trends and the implications for staffing needs within the social service subsystem: Provision of services to the elderly. In T. McClam & M. Woodside (Eds.), *Human service challenges in the 21st century* (pp. 253–262).

Saad, L. (2006). *Gallup poll: Americans at odds over gay rights.* Retrieved from http://www.gallup.com/poll/23140/Americans-Odds-Over-Gay-Rights.aspx

Saad, L. (2008). *Gallup poll: Americans evenly divided on morality of homosexuality.* Retrieved from http://www.gallup.com/poll/108115/Americans-Evenly-Divided-Morality-Homosexuality.aspx

Sandhu, D. S. (1997). Psychocultural profiles of Asian and Pacific Islander Americans: Implications for counseling and psychotherapy. *Journal of Multicultural Counseling and Development, 25*(1), 7–22.

Santrock, J. W. (2008). *Life-span development* (12th ed.). Boston, MA: McGraw-Hill.

Santrock, J. W. (2009). *A topical approach to life-span development* (5th ed.). Boston, MA: McGraw-Hill.

Saravi, F. (2007). The elusive search for a "gay gene." In D. S. Sergio (Ed.), *Tall tales about the mind & brain: Separating fact from fiction* (pp. 461–477). New York: Oxford University Press.

Satir, V. (1967). *Conjoint family therapy.* Palo Alto, CA: Science and Behavior Books.

Satir, V. (1972a). Family systems and approaches to family therapy. In G. D. Erickson & T. P. Hogan (Eds.), *Family therapy: An introduction to theory and technique* (2nd ed., pp. 211–225). Pacific Grove, CA: Brooks/Cole. (Original work published 1967)

Satir, V. (1972b). *Peoplemaking.* Palo Alto, CA: Science and Behavior Books.

Schaefle, S., Smaby, M., Maddux, C., & Cates, J. (2005). Counseling skills attainment, retention, and transfer as measured by the skilled counseling scale. *Counselor Education and Supervision, 44*(4), 280–292.

Schmidt, J. J. (1999). Two decades of CACREP and what do we know? *Counselor Education and Supervision, 39*(1), 34–45.

Schneider, W., & Bullock, M. (2009). *Human development from early childhood to early adulthood: Findings from a 20 year longitudinal study.* New York: Psychology Press.

Schwiebert, V. L., Myers, J. E., & Dice, C. (2000). Ethical guidelines for counselors working with older adults. *Journal of Counseling and Development, 78,* 123–129.

Seem, S. R., & Johnson, E. (1998). Gender bias among counseling trainees: A study of case conceptualization. *Counselor Education and Supervision, 37,* 257–268.

Seligman, L. (2004). *Diagnosis and treatment planning in counseling* (3rd ed.). New York: Kluwer Academic/Plenum Press.

Selye, H. (1956). *The stress of life.* New York: McGraw-Hill.

Selye, H. (1974). *Stress without distress.* New York: Lippincott.

Sewell, H. (2009). *Working with ethnicity, race and culture in mental health.* Philadelphia, PA: Jessica Kingsley Publishers.

Sheehy, G. (1976). *Passages: Predictable crises of adult life.* New York: Bantam Books.

Skinner, B. F. (1938). *The behavior of organisms: An experimental analysis.* New York: Appleton.

Skinner, B. F. (1953). *Science and human behavior.* New York: Macmillan.

Skinner, B. F. (1971). *Beyond freedom and dignity.* New York: Knopf.

Skynner, A. C. (1976). *Systems of marital and family psychotherapy.* New York: Brunner/Mazel.

Skynner, A. C. R. (1981). An open-systems, group-analytic approach to family therapy. In A. S. Gurman & D. P. Kniskern (Eds.), *Handbook of family therapy* (pp. 39–84). New York: Brunner/Mazel.

Smart, J. (2009). Counseling individuals with disabilities. In I. Marini & M. A. Stebnicki (Eds.), *The professional counselor's desk reference* (pp. 639–646). New York: Springer.

Sokal, M. M. (1992). Origins and early years of the American Psychological Association, 1890–1906. *American Psychologist, 47*(2), 111–122. doi: 10.1037/0003-066X.47.2.111

Sommer, B., & Sommer, R. (2002). *A practical guide to behavioral research: Tools and techniques* (5th ed.). New York: Oxford University Press.

Sommer, C. A. (2008). Vicarious traumatization, trauma-sensitive supervision, and counselor preparation. *Counselor Education and Supervision, 48,* 61–71.

Sommers-Flanagan, J., & Sommers-Flanagan, R. (2009). *Clinical interviewing* (4th ed.). Hoboken, NJ: John Wiley & Sons.

Southern, J. A., Erford, B. T., Vernon, A., & Davis-Gage, D. (2011). The value of group work: Functional group models and historical perspective. In B. T. Erford (Ed.), *Group work: Processes and applications* (pp. 1–19). New York: Pearson.

Southern Regional Educational Board. (1969). *Roles and functions for different levels of mental health workers.* Atlanta, GA: Author.

Spillman, L. (2007). Culture. In G. Ritzer (Ed.), *Blackwell encyclopedia of sociology.* Retrieved from www.blackwellreference.com/subscriber/tocnode?d=g9781405124331_chunk_g97814051243319_ss1-183

Spruill, D. A., & Benshoff, J. M. (2000). Developing a personal theory of counseling: A theory building model for counselor trainees. *Counselor Education and Supervision, 40,* 70–80.

Stearns, S. C., Allal, N., & Mace, R. (2008). Life history theory and human development. In C. Crawford & D. Krebs (Eds.), *Foundations of evolutionary psychology* (pp. 47–70). New York: Lawrence Erlbaum, Associates.

Steinem, G. (1992). *Revolution from within: A book on self-esteem.* Boston, MA: Little, Brown.

Steinhaus, D. A., Harley, D. A., & Rogers, J. (2004). Homelessness and people with affective disorders and other mental illnesses. *Journal of Applied Rehabilitation Counseling, 35*(1), 36–40.

Stickle, F., & Onedera, J. (2006). Teaching gerontology in counselor education. *Educational Gerontology, 32*(4), 247–259. doi:10.1080/03601270500493974

Stricker, G., & Gold, J. (2006). *A casebook of psychotherapy integration.* Washington, DC: American Psychological Association.

Stricker, L. J., & Burton, N. W. (1996). Using the SAT and high school record in academic guidance. *Educational and Psychological Measurement, 56*(4), 626–641.

Strong, S. R. (1991). Theory-driven science and naïve empiricism in counseling psychology. *Journal of Counseling Psychology, 38*(2), 204–210.

Substance Abuse and Mental Health Services Administration. (2010). *Homelessness resource center: Learn, connect, share.* Retrieved from http://homeless.samhsa.gov/Resource/View.aspx?id=48800

Sue, D. W. (1992). The challenge of multiculturalism: The road less traveled. *American Counselor, 1*(1), 6–15.

Sue, D. W. (2010). *Microaggressions in everyday life: Race, gender, and sexual orientation.* New York: Wiley.

Sue, D. W., & Sue, D. (2008). *Counseling the culturally diverse: Theory and practice* (5th ed.). New York: Wiley.

Sue, D. W., & Torino, G. C. (2005). Racial-cultural competences: Awareness, knowledge and skills. In R. T. Carter (Ed.), *Handbook of racial-cultural psychology and counseling: Theory and research* (pp. 3–18). Hoboken, NJ: Wiley.

Suzuki, L. A., Kugler, J. F., & Aguiar, L. J. (2005). Assessment practices in racial-cultural psychology. In R. T. Carter (Ed.), *Handbook of racial-cultural psychology and counseling: Theory and research* (Vol. 2, pp. 297–315). Hoboken, NJ: John Wiley.

Sweeney, T. J. (1991). Counselor credentialing: Purpose and origin. In F. O. Bradley (Ed.), *Credentialing in counseling* (pp. 81–85). Alexandria, VA: Association for Counselor Education and Supervision.

Sweeney, T. J. (1992). CACREP: Precursors, promises, and prospects. *Journal of Counseling and Development, 70,* 667–672.

Swenson, L. C. (1997). *Psychology and law for the helping professions* (2nd ed.). Pacific Grove, CA: Brooks/Cole.

Szymanski, D. (2008). Lesbian, gay, bisexual, and transgendered clients. In G. McAuliffe (Ed.), *Culturally alert counseling: A comprehensive introduction* (pp. 466–505). Thousand Oaks, CA: Sage Publications.

Tafoya, T. (1996). *New heights in human services: Multiculturalism.* Keynote address at National Organization of Human Services Annual Conference, St. Louis, MO.

Tarasoff et al. v. Regents of University of California, 529 P.2d 553 (Calif. 1974), vacated, reheard en banc, and affirmed 551 P.2d 334 (1976).

Taylor, M., Bradley, V., & Warren, R. (Eds.). (1996). *The community support skill standards: Tools for managing change and achieving outcomes: Skill standards for direct service workers in the human services.* Cambridge, MA: Human Services Research Institute.

The Pew Forum on Religion and Public Life. (2009). *Results from the 2009 annual religion and public life survey.* Retrieved from http://people-press.org/reports/pdf/542.pdf

Toporek, R. L., Lewis, J. A., & Crethar, H. C. (2009). Promoting systemic change through the ACA advocacy competencies. *Journal of Counseling and Development, 87,* 260–269.

Tuckman, B. W. (1965). Developmental sequence in small groups. *Psychological Bulletin, 63*(6): 384–99. doi:10.1037/h0022100.

Tuckman, B. W., & Jensen, M. A. C. (1977). Stages of small-group development revisited. *Group & Organization Studies, 2*(4), 419–427.

Turner, L. H., & West, R. (2006). *Perspectives on family communication* (3rd ed.). Boston, MA: McGraw-Hill.

U.S. Census Bureau. (2003). *No. HS-E population by age: 1900 to 2002.* Retrieved from http://www.census.gov/statab/hist/HS-03.pdf

U.S. Census Bureau. (2008a). *Americans with disabilities: 2005.* Retrieved from http://www.census.gov/prod/2008pubs/p70-117.pdf

U.S. Census Bureau. (2008b). *An older more diverse nation by midcentury.* Retrieved from http://www.census.gov/newsroom/releases/archives/population/cb08-123.html

U.S. Census Bureau. (2009a). *Annual estimates of the resident population by sex, race, and Hispanic origin for the United States: April 1, 2000 to July 1, 2009* (NC-EST2009-03). Retrieved from http://www.census.gov/popest/national/asrh/NC-EST2009-srh.html

U.S. Census Bureau. (2009b). *Income, poverty, and health insurance coverage in the United States: 2008.* Retrieved from http://www.census.gov/prod/2009pubs/p60-236.pdf

U.S. Census Bureau. (2010a). *Poverty: Highlights.* Retrieved from http://www.census.gov/hhes/www/poverty/about/overview/index.html

U.S. Census Bureau. (2010b). *Race and Hispanic origin of the foreign-born population in the United States: 2007.* Retrieved from http://www.census.gov/prod/2010pubs/acs-11.pdf

U.S. Census Bureau. (2011). *Health and nutrition: Table 128. Hospitals—Summary characteristics: 1990 to 2008.* Retrieved from http://www.census.gov/compendia/statab/2011/tables/11s0168.pdf

U.S. Department of Commerce. (2000). *Percent of U.S. households with a computer and Internet access.* Retrieved from http://www.ntia.doc.gov/ntiahome/fttn00/chartscontents.html

U.S. Department of Education. (2011). *Family Education Rights and Privacy Act (FERPA).* Retrieved from http://www2.ed.gov/policy/gen/guid/fpco/ferpa/index.html

U.S. Department of Health and Human Services. (2001). *Mental health: Culture, race, and ethnicity: A supplement to mental health: A report to the Surgeon General.* Retrieved from http://www.ncbi.nlm.nih.gov/books/NBK44243/

U.S. Department of Health and Human Services. (2009). *Drug and alcohol treatment.* Retrieved from http://www.oas.samhsa.gov/tx.htm#N

U.S. Department of Health and Human Services. (2010). *Results from the 2009 national survey on drug use and health: Volume I. Summary of national findings.* Retrieved from http://www.oas.samhsa.gov/NSDUH/2k9NSDUH/2k9ResultsP.pdf

U.S. Department of Health and Human Services. (2011). *Health, United States, 2010: With special feature on death and dying.* Retrieved from http://www.cdc.gov/nchs/data/hus/hus10.pdf#001

U.S. Department of Health and Human Services. (n.d.). *Understanding health information privacy.* Retrieved from http://www.hhs.gov/ocr/privacy/hipaa/understanding/index.html

U.S. Department of Housing and Urban Development. (2011). *Mckinney-Vento Act.* Retrieved from http://portal.hud.gov/hudportal/HUD?rc=/program_offices/comm_planning/homeless/lawsandregs/mckv

U.S. Department of Justice. (2004). *Freedom of information act guide.* Retrieved from http://www.usdoj.gov/oip/introduc.htm

U.S. Department of Justice. (2008). *Hate crime statistics.* Retrieved from http://www.fbi.gov/ucr/hc2008/data/table_01.html

U.S. Department of Labor. (2010–2011a). *Occupational outlook handbook, 2010-2011: Counselors.* Retrieved from http://www.bls.gov/OCO/ocos067.htm

U.S. Department of Labor. (2010–2011b). *Occupational outlook handbook, 2010-2011: Social and human service assistants.* Retrieved from http://www.bls.gov/oco/ocos059.htm

U.S. Department of Labor. (2010–2011c). *Occupational outlook handbook, 2010-2011: Social and human service assistants: Nature of work.* Retrieved from http://www.bls.gov/oco/ocos059.htm#projections_data

U.S. Department of Labor. (2010–2011d). *Occupational outlook handbook, 2010-2011: Social and human service assistants: Projections data.* Retrieved from http://www.bls.gov/oco/ocos059.htm#projections_data

U.S. Department of Labor. (n.d.). *Help navigating DOL laws and regulations.* Retrieved from http://www.dol.gov/compliance/

UNAIDS. (2010). *Global report: UNAIDS report on the global AIDS epidemic: 2010.* Retrieved from http://www.unaids.org/globalreport/

Urofsky, R. I., Engels, D. W., & Engebretson, K. (2008). Kitchener's principle ethics: Implications for counseling practice and research. *Counseling and Values, 53,* 67–78. doi:10.1037/h0069608

Van Nuys, D. (2007). *An interview with William Glasser, MD and Carleen Glasser on happier marriages.* Retrieved from http://www.mentalhelp.net/poc/view_doc.php?ype=weblog&id=283&wlid=9&cn=289

Videbeck, S. L. (2011). *Psychiatric mental health nursing* (5th ed.). New York/Washington, DC: Lippincott, Williams, & Wilkins/American Psychiatric Press.

Vander Kolk, C. J. (1990). *Introduction to group counseling and psychotherapy.* Prospect Heights, IL: Waveland Press.

von Bertalanffy, L. (1934). *Modern theories of development: An introduction to theoretical biology.* London: Oxford University Press.

von Bertalanffy, L. (1968). *General systems theory.* New York: Braziller.

Wallerstein, J. S., & Blakeslee, S. (2004). *Second chances: Men, women, and children a decade after divorce* (Rev. ed.). New York: Houghton Mifflin.

Walsh, J. (2000). *Clinical case management with persons having mental illness: A relationship-based perspective.* Belmont, CA: Brooks/Cole.

Walsh, W. B., & Betz, N. E. (2001). *Tests and assessment* (4th ed.). Upper Saddle River, NJ: Prentice Hall.

Wampold, B. E. (2010a). *The basics of psychotherapy: An introduction to theory and practice.* Washington, DC: American Psychological Association.

Wampold, B. E. (2010b). *The great psychotherapy debate: Models, methods, and findings.* Mahwah, NJ: Lawrence Erlbaum Associates.

Wampold, B. E. (2010c). The research evidence for common factors models: A historically situated perspective. In B. L. Duncan, S. D. Miller, B. E. Wampold, & M. A. Hubble (Eds.), *The heart and soul of change* (2nd ed., pp. 49–82). Washington, DC: American Psychological Association.

Wark, L. (2008). The advocacy project. *Human Service Education, 27,* 69–82.

Wark, L. (2010). The ethical standards for human service professionals: Past and future. *Journal of Human Services, 30,* 18–22.

Watson, J. B. (1925). *Behaviorism.* New York: Norton.

Watson, J. B., & Raynor, R. (1920). Conditioned emotional reactions. *Journal of Experimental Psychology, 3,* 1–14. doi:10.1037/h0069608

Weil, A. (2009). *Why our health matters: A vision of medicine that can transform our future.* New York: Hudson Street Press.

Welfel, E. R. (2010). *Ethics in counseling and psychotherapy: Standards, research, and emerging* issues (4th ed.), Pacific Grove, CA: Brooks/Cole.

Wertheimer, M. (2000). *A brief history of psychology* (4th ed.). New York: Harcourt College Publishers.

Wexler, D. B. (2009). *Men in therapy: New approaches for effective treatment.* New York: W. W. Norton.

Whiston, S. C., & Coker, J. K. (2000). Reconstructing clinical training: Implications from research. *Counselor Education and Supervision, 39,* 228–253.

Whitaker, C. (1976). The hindrance of theory in clinical work. In P. J. Guerin (Ed.), *Family therapy* (pp. 154–164). New York: Gardner Press.

White, M. (1995). *Re-authoring lives: Interviews and essays.* Adelaide, South Australia: Dulwich Centre Publications.

White, M., & Epston, D. (1990). *Narrative means to therapeutic ends.* New York: Norton.

Whitfield, W., McGrath, P., & Coleman, V. (1992, October). *Increasing multicultural sensitivity and awareness.* Symposium presented at the annual conference of the National Organization for Human Service Education, Alexandria, VA.

Willis, L., & Wilkie, L. (2009). Digital career portfolios: Expanding institutional opportunities. *Journal of Employment Counseling, 46*(2), 73.

Woititz, J. G. (2002). *The complete ACOA sourcebook.* Deerfield Beach, FL: Health Communications.

Wolpe, J. (1958). *Psychotherapy by reciprocal inhibition.* Stanford, CA: Stanford University Press.

Wolpe, J. (1969). *The practice of behavior therapy.* New York: Pergamon Press.

Wong, D. F. K. (2006). *Clinical case management for people with mental illness: A biopsychosocial vulnerability-stress model.* Binghamton, NY: Haworth Press.

Wong-Wylie, G. (2003). Preserving hope in the duty to protect: Counselling clients with HIV or AIDS. *Canadian Journal of Counselling, 27*(1), 35–43.

Woodside, M. R., & McClam, T. (2006). *Generalist case management: A method of human service delivery* (3rd ed.). Belmont, CA: Brooks/Cole.

Yalom, I. D. (2005). *The theory and practice of group psychotherapy* (5th ed.). New York: Basic Books.

Yarhouse, M. A. (2003). Working with families affected by HIV/AIDS. *The American Journal of Family Therapy, 31,* 125–137.

Yeh, C. J., & Hwang, M. Y. (2000). Interdependence in ethnic identity and self: Implications for theory and practice. *Journal of Counseling and Development, 78,* 420–429.

Zuckerman, E. (2008). *The paper office: Forms, guidelines, and resources to make your practice work ethically, legally, and profitably* (4th ed.). New York: Guilford.

Zur, O. (2007). *Boundaries in psychotherapy: Ethical and clinical explorations.* Washington, DC: American Psychological Association.

Zur, O. (2009). Therapist self-disclosure: Standard of care, ethical considerations, and therapeutic context. In A. Bloomgarden & R. B. Mennuti (Ed.), *Psychotherapist revealed: Therapists speak about self-disclosure in psychotherapy* (pp. 31–51). New York: Taylor and Francis Group.

Zwelling, S. S. (1990). *Quest for a cure: The public hospital in Williamsburg, Virginia, 1773-1885.* Williamsburg, VA: Colonial Williamsburg Foundation.

Name Index

Subject Index

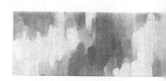

CPSIA information can be obtained
at www.ICGtesting.com
Printed in the USA
FFOW03n1257200815
16212FF

Red Hat Linux 6.0

The Official Red Hat Linux Installation Guide

Red Hat Software, Inc.
Durham, North Carolina